an introduction to orthodontics

an introduction
to orthodontics

FOURTH EDITION

Laura Mitchell MBE

MDS, BDS, FDSRCPS (Glasg), FDSRCS (Eng), FGDP (UK),
D. Orth RCS (Eng), M. Orth RCS (Eng)
Consultant Orthodontist, St. Luke's Hospital, Bradford
Honorary Senior Clinical Lecturer, Leeds Dental Institute, Leeds

With contributions from

Simon J. Littlewood

MDSc, BDS, FDS (Orth) RCPS (Glasg), M. Orth RCS (Edin),
FDSRCS (Eng)
Consultant Orthodontist, St. Luke's Hospital, Bradford
Honorary Senior Clinical Lecturer, Leeds Dental Institute, Leeds

Zararna L. Nelson-Moon

MSc, PhD, BDS, FDS (Orth) RCS (Eng), M. Orth RCS (Eng)
Consultant Orthodontist and Honorary Senior Clinical Lecturer
Leeds Dental Institute, Leeds

Fiona Dyer

MMedSci, BChD, FDS (Orth) RCS (Eng), M. Orth RCS (Eng),
FDS RCS (Eng)
Consultant Orthodontist and Honorary Clinical Lecturer
Charles Clifford Dental Hospital, Sheffield

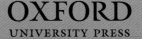

OXFORD
UNIVERSITY PRESS

OXFORD
UNIVERSITY PRESS

Great Clarendon Street, Oxford OX2 6DP,
United Kingdom

Oxford University Press is a department of the University of Oxford.
It furthers the University's objective of excellence in research, scholarship,
and education by publishing worldwide. Oxford is a registered trade mark of
Oxford University Press in the UK and in certain other countries

This edition published 2013

First edition published 1996

Second edition published 2001

Third edition published 2007

Impression: 1

British Library Cataloguing in Publication Data

Data available

Library of Congress Cataloging in Publication

Library of Congress Control Number 2012944035

ISBN 978-0-19-959471-9

Printed in China by
C&C Offset Printing Co. Ltd

Preface for fourth edition

I would like to thank the readers of previous editions and in particular those that have passed on their suggestions for this the fourth edition.

Online Resource Centre

References for this chapter can also be found at: www.oxfordtextbooks.co.uk/orc/mitchell4e/.

Where possible, these are presented as active links which direct you to the electronic version of the work, to help facilitate onward study. If you are a subscriber to that work (either individually or through an institution), and depending on your level of access, you may be able to peruse an abstract or the full article if available.

Acknowledgements

It is difficult to know where to start in terms of thanking those that have assisted with this new edition. However, without the help and hard work of my co-authors, in particular Simon Littlewood, a fourth edition would not have been possible. I should also mention our colleagues and the support staff of the units at which we work for their assistance in getting good quality illustrations and also for their forbearance during the time of writing.

I would like to acknowledge Joanne Birdsall who kindly assisted Fiona Dyer with the preparation of Chapter 15.

The functional appliances illustrated in Chapter 19 were produced by the Senior Orthodontic technician at St. Luke's Hospital Bradford, Nigel Jacques and are testament to his consistently good laboratory work.

I would also like to thank the staff of Oxford University Press for their help and patience.

Finally, once again, I have to pay tribute to the support and encouragement of my husband without which, another edition would not have been possible. Thank you.

Brief contents

Detailed contents

1

The rationale for orthodontic treatment

Chapter contents

1.1 Definition

Orthodontics is that branch of dentistry concerned with facial growth, with development of the dentition and occlusion, and with the diagnosis, interception, and treatment of occlusal anomalies.

1.2 Prevalence of malocclusion

Numerous surveys have been conducted to investigate the prevalence of malocclusion. It should be remembered that the figures for a particular occlusal feature or dental anomaly will depend upon the size and composition of the group studied (for example age and racial characteristics), the criteria used for assessment, and the methods used by the examiners (for example whether radiographs were employed).

The figures for 12-year-olds in the 2003 United Kingdom Child Dental Health Survey in are given in Table 1.1. It is estimated that in the UK approximately 45% of 12-year-olds have a definite need for orthodontic treatment.

Now that a greater proportion of the population is keeping their teeth for longer, orthodontic treatment has an increasing adjunctive role prior to restorative work. In addition, there is an increasing acceptability of orthodontic appliances with the effect that many adults who did not have treatment during adolescence are now seeking treatment.

Table 1.1 UK child dental health survey 2003

In the 12-year-old age band:	
Children undergoing orthodontic treatment at the time of the survey	8%
Children not undergoing treatment – in need of treatment (IOTN dental health component)	26%
No orthodontic need (NB includes children who have had treatment in past)	57%

1.3 Need for treatment

It is perhaps pertinent to begin this section by reminding the reader that malocclusion is one end of the spectrum of normal variation and is not a disease.

Ethically, no treatment should be embarked upon unless a demonstrable benefit to the patient is feasible. In addition, the potential advantages should be viewed in the light of possible risks and side-effects, including failure to achieve the aims of treatment. Appraisal of these factors is called risk–benefit analysis and, as in all branches of medicine and dentistry, needs to be considered before treatment is commenced for an individual patient (Box 1.1). In parallel, financial constraints coupled with the increasing costs of health care have led to an increased focus upon the cost–benefit ratio of treatment. Obviously the threshold for treatment and the amount of orthodontic intervention will differ between a system that is primarily funded by the state and one that is private or based on insurance schemes.

The decision to embark upon a course of treatment will be influenced by the perceived benefits to the patient balanced against the risks of appliance therapy and the prognosis for achieving the aims of treatment

Box 1.1 Decision to treat

The decision to treat depends upon

Benefits of treatment	versus	Risks
Improved function		*Worsening of dental health (e.g. caries)*
Improved aesthetics		*Failure to achieve aims of treatment*
Psychological benefits		

successfully. In this chapter we consider each of these areas in turn, starting with the results of research into the possible benefits of orthodontic treatment upon dental health and psychological well-being.

1.3.1 Dental health

Caries

Research has failed to demonstrate a significant association between malocclusion and caries, whereas diet and the use of fluoride toothpaste are correlated with caries experience. However, clinical experience suggests that in susceptible children with a poor diet, malalignment may reduce the potential for natural tooth-cleansing and increase the risk of decay.

Periodontal disease

The association between malocclusion and periodontal disease is weak, as research has shown that individual motivation has more impact than tooth alignment upon effective tooth brushing. Certainly, good toothbrushers are motivated to brush around irregular teeth, whereas in the individual who brushes infrequently their poor plaque control is clearly of more importance. Nevertheless, it would seem logical that in the middle of this range that, irregular teeth would hinder effective brushing. In addition, certain occlusal anomalies may prejudice periodontal support. Crowding may lead to one or more teeth being squeezed buccally or lingually out of their investing bone, resulting in a reduction of periodontal support. This may also occur in a Class III malocclusion where the lower incisors in crossbite are pushed labially, contributing to gingival recession. Traumatic overbites can also lead to increased loss of periodontal support and therefore are another indication for orthodontic intervention (see also Box 1.2).

Finally, an increased dental awareness has been noted in patients following orthodontic treatment, and this may be of long-term benefit to oral health.

Trauma to the anterior teeth

Any practitioner who treats children will confirm the association between increased overjet and trauma to the upper incisors. A systematic review found that individuals with an overjet in excess of 3 mm had more than double the risk of injury.

Overjet is a greater contributory factor in girls than boys even though traumatic injuries are more common in boys. Other studies have shown that the risk is greater in patients with incompetent lips.

Masticatory function

Patients with anterior open bites (AOB) and those with markedly increased or reverse overjets often complain of difficulty with eating, particularly when incising food. Classically patients with AOB complain that they have to avoid sandwiches containing lettuce or cucumber. Patients with severe hypodontia also may experience problems with eating.

Speech

The soft tissues show remarkable adaptation to the changes that occur during the transition between the primary and mixed dentitions, and when the incisors have been lost owing to trauma or disease. In the main, speech is little affected by malocclusion, and correction of an occlusal anomaly has little effect upon abnormal speech. However, if a patient cannot attain contact between the incisors anteriorly, this may contribute to the production of a lisp (interdental stigmatism).

Tooth impaction

Unerupted teeth may rarely cause pathology (Fig. 1.1). Unerupted impacted teeth, for example maxillary canines, may cause resorption of the roots of adjacent teeth. Dentigerous cyst formation can occur

> **Box 1.2 Those occlusal anomalies for which there is evidence to suggest an adverse effect upon the longevity of the dentition, indicating that their correction would benefit long-term dental health**
>
> - Increased overjet
> - Increased traumatic overbites
> - Anterior crossbites (where causing a decrease in labial periodontal support of affected lower incisors)
> - Unerupted impacted teeth (where there is a danger of pathology)
> - Crossbites associated with mandibular displacement

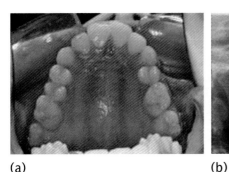
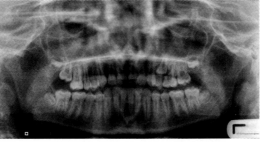
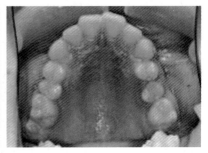

(a)   (b)   (c)

Fig. 1.1 Patient aged 11 years with asymptomatic resorption of the upper left first permanent molar by the upper left second premolar. Following extraction of the first permanent molar the second premolar erupted uneventfully (a); (b) at presentation; (c) 6 months after the extraction of the upper first permanent molar.

around unerupted third molars or canine teeth. Supernumerary teeth may also give rise to problems, most importantly where their presence prevents normal eruption of an associated permanent tooth or teeth.

Temporomandibular joint dysfunction syndrome

This topic is considered in more detail in Section 1.7.

1.3.2 Psychosocial well-being

While it is accepted that dentofacial anomalies and severe malocclusion do have a negative effect on the psychological well-being and self-esteem of the individual, the impact of more minor occlusal problems is more variable and is modified by social and cultural factors. Research has shown that an unattractive dentofacial appearance does have a negative effect on the expectations of teachers and employers. However, in this respect, background facial appearance would appear to have more impact than dental appearance.

A patient's perception of the impact of dental variation upon his or her self-image is subject to enormous diversity and is modified by cultural and racial influences. Therefore, some individuals are unaware of marked malocclusions, whilst others complain bitterly about very minor irregularities.

The dental health component of the Index of Orthodontic Treatment Need was developed to try and quantify the impact of a particular malocclusion upon long-term dental health. The index also comprises an aesthetic element which is an attempt to quantify the aesthetic handicap that a particular arrangement of the teeth poses for a patient. Both aspects of this index are discussed in more detail in Chapter 2.

The psychosocial benefits of treatment are however countered to a degree by the visibility of appliances during treatment and their effect upon the self-esteem of the individual. In other words a child who is being teased about their teeth will probably also be teased about braces.

1.4 Demand for treatment

After working with the general public for a short period of time, it can readily be appreciated that demand for treatment does not necessarily reflect need for treatment. Some patients are very aware of mild rotations of the upper incisors, whilst others are blithely unaware of markedly increased overjets. It has been demonstrated that awareness of tooth alignment and malocclusion, and willingness to undergo orthodontic treatment, are greater in the following groups:

- females
- higher socio-economic families/groups
- in areas which have a smaller population to orthodontist ratio, presumably because appliances become more accepted

One interesting example of the latter has been observed in countries where provision of orthodontic treatment is mainly privately funded, for example, the USA, as orthodontic appliances are now perceived as a 'status symbol'.

With the increasing dental awareness shown by the public and the increased acceptability of appliances, the demand for treatment is increasing rapidly, particularly among the adult population who may not have had ready access to orthodontic treatment as children. This has also been fuelled by the increased availability of less visible appliances including ceramic brackets and lingual fixed appliances. In addition, increased dental awareness also means that patients are seeking a higher standard of treatment result. These combined pressures place considerable strain upon the limited resources of state-funded systems of care. As it appears likely that the demand for treatment will continue to escalate, some form of rationing of state-funded treatment is inevitable and is already operating in some countries. In Sweden for example, the contribution made by the state towards the cost of treatment is based upon need for treatment as determined by the Swedish Health Board's Index (see IOTN in Chapter 2).

1.5 The disadvantages and potential risks of orthodontic treatment

Like any other branch of medicine or dentistry, orthodontic treatment is not without potential risks (see Table 1.2).

1.5.1 Root resorption

It is now accepted that some root resorption is inevitable as a consequence of tooth movement (see also Box 1.3). On average, during the course of a conventional 2-year fixed-appliance treatment around 1 mm of root length will be lost (this amount is not clinically significant). However, this mean masks a wide range of individual variation, as some patients appear to be more susceptible and undergo more marked root resorption. Evidence would suggest a genetic basis in these cases.

> **Box 1.3 Recognized risk factors for root resorption during orthodontic treatment**
>
> - Shortened roots with evidence of previous root resorption
> - Pipette-shaped or blunted roots
> - Teeth which have suffered a previous episode of trauma
> - Iatrogenic – use of excessive forces; intrusion; prolonged treatment time

Table 1.2 Potential risks of orthodontic treatment

Problem	Avoidance/Management of risk
Demineralisation	Dietary advice, improve oral hygiene, increase availability of fluoride
	Abandon treatment
Periodontal attachment loss	Improve oral hygiene. Avoid moving teeth out of alveolar bone
Root resorption	Avoid treatment in patients with resorbed, blunted, or pipette-shaped roots
Loss of vitality	If history of previous trauma to incisors, counsel patient
Relapse	Avoidance of unstable tooth positions at end of treatment
	Retention

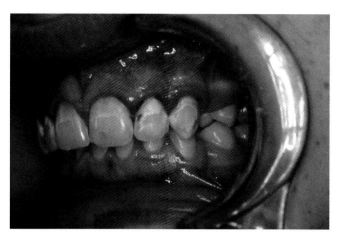

Fig. 1.2 Demineralization.

1.5.2 Loss of periodontal support

As a result of reduced access for cleansing, an increase in gingival inflammation is commonly seen following the placement of fixed appliances. This normally reduces or resolves following removal of the appliance, but some apical migration of periodontal attachment and alveolar bony support is usual during a 2-year course of orthodontic treatment. In most patients this is minimal, but if oral hygiene is poor, particularly in an individual susceptible to periodontal disease, more marked loss may occur.

Removable appliances may also be associated with gingival inflammation, particularly of the palatal tissues, in the presence of poor oral hygiene.

1.5.3 Demineralisation

Caries or demineralisation occurs when a cariogenic plaque occurs in association with a high-sugar diet. The presence of a fixed appliance predisposes to plaque accumulation as tooth cleaning around the components of the appliance is more difficult. Demineralisation during treatment with fixed appliances is a real risk, with a reported prevalence of between 2 and 96 per cent (see Chapter 18, Section 18.7). Although there is evidence to show that the lesions regress following removal of the appliance, patients may still be left with permanent 'scarring' of the enamel (Fig. 1.2).

1.5.4 Soft tissue damage

Traumatic ulceration can occur during treatment with both fixed and removable appliances, although it is more commonly seen in association with the former as a removable appliance which is uncomfortable is usually removed.

1.5.5 Pulpal injury

Over-enthusiastic apical movement can lead to a reduction in blood supply to the pulp and even pulpal death. Teeth which have undergone a previous episode of trauma appear to be particularly susceptible, probably because the pulpal tissues are already compromised.

1.6 The effectiveness of treatment

The decision to embark upon orthodontic treatment must also consider the effectiveness of appliance therapy in correcting the malocclusion of the individual concerned. This has several aspects.

- Are the tooth movements planned attainable? This is considered in more detail in Chapter 7 but, in brief, tooth movement is only feasible within the constraints of the skeletal and growth patterns of the individual patient. The wrong treatment plan, or failure to anticipate adverse growth changes, will reduce the chances of success. In addition, the probable stability of the completed treatment needs to be considered. If a stable result is not possible, do the benefits conferred by proceeding justify prolonged retention, or the possibility of relapse?

- There is a wealth of evidence to show that orthodontic treatment is more likely to achieve a pleasing and successful result if fixed appliances are used, and if the operator has had some postgraduate training in orthodontics.

- Patient co-operation. A successful outcome is dependent upon patient compliance with attending appointments, looking after their teeth and appliance and with wearing auxiliaries e.g. elastics. A patient is more likely to co-operate if they fully understand the process and their role in it from the outset i.e. during the consent process.

Table 1.3 Failure to achieve treatment objectives

Operator factors	Patient factors
Errors of diagnosis	Poor oral hygiene/diet
Errors of treatment planning	Failure to wear appliances/elastics
Anchorage loss	Repeated appliance breakages
Technique errors	Failed appointments

The likelihood that orthodontic treatment will benefit a patient is increased if the malocclusion is severe, the patient is well-motivated and appliance therapy is planned and carried out by an experienced orthodontist. The likelihood of gain is reduced if the malocclusion is mild and treatment is undertaken by an inexperienced operator.

In essence, it may be better not to embark on treatment at all, rather than run the risk of failing to achieve a worthwhile improvement (Table 1.3).

1.7 The temporomandibular joint and orthodontics

The aetiology and management of temporomandibular joint dysfunction syndrome (TMD) have aroused considerable controversy in all branches of dentistry. The debate has been particularly heated regarding the role of orthodontics, with some authors claiming that orthodontic treatment can cause TMD, whilst at the same time others have advocated appliance therapy in the management of the condition.

There are a number of factors that have contributed to the confusion surrounding TMD. The objective view is that TMD comprises a group of related disorders of multifactorial aetiology. Psychological, hormonal, genetic, traumatic, and occlusal factors have all been implicated. Recent research has shown that depression, stress and sleep disorders are major factors in the aetiology of TMD. It is also accepted that parafunctional activity, for example bruxism, can contribute to muscle pain and spasm. Success has been claimed for a wide assortment of treatment modalities, reflecting both the multifactorial aetiology and the self-limiting nature of the condition. Given this, it is wise to try irreversible approaches in the first instance. The reader is directed to look at two recent Cochrane reviews (see Relevant Cochrane reviews and Further reading) on the use of stabilization splints and occlusal adjustment.

1.7.1 Orthodontic treatment as a contributory factor in TMD

A survey of the literature reveals that those articles claiming that orthodontic treatment (with or without extractions) can contribute to the development of TMD are predominantly of the viewpoint (based on the authors' opinion) and case report type. In contrast, controlled longitudinal studies have indicated a trend towards a lower incidence of the symptoms of TMD among post-orthodontic patients compared with matched groups of untreated patients.

The consensus view is that orthodontic treatment, either alone or in combination with extractions, does not 'cause' TMD.

1.7.2 The role of orthodontic treatment in the prevention and management of TMD

Some authors maintain that minor occlusal imperfections lead to abnormal paths of closure and/or bruxism, which then result in the development of TMD. If this were the case, then given the high incidence of malocclusion in the population (50–75 per cent), one would expect a higher prevalence of TMD. A number of carefully controlled longitudinal studies have been carried out in North America, and these have found no relationship between the signs and symptoms of TMD and the presence of non-functional occlusal contacts or mandibular displacements. However, other studies have found a weak association between TMD and some types of malocclusion including Class II skeletal pattern (especially associated with a retrusive mandible); Class III; anterior open bite; crossbite and asymmetry.

A review of the current literature would indicate that orthodontic treatment does not 'cure' TMD. It is important to advise patients of this, particularly those who present reporting TMD symptoms, and to note this in their records.

Whilst current evidence indicates that orthodontic treatment is not a contributory factor and also does not cure the TMD, it is advisable to carry out a TMD screen for all potential orthodontic patients. At the very least this should include questioning patients about symptoms; an examination of the temporomandibular joint and associated muscles and recording the range of opening and movement (see Chapter 5). If signs or symptoms of TMD are found then it may be wise to refer the patient for a comprehensive assessment and specialist management before embarking on orthodontic treatment.

Key points

- The decision to undertake orthodontic treatment or not is essentially a risk–benefit analysis where the perceived benefits in commencing treatment at that time outweigh the potential risks.
- If there is any uncertainty as to whether the patient will co-operate and/or benefit from treatment, then it is advisable not to proceed at that time.

Relevant Cochrane reviews:

Occlusal adjustment for treating and preventing temporomandibular joint disorders

Koh, H. *et al.* (2009)

http://onlinelibrary.wiley.com/o/cochrane/clsysrev/articles/CD003812/frame.html

The authors concluded that there is an absence of evidence, from RCTs, that occlusal adjustment treats or prevents TMD. Occlusal adjustment cannot be recommended for the management or prevention of TMD.

Orthodontics for treating temporomandibular joint (TMJ) disorders

Luther, F. *et al.* (2010).

http://onlinelibrary.wiley.com/o/cochrane/clsysrev/articles/CD006541/frame.html

The conclusion was there are insufficient research data on which to base our clinical practice on the relationship of active orthodontic intervention and TMD.

Stabilisation splint therapy for temporomandibular pain dysfunction syndrome.

Al-Ani, M.Z. *et al.* (2009).

http://onlinelibrary.wiley.com/o/cochrane/clsysrev/articles/CD002778/frame.html

There is insufficient evidence either for or against the use of stabilisation splint therapy for the treatment of temporomandibular pain dysfunction syndrome.

Principal sources and further reading

American Journal of Orthodontics and Dentofacial Orthopedics, **101**(1), (1992).

This is a special issue dedicated to the results of several studies set up by the American Association of Orthodontists to investigate the link between orthodontic treatment and the temporomandibular joint.

Chestnutt, I. G., Burden, D. J., Steele, J. G., Pitts, N. B., Nuttall, N. M., and Morris, A. J. (2006). The orthodontic condition of children in the United Kingdom, 2003. *British Dental Journal*, **200**, 609–12.

Davies, S. J., Gray, R. M. J., Sandler, P. J., and O'Brien, K. D. (2001). Orthodontics and occlusion. *British Dental Journal*, **191**, 539–49.

This concise article is part of a series of articles on occlusion. It contains an example of an articulatory examination.

Egermark, I., Magnusson, T., and Carlsson, G. E. (2003). A 20-year follow-up of signs and symptoms of temporomandibular disorders in subjects with and without orthodontic treatment in childhood. *Angle Orthodontist*, **73**, 109–15.

A long-term cohort study which found no statistically-significant difference in TMD signs and symptoms between subjects with or without previous experience of orthodontic treatment.

Holmes, A. (1992). The subjective need and demand for orthodontic treatment. *British Journal of Orthodontics*, **19**, 287–97.

Joss-Vassalli, I., Grebenstein, C., Topouzelis, N., Sculean, A. and Katsaros, C. (2010). Orthodontic therapy and gingival recession: a systematic review. *Orthodontics and Craniofacial Research*, **13**, 127–41.

Luther, F. (2007). TMD and occlusion part I. Damned if we do? Occlusion the interface of dentistry and orthodontics. *British Dental Journal*, **13**, 202.

Luther, F. (2007). TMD and occlusion part II. Damned if we don't? Functional occlusal problems: TMD epidemiology in a wider context. *British Dental Journal*, **13**, 202.

These 2 articles are well worth reading.

Maaitah, E. F., Adeyami, A. A., Higham, S. M., Pender, N. and Harrison, J. E. (2011). Factors affecting demineralization during orthodontic treatment: A post-hoc analysis of RCT recruits. *American Journal of Orthodontics and Dentofacial Orthopedics*, **139**, 181–91.

A useful study which concludes that pre-treatment age, oral hygiene and status of the first permanent molars can be used as a guide to the likelihood of decalcification occurring during treatment.

Mizrahi, E. (2010). Risk management in clinical practice. Part 7. Dento-legal aspects of orthodontic practice. *British Dental Journal*, **209**, 381–90.

Murray, A. M. (1989). Discontinuation of orthodontic treatment: a study of the contributing factors. *British Journal of Orthodontics*, **16**, 1–7.

Nguyen, Q. V., Bezemer, P. D., Habets, L., and Prahl-Andersen, B. (1999). A systematic review of the relationship between overjet size and traumatic dental injuries. *European Journal of Orthodontics*, **21**, 503–15.

Office for National Statistics (2004). *Children's dental health in the United Kingdom 2003*. Office for National Statistics, London.

Shaw, W. C., O'Brien, K. D., Richmond, S., and Brook, P. (1991). Quality control in orthodontics: risk/benefit considerations. *British Dental Journal*, **170**, 33–7.

A rather pessimistic view of orthodontics.

Weltman, B., Vig, K. W., Fields, H. W., Shanker, S. and Kaizar, E. E. (2010). Root resorption associated with orthodontic tooth movement: a systematic review. *American Journal of Orthodontics and Dentofacial Orthopedics*, **137**, 462–76.

Wheeler, T. T., McGorray, S. P., Yurkiewicz, L., Keeling, S. D., and King, G. J. (1994). Orthodontic treatment demand and need in third and fourth grade schoolchildren. *American Journal of Orthodontics and Dentofacial Orthopedics*, **106**, 22–33.

Contains a good discussion on the need and demand for treatment.

See also:

Readers' forum (December 2011) *American Journal of Orthodontics and Dentofacial Orthopedics*, **138**, 690–6.

An interesting and informative read on decalcification during orthodontic treatment.

The British Orthodontic Society also do an excellent Advice Sheet entitled 'Temporomandibular disorders (TMD) and the orthodontic patient' which unfortunately is only available to members (so you may need to track down a BOS member and ask nicely!).

References for this chapter can also be found at: www.oxfordtextbooks.co.uk/orc/mitchell4e/. Where possible, these are presented as active links which direct you to the electronic version of the work, to help facilitate onward study. If you are a subscriber to that work (either individually or through an institution), and depending on your level of access, you may be able to peruse an abstract or the full article if available.

2

The aetiology and classification of malocclusion

Chapter contents

2.1 The aetiology of malocclusion

The aetiology of malocclusion is a fascinating subject about which there is still much to elucidate and understand. At a basic level, malocclusion can occur as a result of genetically determined factors, which are inherited, or environmental factors, or more commonly a combination of both inherited and environmental factors acting together. For example, failure of eruption of an upper central incisor may arise as a result of dilaceration following an episode of trauma during the deciduous dentition which led to intrusion of the primary predecessor – an example of environmental aetiology. Failure of eruption of an upper central incisor can also occur as a result of the presence of a supernumerary tooth – a scenario which questioning may reveal also affected the patient's parent, suggesting an inherited problem. However, if in the latter example caries (an environmental factor) has led to early loss of many of the deciduous teeth then forward drift of the first permanent molar teeth may also lead to superimposition of the additional problem of crowding.

While it is relatively straightforward to trace the inheritance of syndromes such as cleft lip and palate (see Chapter 22), it is more difficult to determine the aetiology of features which are in essence part of normal variation, and the picture is further complicated by the compensatory mechanisms that exist. Evidence for the role of inherited factors in the aetiology of malocclusion has come from studies of families and twins. The facial similarity of members of a family, for example the prognathic mandible of the Hapsburg royal family, is easily appreciated. However, more direct testimony is provided in studies of twins and triplets, which indicate that skeletal pattern and tooth size and number are largely genetically determined.

Examples of environmental influences include digit-sucking habits and premature loss of teeth as a result of either caries or trauma. Soft tissue pressures acting upon the teeth for more than 6 hours per day can also influence tooth position. However, because the soft tissues including the lips are by necessity attached to the underlying skeletal framework, their effect is also mediated by the skeletal pattern.

Crowding is extremely common in Caucasians, affecting approximately two-thirds of the population. As was mentioned above, the size of the jaws and teeth are mainly genetically determined; however, environmental factors, for example premature deciduous tooth loss, can precipitate or exacerbate crowding. In evolutionary terms both jaw size and tooth size appear to be reducing. However, crowding is much more prevalent in modern populations than it was in prehistoric times. It has been postulated that this is due to the introduction of a less abrasive diet, so that less interproximal tooth wear occurs during the lifetime of an individual. However, this is not the whole story, as a change from a rural to an urban life-style can also apparently lead to an increase in crowding after about two generations.

Although this discussion may at first seem rather theoretical, the aetiology of malocclusion is a vigorously debated subject. This is because if one believes that the basis of malocclusion is genetically determined, then it follows that orthodontics is limited in what it can achieve. However, the opposite viewpoint is that every individual has the potential for ideal occlusion and that orthodontic intervention is required to eliminate those environmental factors that have led to a particular malocclusion. Research suggests that for the majority of malocclusions the aetiology is multifactorial with polygenic inheritance, and orthodontic treatment can effect only limited skeletal change. Therefore, as a patient's skeletal and growth pattern is largely genetically determined, if orthodontic treatment is to be successful clinicians must recognize and work within those parameters (see also Box 2.1).

When planning treatment for an individual patient it is often helpful to consider the role of the following in the aetiology of their malocclusion. Further discussion of these factors will be considered in the forthcoming chapters covering the main types of malocclusion:

(1) Skeletal pattern – in all three planes of space

(2) Soft tissues

(3) Dental factors

Of necessity, the above is a brief summary, but it can be appreciated that the aetiology of malocclusion is a complex subject, much of which is still not fully understood. The reader seeking more information is advised to consult the publications listed in the section on Further reading.

Box 2.1 Functional occlusion

- An occlusion which is free of interferences to smooth gliding movements of the mandible with no pathology
- Orthodontic treatment should aim to achieve a functional occlusion
- BUT lack of evidence to indicate that if an ideal functional occlusion is not achieved that there are deleterious long-term effects on the TMJs

2.2 Classifying malocclusion

The categorization of a malocclusion by its salient features is helpful for describing and documenting a patient's occlusion. In addition, classifications and indices allow the prevalence of a malocclusion within a population to be recorded, and also aid in the assessment of need, difficulty, and success of orthodontic treatment.

Malocclusion can be recorded qualitatively and quantitatively. However, the large number of classifications and indices which have been devised are testimony to the problems inherent in both these approaches. All have their limitations, and these should be borne in mind when they are applied (Box 2.2).

2.2.1 Qualitative assessment of malocclusion

Essentially, a qualitative assessment is descriptive and therefore this category includes the diagnostic classifications of malocclusion. The main drawback to a qualitative approach is that malocclusion is a continuous variable so that clear cut-off points between different categories do not always exist. This can lead to problems when classifying borderline malocclusions. In addition, although a qualitative classification is a helpful shorthand method of describing the salient features of a malocclusion, it does not provide any indication of the difficulty of treatment.

Qualitative evaluation of malocclusion was attempted historically before quantitative analysis. One of the better known classifications was devised by Angle in 1899, but other classifications are now more widely used, for example the British Standards Institute (1983) classification of incisor relationship.

2.2.2 Quantitative assessment of malocclusion

In quantitative indices two differing approaches can be used:

- Each feature of a malocclusion is given a score and the summed total is then recorded (e.g. the PAR Index).
- The worst feature of a malocclusion is recorded (e.g. the Index of Orthodontic Treatment Need).

> **Box 2.2 Important attributes of an index**
>
> - **Validity** — Can the index measure what it was designed to measure?
> - **Reproducibility** — Does the index give the same result when recorded on two different occasions and by different examiners?

2.3 Commonly used classifications and indices

2.3.1 Angle's classification

Angle's classification was based upon the premise that the first permanent molars erupted into a constant position within the facial skeleton, which could be used to assess the anteroposterior relationship of the arches. In addition to the fact that Angle's classification was based upon an incorrect assumption, the problems experienced in categorizing cases with forward drift or loss of the first permanent molars have resulted in this particular approach being superseded by other classifications. However, Angle's classification is still used to describe molar relationship, and the terms used to describe incisor relationship have been adapted into incisor classification.

Angle described three groups (Fig. 2.1):

- *Class I or neutrocclusion* — the mesiobuccal cusp of the upper first molar occludes with the mesiobuccal groove of the lower first molar. In practice discrepancies of up to half a cusp width either way were also included in this category.
- *Class II or distocclusion* — the mesiobuccal cusp of the lower first molar occludes distal to the Class I position. This is also known as a postnormal relationship.
- *Class III or mesiocclusion* — the mesiobuccal cusp of the lower first molar occludes mesial to the Class I position. This is also known as a prenormal relationship.

2.3.2 British Standards Institute classification

This is based upon incisor relationship and is the most widely used descriptive classification. The terms used are similar to those of Angle's classification, which can be a little confusing as no regard is taken of molar relationship. The categories defined by British Standard 4492 are shown in Box 2.3 below (see also Figs 2.2, 2.3, 2.4, 2.5):

As with any descriptive analysis it is difficult to classify borderline cases. Some workers have suggested introducing a Class II intermediate category for those cases where the upper incisors are upright and the overjet increased to between 4 and 6 mm. However, this suggestion has not gained widespread acceptance.

2.3.3 Summers occlusal index

This index was developed by Summers, in the USA, during the 1960s. It is popular in America, particularly for research purposes. Good reproducibility has been reported and it has also been employed to determine the success of treatment with acceptable results. The index scores nine defined parameters including molar relationship, overbite, overjet, posterior crossbite, posterior open bite, tooth displacement, midline relation, maxillary median diastema, and absent upper incisors. Allowance is made for different stages of development by varying the weighting applied to certain parameters in the deciduous, mixed, and permanent dentition.

Box 2.3 British Standards incisor classification

- *Class I* — the lower incisor edges occlude with or lie immediately below the cingulum plateau of the upper central incisors.
- *Class II* — the lower incisor edges lie posterior to the cingulum plateau of the upper incisors. There are two subdivisions of this category:

  Division 1 — the upper central incisors are proclined or of average inclination and there is an increase in overjet.

  Division 2 — The upper central incisors are retroclined. The overjet is usually minimal or may be increased.
- *Class III* — The lower incisor edges lie anterior to the cingulum plateau of the upper incisors. The overjet is reduced or reversed.

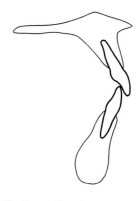

Fig. 2.2 Incisor classification — Class I.

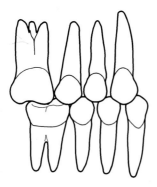

Class I

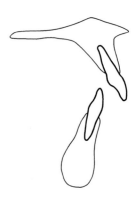

Fig. 2.3 Incisor classification — Class II division 1.

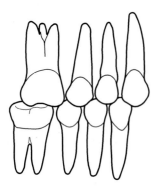

Class II

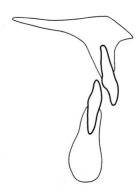

Fig. 2.4 Incisor classification — Class II division 2.

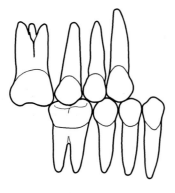

Class III

Fig. 2.1 Angle's classification.

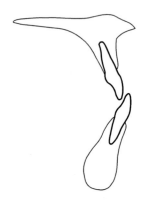

Fig. 2.5 Incisor classification — Class III.

2.3.4 Index of Orthodontic Treatment Need (IOTN)

The Index of Orthodontic Treatment Need was developed as a result of a government initiative. The purpose of the index was to help determine the likely impact of a malocclusion on an individual's dental health and psychosocial well-being. It comprises two elements.

Dental health component

This was developed from an index used by the Dental Board in Sweden designed to reflect those occlusal traits which could affect the function and longevity of the dentition. The single worst feature of a malocclusion is noted (the index is not cumulative) and categorized into one of five grades reflecting need for treatment (Table 2.1):

- *Grade 1* — no need
- *Grade 2* — little need
- *Grade 3* — moderate need
- *Grade 4* — great need
- *Grade 5* — very great need

A ruler has been developed to help with assessment of the dental health component (reproduced with the kind permission of UMIP Ltd. in Fig. 2.6), and these are available commercially. As only the single worst feature is recorded, an alternative approach is to look consecutively for the following features (known as MOCDO):

- Missing teeth
- Overjet
- Crossbite
- Displacement (contact point)
- Overbite

Aesthetic component

This aspect of the index was developed in an attempt to assess the aesthetic handicap posed by a malocclusion and thus the likely psychosocial impact upon the patient – a difficult task (see Chapter 1). The aesthetic component comprises a set of ten standard photographs (Fig. 2.7), which are also graded from score 1, the most aesthetically pleasing, to score 10, the least aesthetically pleasing. Colour photographs are available for assessing a patient in the clinical situation and black-and-white photographs for scoring from study models alone. The patient's teeth (or study models), in occlusion, are viewed from the anterior aspect and the appropriate score determined by choosing the photograph that is thought to pose an equivalent aesthetic handicap. The scores are categorized according to need for treatment as follows:

- score 1 or 2 — none
- score 3 or 4 — slight
- score 5, 6, or 7 — moderate/borderline
- score 8, 9, or 10 — definite

An average score can be taken from the two components, but the dental health component alone is more widely used. The aesthetic component has been criticized for being subjective – particular difficulty is experienced in accurately assessing Class III malocclusions or anterior open bites, as the photographs are composed of Class I and Class II cases, but studies have indicated good reproducibility.

2.3.5 Peer Assessment Rating (PAR)

The PAR index was developed primarily to measure the success (or otherwise) of treatment. Scores are recorded for a number of parameters (listed below), before and at the end of treatment using study models. Unlike IOTN, the scores are cumulative; however, a weighting is accorded to each component to reflect current opinion in the UK as to their relative importance. The features recorded are listed below, with the current weightings in parentheses:

- crowding — by contact point displacement ($\times 1$)
- buccal segment relationship — in the anteroposterior, vertical, and transverse planes ($\times 1$)
- overjet ($\times 6$)
- overbite ($\times 2$)
- centrelines ($\times 4$)

The difference between the PAR scores at the start and on completion of treatment can be calculated, and from this the percentage change in PAR score, which is a reflection of the success of treatment, is derived. A high standard of treatment is indicated by a mean percentage reduction of greater than 70 per cent. A change of 30 per cent or less indicates that no appreciable improvement has been achieved. The size of the PAR score at the beginning of treatment gives an indication of the severity of a malocclusion. Obviously it is difficult to achieve a significant reduction in PAR in cases with a low pretreatment score.

2.3.6 Index of Complexity, Outcome and Need (ICON)

This new index incorporates features of both the Index of Orthodontic Need (IOTN) and the Peer Assessment Rating (PAR). The following are scored and then each score is multiplied by its weighting:

- Aesthetic component of IOTN ($\times 7$)
- Upper arch crowding/spacing ($\times 5$)
- Crossbite ($\times 5$)
- Overbite/open bite ($\times 4$)
- Buccal segment relationship ($\times 3$)

The total sum gives a pretreatment score, which is said to reflect the need for, and likely complexity of, the treatment required. A score of more than 43 is said to indicate a demonstrable need for treatment. Following treatment the index is scored again to give an improvement grade and thus the outcome of treatment.

Improvement grade = pre-treatment score − (4 × post-treatment score)

This ambitious index has been criticized for the large weighting given to the aesthetic component and has not yet gained widespread acceptability.

Table 2.1 The Index of Orthodontic Treatment Need (Reproduced with the kind permission of UMIP Ltd.)

Grade 5 (Very Great)

5a	Increased overjet greater than 9 mm
5h	Extensive hypodontia with restorative implications (more than one tooth missing in any quadrant) requiring pre-restorative orthodontics
5i	Impeded eruption of teeth (with the exception of third molars) due to crowding, displacement, the presence of supernumerary teeth, retained deciduous teeth, and any pathological cause
5m	Reverse overjet greater than 3.5 mm with reported masticatory and speech difficulties
5p	Defects of cleft lip and palate
5s	Submerged deciduous teeth

Grade 4 (Great)

4a	Increased overjet 6.1–9 mm
4b	Reversed overjet greater than 3.5 mm with no masticatory or speech difficulties
4c	Anterior or posterior crossbites with greater than 2 mm discrepancy between retruded contact position and intercuspal position
4d	Severe displacement of teeth, greater than 4 mm
4e	Extreme lateral or anterior open bites, greater than 4 mm
4f	Increased and complete overbite with gingival or palatal trauma
4h	Less extensive hypodontia requiring pre-restorative orthodontic space closure to obviate the need for a prosthesis
4l	Posterior lingual crossbite with no functional occlusal contact in one or both buccal segments
4m	Reverse overjet 1.1–3.5 mm with recorded masticatory and speech difficulties
4t	Partially erupted teeth, tipped and impacted against adjacent teeth
4x	Supplemental teeth

Grade 3 (Moderate)

3a	Increased overjet 3.6–6 mm with incompetent lips
3b	Reverse overjet 1.1–3.5 mm
3c	Anterior or posterior crossbites with 1.1–2 mm discrepancy
3d	Displacement of teeth 2.1–4 mm
3e	Lateral or anterior open bite 2.1–4 mm
3f	Increased and complete overbite without gingival trauma

Grade 2 (Little)

2a	Increased overjet 3.6–6 mm with competent lips
2b	Reverse overjet 0.1–1 mm
2c	Anterior or posterior crossbite with up to 1 mm discrepancy between retruded contact position and intercuspal position
2d	Displacement of teeth 1.1–2 mm
2e	Anterior or posterior open bite 1.1–2 mm
2f	Increased overbite 3.5 mm or more, without gingival contact
2g	Prenormal or postnormal occlusions with no other anomalies; includes up to half a unit discrepancy

Grade 1 (None)

1	Extremely minor malocclusions including displacements less than 1 mm

	3				5 Defect of CLP	3 O.B. with NO G + P trauma	Displacement

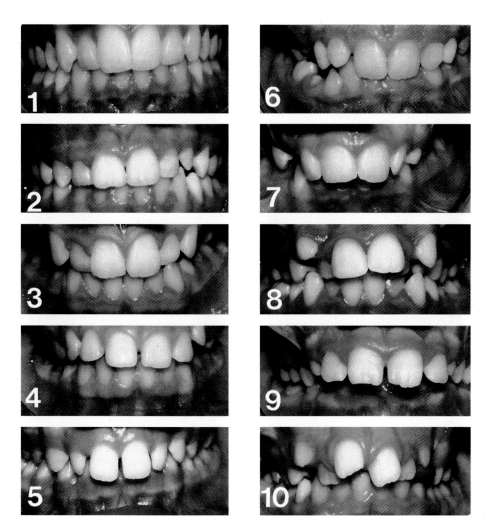

Figure content area showing an IOTN ruler table:

0	3 i 2 c	4		5	5 Defect of CLP 5 Non-eruption of teeth 5 Extensive hypodontia 4 Less extensive hypodontia 4 Crossbite >2 mm discrepancy 4 Scissors bite 4 O.B. with G + P trauma	3 O.B. with NO G + P trauma 3 Crossbite 1.2 mm discrepancy 2 O.B. > 2 Dev. From full interdig 2 Crossbite < 1 mm discrepancy ***IOTN Manchester (clinical)***	Displacement open bite V | | | ' 4 3 2 1
2							
3		4					
4	ms	-	5				

Fig. 2.6 IOTN ruler (Copyright © The University of Manchester 2005. All rights reserved).

Fig. 2.7 Aesthetic component of IOTN (the Aesthetic Component was originally described as 'SCAN' and was first published in 1987 by Evans, R. and Shaw, W. C. (1987). A preliminary evaluation of an illustrated scale for rating dental attractiveness. *European Journal of Orthodontics*, **9**, 314–8.

2.4 Andrews' six keys

Andrews analysed 120 'normal' occlusions to evaluate those features which were key to a good occlusion (it has been pointed out that these occlusions can more correctly be described as 'ideal'). He found six features, which are described in Box 2.4. These six keys are not a method of classifying occlusion as such, but serve as a goal. Occasionally at the end of treatment it is not possible to achieve a good Class I occlusion – in such cases it is helpful to look at each of these features in order to evaluate why.

Andrews used this analysis to develop the first pre-adjusted bracket system, which was designed to place the teeth (in three planes of space) to achieve his six keys (see Box 2.4). This prescription is called the Andrews' bracket prescription. For further details of pre-adjusted systems see Chapter 18.

Box 2.4 Andrews' six keys

Correct molar relationship: the mesiobuccal cusp of the upper first molar occludes with the groove between the mesiobuccal and middle buccal cusp of the lower first molar. The distobuccal cusp of the upper first molar contacts the mesiobuccal cusp of the lower second molar

Correct crown angulation: all tooth crowns are angulated mesially

Correct crown inclination: incisors are inclined towards the buccal or labial surface. Buccal segment teeth are inclined lingually. In the lower buccal segments this is progressive

No rotations

No spaces

Flat occlusal plane

Principal sources and further reading

Andrews, L. F. (1972). The six keys to normal occlusion. *American Journal of Orthodontics*, **62**, 296–309.

Angle, E. H. (1899). Classification of malocclusion. *Dental Cosmos*, **41**, 248–64.

British Standards Institute (1983). *Glossary of Dental Terms (BS 4492)*, BSI, London.

Daniels, C. and Richmond, S. (2000). The development of the Index of Complexity, Outcome and Need (ICON). *Journal of Orthodontics*, **27**, 149–62.

Harradine, N. W. T., Pearson, M. H., and Toth, B. (1998). The effect of extraction of third molars on late lower incisor crowding: A randomized controlled clinical trial. *British Journal of Orthodontics*, **25**, 117–22.

Markovic, M. (1992). At the crossroads of oral facial genetics. *European Journal of Orthodontics*, **14**, 469–81.

A fascinating study of twins and triplets with Class II/2 malocclusions.

Mossey, P. A. (1999). The heritability of malocclusion. *British Journal of Orthodontics*, **26**, 103–13, 195–203.

Proffit, W. R. (1978). Equilibrium theory revisited: factors influencing position of the teeth. *Angle Orthodontist*, **48**, 175–186.

Further reading for those wishing to learn more.

Richmond, S., Shaw, W. C., O'Brien, K. D., Buchanan, I. B., Jones, R., Stephens, C. D., *et al.* (1992). The development of the PAR index (Peer Assessment Rating): reliability and validity. *European Journal of Orthodontics*, **14**, 125–39.

The PAR index, part 1.

Richmond, S., Shaw, W. C., Roberts, C. T., and Andrews, M. (1992). The PAR index (Peer Assessment Rating): methods to determine the outcome of orthodontic treatment in terms of improvements and standards. *European Journal of Orthodontics*, **14**, 180–7.

The PAR index, part 2.

Summers, C. J. (1971). A system for identifying and scoring occlusal disorders. *American Journal of Orthodontics*, **59**, 552–67.

For readers requiring further information on Summers' occlusal index.

Shaw, W. C., O'Brien, K. D., and Richmond, S. (1991). Quality control in orthodontics: indices of treatment need and treatment standards. *British Dental Journal*, **170**, 107–12.

An interesting paper on the role of indices, with good explanations of the IOTN and the PAR index.

Tang, E. L. K. and Wei, S. H. Y. (1993). Recording and measuring malocclusion: a review of the literature. *American Journal of Orthodontics and Dentofacial Orthopedics*, **103**, 344–51.

Useful for those researching the subject.

References for this chapter can also be found at www.oxfordtextbooks.co.uk/orc/mitchell4e/. Where possible, these are presented as active links which direct you to the electronic version of the work, to help facilitate onward study. If you are a subscriber to that work (either individually or through an institution), and depending on your level of access, you may be able to peruse an abstract or the full article if available.

3 Management of the developing dentition

Many dental practitioners find it difficult to judge when to intervene in a developing malocclusion and when to let nature take its course. This is because experience is only gained over years of careful observation and decisions to intercede are often made in response to pressure exerted by the parents 'to do something'. It is hoped that this chapter will help impart some of the former, so that the reader is better able to resist the latter.

3.1 Normal dental development

It is important to realize that 'normal' in this context means average, rather than ideal. An appreciation of what constitutes the range of normal development is essential. One area in which this is particularly pertinent is eruption times (Table 3.1).

3.1.1 Calcification and eruption times

Knowledge of the calcification times of the permanent dentition is invaluable if one wishes to impress patients and colleagues. It is also helpful for assessing dental as opposed to chronological age; for determining whether a developing tooth not present on radiographic examination can be considered absent; and for estimating the timing of any possible causes of localized hypocalcification or hypoplasia (termed in this situation chronological hypoplasia).

3.1.2 The transition from primary to mixed dentition

The eruption of a baby's first tooth is heralded by the proud parents as a major landmark in their child's development. This milestone is described in many baby-care books as occurring at 6 months of age, which can lead to unnecessary concern as it is normal for the mandibular incisors to erupt at any time in the first year. Dental textbooks often dismiss 'teething', ascribing the symptoms that occur at this time to the diminution of maternal antibodies. Any parent will be able to correct this fallacy!

Eruption of the primary dentition (Fig. 3.1) is usually completed around 3 years of age. The deciduous incisors erupt upright and spaced – a lack of spacing strongly suggests that the permanent successors will be crowded. Overbite reduces throughout the primary dentition until the incisors are edge to edge, which can contribute to marked attrition.

The mixed dentition phase is usually heralded by the eruption of either the first permanent molars or the lower central incisors. The lower labial segment teeth erupt before their counterparts in the upper arch and develop lingual to their predecessors. It is usual for there to be some crowding of the permanent lower incisors as they emerge into the mouth, which reduces with intercanine growth. As a result the lower incisors often erupt slightly lingually placed and/or rotated (Fig. 3.2), but will usually align spontaneously if space becomes available. If the arch is inherently crowded, this space shortage will not resolve with intercanine growth.

Table 3.1 Average calcification and eruption times

	Calcification commences (weeks *in utero*)	Eruption (months)
Primary dentition		
Central incisors	12–16	6–7
Lateral incisors	13–16	7–8
Canines	15–18	18–20
First molars	14–17	12–15
Second molars	16–23	24–36

Root development complete 1–1½ years after eruption

	Calcification commences (months)	Eruption (years)
Permanent dentition		
Mand. central incisors	3–4	6–7
Mand. lateral incisors	3–4	7–8
Mand. canines	4–5	9–10
Mand. first premolars	21–24 ~ 2 years	10–12
Mand. second premolars	27–30 ~ 2½	11–12
Mand. first molars	Around birth	5–6
Mand. second molars	30–36	12–13
Mand. third molars	96–120	17–25
Max. central incisors	3–4	7–8
Max. lateral incisors	10–12	8–9
Max. canines	4–5	11–12
Max. first premolars	18–21	10–11
Max. second premolars	24–27 2y	10–12
Max. first molars	Around birth	5–6
Max. second molars	30–36 2½-3	12–13
Max. third molars	84–108 7-9	17–25

Root development complete 2–3 years after eruption.

The upper permanent incisors also develop lingual to their predecessors. Additional space is gained to accommodate their greater width because they erupt onto a wider arc and are more proclined than the primary incisors. If the arch is intrinsically crowded, the lateral incisors will not be able to move labially following eruption of the central incisors and therefore may erupt palatal to the arch. Pressure from the developing lateral incisor often gives rise to spacing between the central incisors which resolves as the laterals erupt. They in turn are tilted distally by the canines lying on the distal aspect of their root. This latter stage of development used to be described as the 'ugly duckling' stage of development (Fig. 3.3), although it is probably diplomatic to describe it as normal dental development to concerned parents. As the canines

erupt, the lateral incisors usually upright themselves and the spaces close. The upper canines develop palatally, but migrate labially to come to lie slightly labial and distal to the root apex of the lateral incisors. In normal development they can be palpated buccally from as young as 8 years of age.

The combined width of the deciduous canine, first molar, and second molar is greater than that of their permanent successors, particularly in the lower arch. This difference in widths is called the leeway space (Fig. 3.4) and in general is of the order of 1–1.5 mm in the maxilla and 2–2.5 mm in the mandible (in Caucasians). This means that if the deciduous buccal segment teeth are retained until their normal exfoliation time, there will be sufficient space for the permanent canine and premolars.

The deciduous second molars usually erupt with their distal surfaces flush anteroposteriorly. The transition to the stepped Class I molar relationship occurs during the mixed dentition as a result of differential mandibular growth and/or the leeway space.

3.1.3 Development of the dental arches

Intercanine width is measured across the cusps of the deciduous/permanent canines, and during the primary dentition an increase of around 1–2 mm is seen. In the mixed dentition an increase of about 3 mm occurs, but this growth is largely completed around a developmental stage of 9 years with some minimal increase up to age 13 years. After this time a gradual decrease is the norm.

Arch width is measured across the arch between the lingual cusps of the second deciduous molars or second premolars. Between the ages of 3 and 18 years an increase of 2–3 mm occurs; however, for clinical purposes arch width is largely established in the mixed dentition.

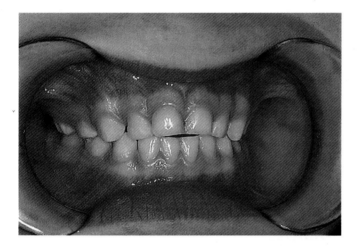

Fig. 3.1 Primary dentition.

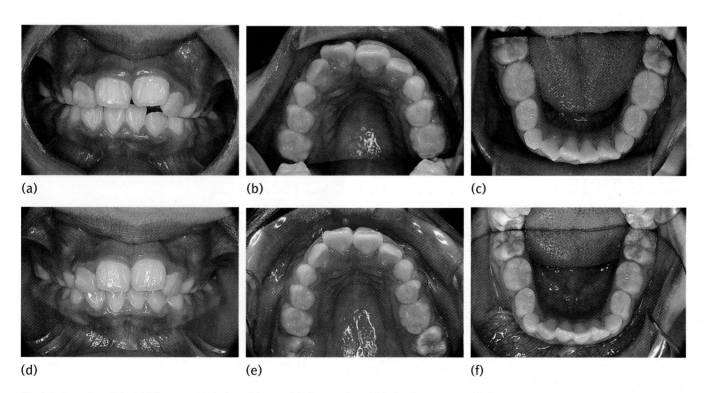

(a)   (b)   (c)

(d)   (e)   (f)

Fig. 3.2 Crowding of the labial segment reducing with growth in intercanine width: (a–c) age 8 years; (d–f) age 9 years.

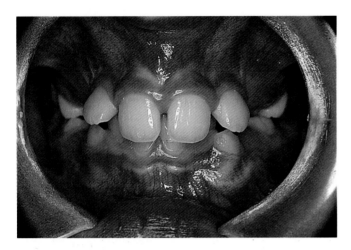

Fig. 3.3 'Ugly duckling' stage.

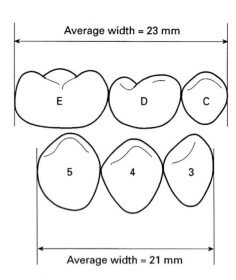

Fig. 3.4 Leeway space.

Arch circumference is determined by measuring around the buccal cusps and incisal edges of the teeth to the distal aspect of the second deciduous molars or second premolars. On average, there is little change with age in the maxilla; however, in the mandible arch circumference decreases by about 4 mm because of the leeway space. In individuals with crowded mouths a greater reduction may be seen.

In summary, on the whole there is little change in the size of the arch anteriorly after the establishment of the primary dentition, except for an increase in intercanine width which results in a modification of arch shape. Growth posteriorly provides space for the permanent molars, and considerable appositional vertical growth occurs to maintain the relationship of the arches during vertical facial growth.

3.2 Abnormalities of eruption and exfoliation

3.2.1 Screening

Early detection of any abnormalities in tooth development and eruption is essential to give the opportunity for interceptive action to be taken. This requires careful observation of the developing dentition for evidence of any problems, for example deviations from the normal sequence of eruption. If an abnormality is suspected then further investigation including radiographs is indicated. Around 9 to 10 years of age it is important to palpate the buccal sulcus for the permanent maxillary canines in order to detect any abnormalities in the eruption path of this tooth.

3.2.2 Natal teeth

A tooth, which is present at birth, or erupts soon after, is described as a natal tooth. These most commonly arise anteriorly in the mandible and are typically a lower primary incisor which has erupted prematurely (Fig. 3.6). Because root formation is not complete at this stage, natal teeth can be quite mobile, but they usually become firmer relatively quickly. If the tooth (or teeth) interferes with breast feeding or is so mobile that there is a danger of inhalation, removal is indicated and this

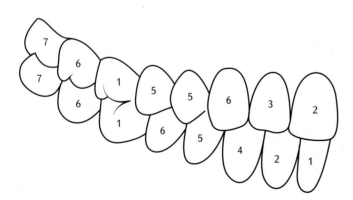

Fig. 3.5 Most common sequence of eruption.

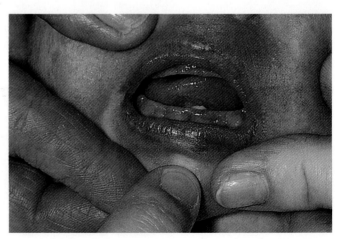

Fig. 3.6 Natal tooth present at birth.

can usually be accomplished with topical anaesthesia. If the tooth is symptomless, it can be left *in situ*.

3.2.3 Eruption cyst

An eruption cyst is caused by an accumulation of fluid or blood in the follicular space overlying the crown of an erupting tooth (Fig. 3.7). They usually rupture spontaneously, but very occasionally marsupialization may be necessary.

3.2.4 Failure of/delayed eruption

There is a wide individual variation in eruption times, which is illustrated by the patients in Fig. 3.8. Where there is a generalized tardiness in tooth eruption in an otherwise fit child, a period of observation is indicated. However, the following may be indicators of some abnormality and therefore warrant further investigation (Fig. 3.9). See also Box 3.1:

- A disruption in the normal sequence of eruption.
- An asymmetry in eruption pattern between contralateral teeth. If a tooth on one side of the arch has erupted and 6 months later there is still no sign of its equivalent on the other side, radiographic examination is indicated.

Localized failure of eruption is usually due to mechanical obstruction – this is advantageous as if the obstruction is removed then the affected tooth/teeth has the potential to erupt. More rarely, there is an abnormality of the eruption mechanism, which results in primary failure of eruption (the tooth does not erupt into the mouth) or arrest of eruption

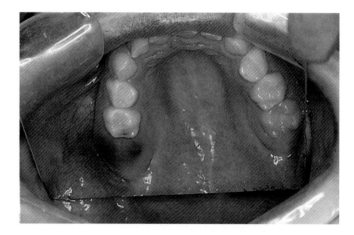

Fig. 3.7 Eruption cyst.

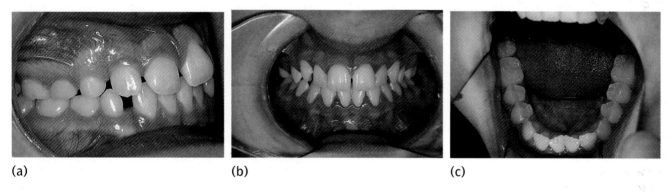

(a) (b) (c)

Fig. 3.8 Normal variation in eruption times: (a) patient aged 12.5 years with deciduous canines and molars still present; (b, c) patient aged 9 years with all permanent teeth to the second molars erupted.

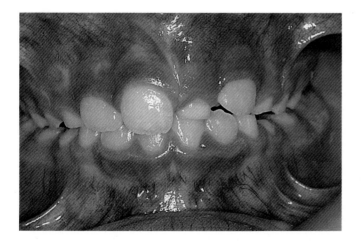

Fig. 3.9 Disruption of normal eruption sequence as 21/2 erupted, but /1 unerupted.

> ### Box 3.1 Causes of delayed eruption
>
> **Generalized causes**
>
> Hereditary gingival fibromatosis
> Down syndrome
> Cleidocranial dysostosis
> Cleft lip and palate
> Rickets
>
> **Localized causes**
>
> Congenital absence
> Crowding
> Delayed exfoliation of primary predecessor
> Supernumerary tooth
> Dilaceration
> Abnormal position of crypt
> Primary failure of eruption

(the tooth erupts, but then fails to keep up with eruption/development). This problem usually affects molar teeth and unfortunately for the individuals concerned, commonly affects more than one molar tooth in a quadrant. Extraction of the affected teeth is often necessary.

3.3 Mixed dentition problems

3.3.1 Premature loss of deciduous teeth

The major effect of early loss of a primary tooth, whether due to caries, premature exfoliation, or planned extraction, is localization of pre-existing crowding. In an uncrowded mouth this will not occur. However, where some crowding exists and a primary tooth is extracted, the adjacent teeth will drift or tilt around into the space provided. The extent to which this occurs depends upon the degree of crowding, the patient's age, and the site. Obviously, as the degree of crowding increases so does the pressure for the remaining teeth to move into the extraction space. The younger the child is when the primary tooth is extracted, the greater is the potential for drifting to ensue. The effect of the site of tooth loss is best considered by tooth type, but it is important to bear in mind the increased potential for mesial drift in the maxilla (see also Box 3.2).

- **Deciduous incisor:** premature loss of a deciduous incisor has little impact, mainly because they are shed relatively early in the mixed dentition.
- **Deciduous canine:** unilateral loss of a primary canine in a crowded mouth will lead to a centreline shift (Fig. 3.10). To avoid this when unilateral premature loss of a deciduous canine is necessary consideration should be given to balancing with the extraction of the contralateral tooth.
- **Deciduous first molar:** unilateral loss of this tooth may result in a centreline shift. In most cases an automatic balancing extraction is not necessary, but the centreline should be kept under observation and, if indicated, a tooth on the opposite side of the arch removed.
- **Deciduous second molar:** if a second primary molar is extracted the first permanent molar will drift forwards (Fig. 3.11). This is particularly marked if loss occurs before the eruption of the permanent tooth and for this reason it is better, if at all possible, to try to preserve the second deciduous molar at least until the first permanent molar has appeared. In most cases balancing or compensating extractions of other sound second primary molars is not necessary unless they are also of poor long-term prognosis.

It should be emphasized that the above are suggestions, not rules, and at all times a degree of common sense and forward planning should be applied – in essence a risk–benefit analysis needs to be worked

through for each child/tooth. For example, if extraction of a carious first primary molar is required and the contralateral tooth is also doubtful, then it might be preferable in the long term to extract both. Also, in children with an absent permanent tooth (or teeth) early extraction of the primary buccal segment teeth may be advantageous to encourage forward movement of the first permanent molars if space closure (rather then space opening) is planned.

The effect of early extraction of a primary tooth on the eruption of its successor is variable and will not necessarily result in a hastening of eruption.

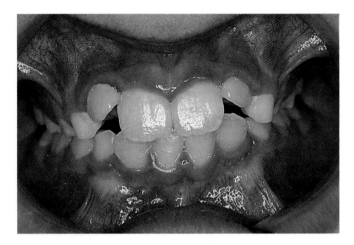

Fig. 3.10 Centreline shift to patient's left owing to early unbalanced loss of lower left deciduous canine.

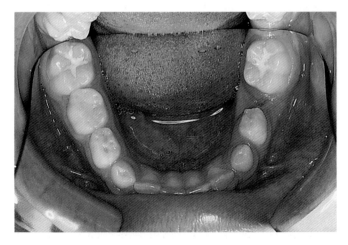

Fig. 3.11 Loss of a lower second deciduous molar leading to forward drift of first permanent molar.

Box 3.2 Balancing and compensating extractions

Balancing extraction is the removal of the contralateral tooth – *rationale is to avoid centreline shift problems*

Compensating extraction is the removal of the equivalent opposing tooth – *rationale is to maintain occlusal relationships between the arches*

Space maintenance

It goes without saying that the best space maintenance is a tooth – particularly as this will preserve alveolar bone. Much has been written in paedodontic texts about using space maintainers to replace extracted deciduous teeth, but in practice most orthodontists avoid this approach in the mixed dentition because of the implications for dental health and to minimize straining patient co-operation (which may be needed for definitive orthodontic treatment later). The exception to this is where preservation of space for a permanent successor will avoid subsequent appliance treatment.

3.3.2 Retained deciduous teeth

A difference of more than 6 months between the shedding of contralateral teeth should be regarded with suspicion. Provided that the permanent successor is present, retained primary teeth should be extracted, particularly if they are causing deflection of the permanent tooth (Fig. 3.12).

3.3.3 Infra-occluded (submerged) primary molars

Infra-occlusion is now the preferred term for describing the process where a tooth fails to achieve or maintain its occlusal relationship with adjacent or opposing teeth. Most infra-occluded deciduous teeth erupt into occlusion but subsequently become 'submerged' because bony growth and development of the adjacent teeth continues (Fig. 3.13). Estimates vary, but this anomaly would appear to occur in around 1–9 per cent of children.

Resorption of deciduous teeth is not a continuous process. In fact, resorption is interchanged with periods of repair, although in most cases the former prevails. If a temporary predominance of repair occurs, this can result in ankylosis and infra-occlusion of the affected primary molar.

The results of recent epidemiological studies have suggested a genetic tendency to this phenomenon and also an association with other dental anomalies including ectopic eruption of first permanent molars, palatal displacement of maxillary canines, and congenital absence of premolar teeth. Therefore, it is advisable to be vigilant in patients exhibiting any of these features.

Where a permanent successor exists the phenomenon is usually temporary, and studies have shown no difference in the age at exfoliation of a submerged primary molar compared with an unaffected contralateral tooth. Therefore extraction of a submerged primary tooth is only necessary under the following conditions:

- There is a danger of the tooth disappearing below gingival level (Fig. 3.14).
- Root formation of the permanent tooth is nearing completion (as eruptive force reduces markedly after this event).

In the buccal segments if the permanent successor is missing preservation of the primary molar will preserve bone, therefore consideration should be given to building up the occlusal surface to maintain occlusal relationships. If this is not practicable then extraction is indicated.

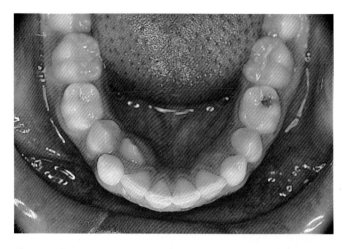

Fig. 3.12 Retained primary tooth contributing to deflection of the permanent successor.

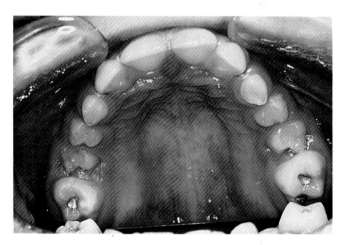

Fig. 3.13 Ankylosed primary molars.

3.3.4 Impacted first permanent molars

Impaction of a first permanent molar tooth against the second deciduous molar occurs in approximately 2–6 per cent of children and is indicative of crowding. It most commonly occurs in the upper arch (Fig. 3.15). Spontaneous disimpaction may occur, but this is rare after 8 years of age. Mild cases can sometimes be managed by tightening a brass separating wire around the contact point between the two teeth over a period of about 2 months. This can have the effect of pushing the permanent molar distally, thus letting it jump free. In more severe cases the impaction can be kept under observation, although extraction of the deciduous tooth may be indicated if it becomes abscessed or the permanent tooth becomes carious and restoration is precluded by poor access. The resultant space loss can be dealt with in the permanent dentition.

3.3.5 Dilaceration

Dilaceration is a distortion or bend in the root of a tooth. It usually affects the upper central and/or lateral incisor.

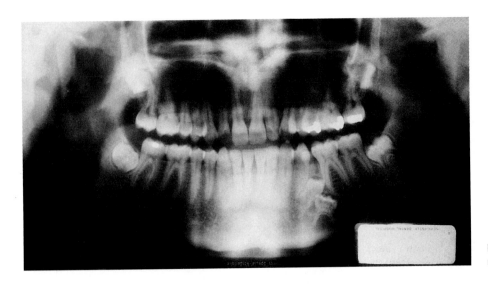

Fig. 3.14 Marked submergence of deciduous molar (with second premolar affected).

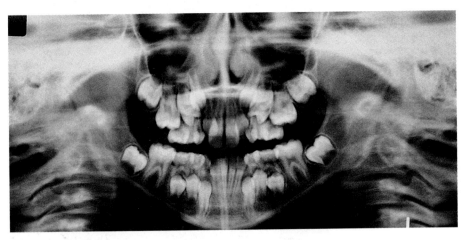

Fig. 3.15 Impacted bilateral upper first permanent molars.

Aetiology

There appears to be two distinct aetiologies:

- Developmental – this anomaly usually affects an isolated central incisor and occurs more often in females than males. The crown of the affected tooth is turned upward and labially and no disturbance of enamel and dentine is seen (Fig. 3.16).

- Trauma – intrusion of a deciduous incisor leads to displacement of the underlying developing permanent tooth germ. Characteristically, this causes the developing permanent tooth crown to be deflected palatally, and the enamel and dentine forming at the time of the injury are disturbed, giving rise to hypoplasia. The sexes are equally affected and more than one tooth may be involved depending upon the extent of the trauma.

Management

Dilaceration usually results in failure of eruption. Where the dilaceration is severe there is often no alternative but to remove the affected tooth. In milder cases it may be possible to expose the crown surgically and apply traction to align the tooth, provided that the root apex will be sited within cancellous bone at the completion of crown alignment.

3.3.6 Supernumerary teeth

A supernumerary tooth is one that is additional to the normal series. This anomaly occurs in the permanent dentition in approximately 2 per cent of the population and in the primary dentition in less than 1 per cent, though a supernumerary in the deciduous dentition is often followed by a supernumerary in the permanent dentition. The aetiology is not completely understood, but appears to have a genetic component. It occurs more commonly in males than females. Supernumerary teeth are also commonly found in the region of the cleft in individuals with a cleft of the alveolus.

Supernumerary teeth can be described according to their morphology or position in the arch.

Morphology

- Supplemental: this type resembles a tooth and occurs at the end of a tooth series, for example an additional lateral incisor, second premolar, or fourth molar (Fig. 3.17).

- Conical: the conical or peg-shaped supernumerary most often occurs between the upper central incisors (Fig. 3.18). It is said to be more commonly associated with displacement of the adjacent teeth, but can also cause failure of eruption or not affect the other teeth.

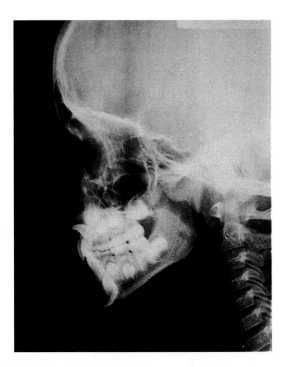

Fig. 3.16 A dilacerated central incisor.

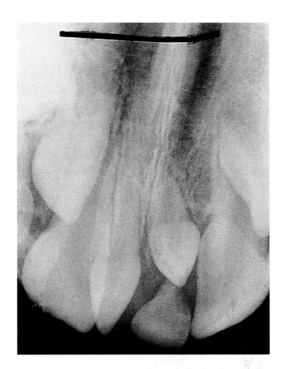

Fig. 3.18 Two conical supernumeraries lying between 1/1 with /A retained.

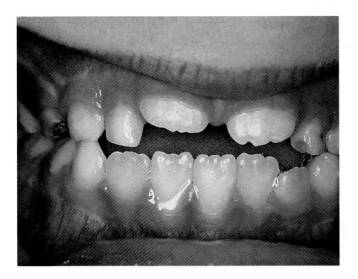

Fig. 3.17 A supplemental lower lateral incisor.

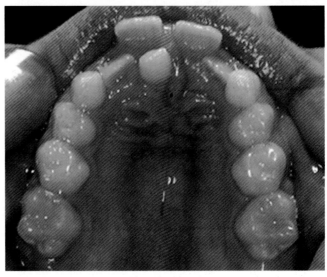

Fig. 3.19 A supernumerary which erupted palatal to upper incisors.

- Tuberculate: this type is described as being barrel-shaped, but usually any supernumerary which does not fall into the conical or supplemental categories is included. Classically, this type is associated with failure of eruption (Fig. 3.19).

- Odontome: this variant is rare. Both compound and complex forms have been described.

Position

Supernumerary teeth can occur within the arch, but when they develop between the central incisors they are often described as a mesiodens. A supernumerary tooth distal to the arch is called a distomolar, and one adjacent to the molars is known as a paramolar. Eighty per cent of supernumeraries occur in the anterior maxilla.

Effects of supernumerary teeth and their management

Failure of eruption

The presence of a supernumerary tooth is the most common reason for the non-appearance of a maxillary central incisor. However, failure of eruption of any tooth in either arch can be caused by a supernumerary.

Management of this problem involves removing the supernumerary tooth and ensuring that there is sufficient space to accommodate the unerupted tooth in the arch. If the tooth does not erupt spontaneously within 1 year, then a second operation to expose it and apply orthodontic traction may be required. Management of a patient with this problem is illustrated in Fig. 3.20.

Displacement

The presence of a supernumerary tooth can be associated with displacement or rotation of an erupted permanent tooth (Fig. 3.21). Management involves firstly removal of the supernumerary, usually followed by fixed appliances to align the affected tooth or teeth. It is said that this type of displacement has a high tendency to relapse following treatment, but this may be a reflection of the fact that the malposition is usually in the form of a rotation or an apical displacement which, in themselves, are particularly liable to relapse.

Crowding

This is caused by the supplemental type and is treated by removing the most poorly formed or more displaced tooth (Fig. 3.22).

No effect

Occasionally a supernumerary tooth (usually of the conical type) is detected as a chance finding on a radiograph of the upper incisor region (Fig. 3.23). Provided that the extra tooth will not interfere with any planned movement of the upper incisors, it can be left *in situ* under radiographic observation. In practice these teeth usually remain symptomless and do not give rise to any problems. Some conical supernumeraries erupt palatally to the upper incisors, in which case their removal is straightforward.

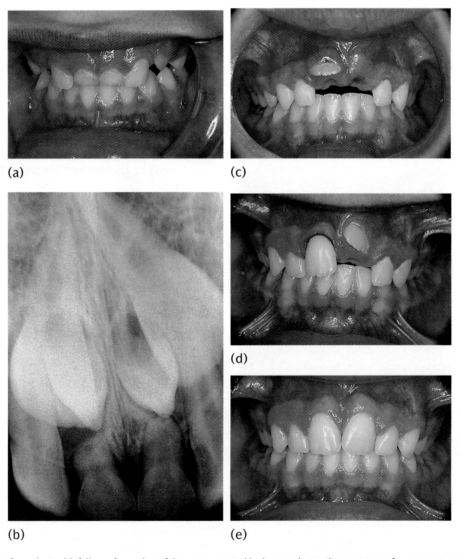

(a)

(c)

(b)

(d)

(e)

Fig. 3.20 Management of a patient with failure of eruption of the upper central incisors owing to the presence of two supernumerary teeth: (a) patient on presentation aged 10 years; (b) radiograph showing unerupted central incisors and associated conical supernumerary teeth; (c) following removal of the supernumerary teeth a URA was fitted to open space for the central incisors, until 1/ erupted 10 months later; (d) 7 months later /1 erupted and a simple appliance was used to align /1; (e) occlusion 3 years after initial presentation.

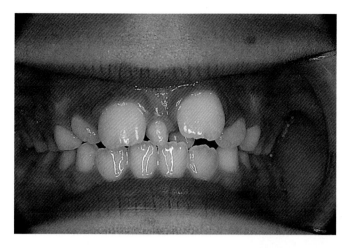

Fig. 3.21 Displacement of 1/1 caused by two erupted conical supernumerary teeth.

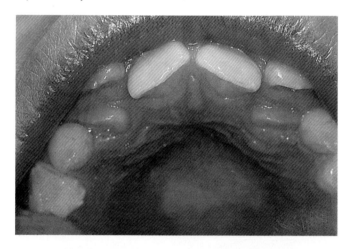

Fig. 3.22 Crowding due to the presence of two supplemental upper lateral incisors.

3.3.7 Habits

The effect of a habit will depend upon the frequency and intensity of indulgence. This problem is discussed in greater detail in Chapter 9, Section 9.1.4.

3.3.8 First permanent molars of poor long-term prognosis

The integrity of the first permanent molars is often compromised due to caries and/or hypoplasia secondary to a childhood illness. Treatment planning for a child with poor-quality first permanent molars is always difficult because several competing factors have to be considered before a decision can be reached for a particular individual. First permanent molars are never the first tooth of choice for extraction as their position within the arch means that little space is provided anteriorly for relief of crowding or correction of the incisor relationship unless appliances are used. Removal of maxillary first molars often compromises anchorage in the upper arch, and a good spontaneous result in the lower arch following extraction of the first molars is rare. However, patients for whom enforced extraction of the first molars is required are often the least able to support complicated treatment. Finally, it has to be remembered that, unless the caries rate is reduced, the premolars may be similarly affected a few years later. Nevertheless, if a two-surface restoration is present or required in the first permanent molar of a child, the prognosis for that tooth and the remaining first molars should be considered as the planned extraction of first permanent molars of poor quality may be preferable to their enforced extraction later on (Fig. 3.24).

Factors to consider when assessing first permanent molars of poor long-term prognosis

It is impossible to produce hard and fast rules regarding the extraction of first permanent molars, and therefore the following should only be considered a starting point:

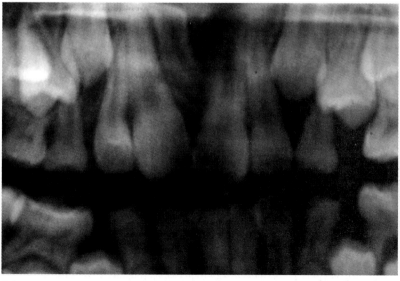

(a)

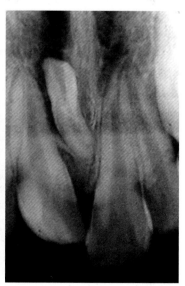

(b)

Fig. 3.23 Chance finding of a supernumerary on routine radiographic examination.

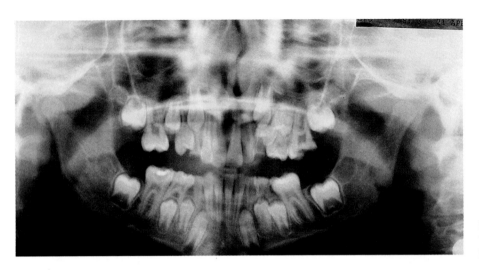

Fig. 3.24 All four first permanent molars were extracted in this patient because of the poor long-term prognosis for 6⌐ and ⌐6.

- Check for the presence of all permanent teeth. If any are absent, extraction of the first permanent molar in that quadrant should be avoided.
- If the dentition is uncrowded, extraction of first permanent molars should be avoided as space closure will be difficult.
- Remember that in the maxilla there is a greater tendency for mesial drift and so the timing of the extraction of upper first permanent molars is less critical if aiming for space closure.
- In the lower arch a good spontaneous result is more likely if:
  (a) the lower second permanent molar has developed as far as its bifurcation;
  (b) the angle between the long axis of the crypt of the lower second permanent molar and the first permanent molar is between 15° and 30°;
  (c) the crypt of the second molar overlaps the root of the first molar (a space between the two reduces the likelihood of good space closure).
- Extraction of the first molars alone will relieve buccal segment crowding, but will have little effect on a crowded labial segment.
- If space is needed anteriorly for the relief of labial segment crowding or for retraction of incisors (i.e. the upper arch in Class II cases or the lower arch in Class III cases), then it may be prudent to delay extraction of the first molar, if possible, until the second permanent molar has erupted in that arch. The space can then be utilized for correction of the labial segment.
- Serious consideration should be given to extracting the opposing upper first permanent molar, should extraction of a lower molar be necessary. If the upper molar is not extracted it will over-erupt and prevent forward drift of the lower second molar (Fig. 3.25).
- A compensating extraction in the lower arch (when extraction of an upper first permanent molar is necessary) should be avoided where possible as a good spontaneous result in the mandibular arch is less likely.
- Impaction of the third permanent molars is less likely, but not impossible, following extraction of the first molar.

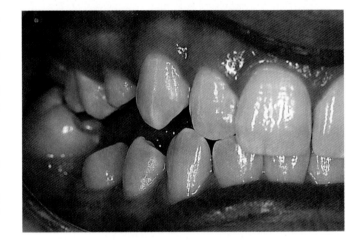

Fig. 3.25 Over-eruption of 6/ preventing forward movement of the lower right second permanent molar.

3.3.9 Median diastema

Prevalence

Median diastema occurs in 98 per cent of 6-year-olds, 49 per cent of 11-year-olds, and 7 per cent of 12–18-year-olds.

Aetiology

Factors, which have been considered to lead to a median diastema include the following:

- physiological (normal dental development)
- small teeth in large jaws (a spaced dentition)
- missing teeth
- midline supernumerary tooth/teeth
- proclination of the upper labial segment
- prominent fraenum

A median diastema is normally present between the maxillary permanent central incisors when they first erupt. As the lateral incisors and then the canines emerge the diastema usually closes. Therefore a midline diastema is a normal feature of the developing dentition; however, if it persists after eruption of the canines, it is unlikely that it will close spontaneously.

In the deciduous dentition the upper midline fraenum runs between the central incisors and attaches into the incisive papilla area. However, as the central incisors move together with eruption of the lateral incisors, it tends to migrate round onto the labial aspect. In a spaced upper arch, or where the upper lateral incisors are missing (see Fig. 8.12), this recession of the fraenal attachment is less likely to occur and in such cases it is obviously not appropriate to attribute the persistence of a diastema to the fraenum itself. However, in a small proportion of cases the upper midline fraenum can contribute to the persistence of a diastema. Factors, which may indicate that this is the case, include the following.

- When the fraenum is placed under tension there is blanching of the incisive papilla.
- Radiographically, a notch can be seen at the crest of the interdental bone between the upper central incisors (Fig. 3.26).
- The anterior teeth may be crowded.

Management

It is advisable to take a periapical radiograph to exclude the presence of a midline supernumerary tooth prior to planning treatment for a midline diastema.

In the developing dentition a diastema of less than 3 mm rarely warrants intervention; in particular, extraction of the deciduous canines should be avoided as this will tend to make the diastema worse. However, if the diastema is greater than 3 mm and the lateral incisors are present, it may be necessary to consider appliance treatment to approximate the central incisors to provide space for the laterals and canines to erupt. However, care should be taken to ensure that the

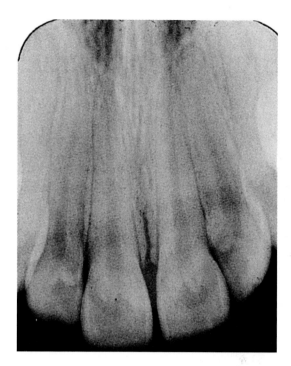

Fig. 3.26 Notch in interdental bone between 1/1 associated with a fraenal insertion running between 1/1 into the incisive papilla.

roots of the teeth being moved are not pressed against any unerupted crowns as this can lead to root resorption. If the crowns of the teeth are tilted distally, an upper removable appliance can be used to approximate the teeth, but usually fixed appliances are required. Closure of a diastema has a notable tendency to relapse, therefore long-term retention is required. This is most readily accomplished by placement of a bonded retainer.

3.4 Planned extraction of deciduous teeth

3.4.1 Serial extraction

Serial extraction was first advocated in 1948 by Kjellgren, a Swedish orthodontist, as a solution to a shortage of orthodontists. Kjellgren hoped that his scheme would facilitate the treatment of patients with straightforward crowding by their own dentists, thus minimizing demands upon the orthodontic service. He suggested the employment of a planned sequence of extractions (initially the deciduous canines, then the deciduous first molars) designed to allow crowded incisor segments to align spontaneously during the mixed dentition by shifting labial segment crowding to the buccal segments where it could be dealt with by first premolar extractions. The disadvantages to this approach are that it involves putting the child through several sequences of extractions and, as intercanine growth is occurring during this time, it is difficult to assess accurately how crowded the dentition will be, at the stage when serial extraction is usually embarked upon. A nice result can be achieved with serial extraction in selected cases,

namely Class I with moderate crowding and all permanent teeth present in a good position, but often this type of case also responds well to extraction of only the first premolars upon eruption – this latter approach eliminates some of the potential pitfalls and diminishes the guesswork involved.

3.4.2 Indications for the extraction of deciduous canines

Nevertheless there are a number of occasions where the timely extraction of the deciduous canines may avoid more complicated treatment later.

- In a crowded upper arch the erupting lateral incisors may be forced palatally. In a Class I malocclusion this will result in a crossbite and in addition the apex of the affected lateral incisor will be palatally positioned, making later correction more difficult. Extraction of the deciduous canines whilst the lateral incisors are erupting often results in their being able to escape spontaneously labially into a better position.

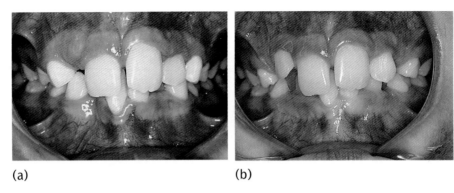

(a)   (b)

Fig. 3.27 (a) In this patient all four deciduous canines were extracted to relieve the labial segment crowding; (b) note how the periodontal condition of the lower right central incisor has improved 6 months later.

- In a crowded lower labial segment one incisor may be pushed through the labial plate of bone, resulting in a compromised labial periodontal attachment. Relief of crowding by extraction of the lower deciduous canines usually results in the lower incisor moving back into the arch and improving periodontal support (Fig. 3.27).
- Extraction of the lower deciduous canines in a Class III malocclusion can be advantageous.

- To provide space for appliance therapy in the upper arch, for example correction of an instanding lateral incisor, or to facilitate eruption of an incisor prevented from erupting by a supernumerary tooth.
- To improve the position of a displaced permanent canine (see Chapter 14).

3.5 What to refer and when

Most orthodontic problems are more appropriately referred and treated in the early permanent dentition. However, earlier referral is indicated:

Deciduous dentition

- Cleft lip and/or palate (if patient not under the care of a cleft team)
- Other craniofacial anomalies (if patient not under the care of a multi-disciplinary team)

Mixed dentition

- Severe Class III skeletal problems which would benefit from orthopaedic treatment
- Delayed eruption of the permanent incisors
- Impaction or failure of eruption of the first permanent molars

- First permanent molars of poor long-term prognosis where forced extraction is being considered
- Marked mandibular displacement on closure and/or anterior cross-bites which compromise periodontal support
- Hypodontia
- Ectopic maxillary canines
- Patients with medical problems where monitoring of the occlusion would be beneficial
- Pathology e.g. cysts

Growth modification in skeletal Class II malocclusions is more successful if carried out in early permanent dentition, therefore referral should be timed accordingly. The exceptions to this are patients with increased overjets who are being psychologically affected by severe teasing and those whose upper incisors are at risk of trauma (usually due to grossly incompetent lips).

Principal sources and further reading

Bishara, S. E. (1997). Arch width changes from 6 weeks to 45 years of age. *American Journal of Orthodontics and Dentofacial Orthopedics*, **111**, 401–9.

British Orthodontic Society (http://www.bos.org.uk) Advice Sheet 7. Dummies and Digit Sucking.

Unfortunately this advice sheet is only available to BOS members so you will need to approach a member to get a copy

Bjerklin, K., Kurol, J., and Valentin, J. (1992). Ectopic eruption of maxillary first permanent molars and association with other tooth and development disturbances. *European Journal of Orthodontics*, **14**, 369–75

The results of this study suggest a link between ectopic eruption of first permanent molars, infra-occlusion of deciduous molars, ectopic maxillary canines and absent premolars. Given this association, the wise practitioner will be alerted to other anomalies in patients presenting with any of these features.

Cobourne, M., Williams, A. and McMullan, R. (2009). A Guideline for first permanent molar extraction in children. Faculty of Dental Surgery of the Royal College of Surgeons of England. (http://www.rcseng.ac.uk/fds/publications-clinical-guidelines/clinical_guidelines/documents/A%20Guideline%20for%20the%20Enforced%20Extraction%20of%20First%20Permanent%20Molars%20in%20Children%20rev%20March%202009.pdf).

An excellent résumé of the available evidence on this important topic.

Foster, T. D. and Grundy, M. C. (1986). Occlusal changes from primary to permanent dentitions. *British Journal of Orthodontics*, **13**, 187–93.

Faculty of Dental Surgery of the Royal College of Surgeons of England Guidelines. (2006) Extraction of primary teeth – Balance and Compensation (http://www.rcseng.ac.uk/fds/publications-clinical-guidelines/clinical_guidelines/documents/extractp.pdf).

Gorlin, R. J., Cohen, M. M., and Levin, L. S. (1990). *Syndromes of the Head and Neck* (3rd edn). Oxford University Press, Oxford.

Source of calcification and eruption dates (and a vast amount of additional information not directly related to this chapter).

Kurol, J. and Bjerklin, K. (1986). Ectopic eruption of maxillary first permanent molars: a review. *Journal of Dentistry for Children*, **53**, 209–15.

All you need to know about impacted first permanent molars.

Kurol, J. and Koch, G. (1985). The effect of extraction of infraoccluded deciduous molars: a longitudinal study. *American Journal of Orthodontics*, **87**, 46–55.

Stewart, D. J. (1978). Dilacerate unerupted maxillary incisors. *British Dental Journal*, **145**, 229–33.

Welbury, R. R., Duggal, M. S. and Hosey, M-T. (2005). *Paediatric Dentistry* (3rd edn). Oxford University Press, Oxford.

Yacoob, O., O'Neill, J., Gregg, T., Noar, J., Cobourne, M. and Morris, D. (2010). Management of unerupted maxillary incisors. Faculty of Dental Surgery of the Royal College of Surgeons of England. (http://www.rcseng.ac.uk/fds/publications-clinical-guidelines/clinical_guidelines/documents/ManMaxIncisors2010.pdf)

The British Orthodontic Society also produced an excellent booklet entitled:

Managing the Developing Occlusion (2010) http://www.bos.org.uk/publicationslinks/Publications+relevant+to+Members/Managing+the+Developing+Occlusion

 References for this chapter can also be found at www.oxfordtextbooks.co.uk/orc/mitchell4e/. Where possible, these are presented as active links which direct you to the electronic version of the work, to help facilitate onward study. If you are a subscriber to that work (either individually or through an institution), and depending on your level of access, you may be able to peruse an abstract or the full article if available.

4

Craniofacial growth, the cellular basis of tooth movement and anchorage

Z. L. Nelson-Moon

Chapter contents

Learning objectives for this chapter

- Explain the processes of craniofacial development, including the role of the cranial neural crest cells
- Describe post-natal craniofacial growth from birth onwards
- Describe the cellular biology of orthodontic tooth movement
- Demonstrate knowledge of the molecular biological processes involved in craniofacial development and orthodontic tooth movement
- Explain the cellular basis of orthodontic anchorage and orthodontically-induced root resorption

---

4.1 Introduction

Growth may be defined as an increase in size by natural development and is the consequence of cellular proliferation and differentiation. An understanding of craniofacial development and growth is essential for the accurate diagnosis and treatment planning of even the most straightforward malocclusion as the majority of orthodontic treatment is still performed on growing individuals – children. Growth can affect the severity of the malocclusion, improving it or worsening it as growth continues; the progress and outcome of orthodontic treatment, and the stability of the orthodontic result. Orthodontic treatment may also have an effect on facial growth.

Craniofacial growth is a complex process involving many interactions between the different bones that make up the skull and between the hard and soft tissues. The processes that control craniofacial growth are not fully understood and are an area of extremely active research globally. However, the descriptions of where growth occurs within a bone and how this relates to changes in bone shape and position have been described for over 200 years.

Orthodontic treatment would not be possible without the ability of the alveolar bone to remodel to allow the teeth and the associated periodontium to move within the alveolus. In the last 25 years, rapid advances in scientific techniques, especially those related to cellular and molecular biology, have ensured a better, albeit not complete, understanding of the cellular responses involved in tooth movement.

This chapter will begin by outlining some essential embryology followed by a description of the manner in which the craniofacial bones grow, the control of craniofacial growth and the ability to predict craniofacial growth. This is followed by a description of the cellular basis for orthodontic tooth movement and the relevance of this to planning orthodontic anchorage requirements.

4.2 Craniofacial embryology

A basic knowledge of craniofacial embryology is important for all dental practitioners, but especially for orthodontists as it gives insight into future craniofacial growth and the possible causes of developmental anomalies of the craniofacial region. Craniofacial anomalies represent three-quarters of all birth defects. However, before discussing the development of the face, an understanding of the role of neural crest and pharyngeal arch development is essential.

4.2.1 Neural crest

Neural crest (NC) is ectomesenchymal tissue arising from the crest of the neural fold (Fig. 4.1) and is considered to be a separate (4th) germ layer that is capable of forming many different cell types (pluripotent) and is highly migratory (Box 4.1). The fact that so many of the tissues of the craniofacial region are derivatives of neural crest means that any errors in specification, migration, proliferation and differentiation of neural crest cells will lead to significant disruption in the development of the structures in this region. Conditions caused by errors with neural crest cells are called neurocristopathies.

Neural crest from the cranial region of the neural tube which is destined to become the hind brain migrates between the ectoderm and mesoderm and expands during migration. However, cranial neural crest cells from different regions (rhombomeres) of the developing hind brain

---

Box 4.1 Derivatives of cranial neural crest cells

Cartilage and bone of the prechordal skull
Meckel's (1st), Reichart's (2nd) and other pharyngeal arch cartilages
Intramembranous bones of the craniofacial skeleton
Odontoblasts
Connective tissue
Dermis of the face and neck
Tendons and fascia of craniofacial voluntary muscles
Meninges of the brain
Neurones of most cranial nerve ganglia
Parafollicular (calcitonin) cells of thyroid gland
Melanocytes

(a)

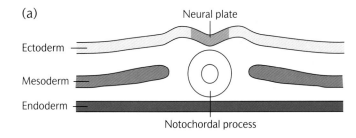

(b)

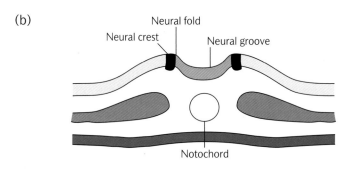

(c)

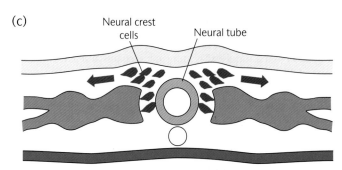

Fig. 4.1 Diagrammatic representation of neural tube and neural crest development. A, Cross section through trilaminar disc at day 18 i.u. The appearance of the neural plate marks the beginning of neural tube development. B and C Development of the neural tube from the neural plate and migration of the neural crest cells from the neural folds. (Redrawn from Meikle, M. C. (2002) *Craniofacial Development, Growth and Evolution*, Bateson Publishing, Norfolk, England).

migrate into specific areas and neural crest derivatives are pre-specified. The patterning of cranial neural crest derivatives is controlled by a number of different homeodomain transcription factors, the genes of which contain a conserved DNA sequence (the homeobox). Transcription factors bind to the DNA of the genes for other proteins and act to up-regulate or down-regulate those genes and, hence, alter protein expression. The presence of homeodomain transcription factors in all animal species indicates the huge importance of these to the existence of the animal.

Migration of cranial neural crest cells to specific regions is dictated by strong attracting and repelling signals from different families of cell signalling molecules and allows the neural crest cells to remain in discrete streams as they migrate to their destination. Once the neural crest cells reach their destination, interaction between the epithelium and the mesenchyme is required for differentiation into particular cell types to take place. The endoderm and ectoderm which cover the pharyngeal and external surfaces respectively of the developing pharyngeal

arches (see Section 4.2.2) produce a range of stimulatory and inhibitory signals, some of which induce the activation of further homeodomain transcription factors. This signalling has a significant epigenetic effect on the neural crest cells and can over-ride their pre-specification under certain conditions.

4.2.2 Pharyngeal arches

Six pairs of pharyngeal arches develop, decreasing in size from cranial to caudal. Development is initiated by migrating neural crest cells interacting with lateral extensions of the endoderm germ layer lining the future pharynx and augmenting the mesodermal core of these extensions. The arches are separated by pharyngeal grooves/clefts externally and pouches internally. Each arch consists of a central cartilage rod that forms the skeleton of the arch (derived from cranial neural crest); a muscular component, with the muscle cells formed from mesoderm and the fascia and tendons from neural crest; a vascular component, and a nervous element which includes sensory and special visceral motor fibres from a cranial nerve which supplies the mucosa and muscle of that arch (Table 4.1).

The signalling that induces the formation of bone and skeletal muscles in the craniofacial region is different from the signalling involved in bone and skeletal muscle formation in the axial skeleton and limb girdles. Neural crest cells are not involved in the formation of bone and muscle outside the craniofacial region. Despite these differences in development, bones and muscles thoughout the body behave in a similar manner post-partum.

4.2.3 Facial development

The development of the face begins at the end of the 4th week *in utero* (i.u.) with the appearance of five prominences around the stomodeum which is the primitive mouth and forms the topographical centre of the developing face. The maxillary swellings can be distinguished lateral, and the mandibular swellings caudal, to the stomodeum. The midline frontonasal process lies rostral to the stomodeum. Between 24 and 28 days i.u. the paired maxillary swellings enlarge and grow ventrally and medially. A pair of ectodermal thickenings called the nasal placodes appear on the frontonasal process and begin to enlarge. From 28–32 days the ectoderm at the centre of each nasal placode invaginates to form a nasal pit, dividing the raised rim of the placode into a lateral nasal process and a medial nasal process. Between 32 and 35 days each medial nasal process begins to migrate towards the other and they merge. The mandibular swellings have now merged to create the primordial lower lip. The nasal pits deepen and fuse to form a single, enlarged, ectodermal nasal sac. From 40–48 days there is lateral and inferior expansion of the now fused medial nasal processes to form the intermaxillary process. The tips of the maxillary swellings grow to meet this process. The intermaxillary process gives rise to the bridge and septum of the nose. From 7–10 weeks the ectoderm and mesoderm of the frontonasal process and the intermaxillary process proliferate, forming a midline nasal septum. This divides the nasal cavity into two nasal passages which open into the pharynx, behind the secondary palate, through the definitive choana. The philtrum is now formed by merging of the paired maxillary processes in front of the intermaxillary process, and the lateral

Table 4.1 Derivatives of first and second pharyngeal arches

Arch	Muscles	Nerves	Skeleton
First arch	Muscles of mastication	Trigeminal (V) – maxillary and mandibular divisions	All the facial bones
	Mylohyoid		Incus, malleus
	Anterior digastirc		Sphenomandibular ligament
	Tensor veli palatini		Mandible
	Tensor tympani		
Second arch	Muscles of facial expression	Facial (VII)	Stapes
	Posterior digastric		Styloid process
	Stylohyoid		Stylohyoid ligament
	Stapedius		Lesser horn and upper part of body of hyoid
	Levator veli palatini		

portions of the maxillary and mandibular swellings merge to create the cheeks and reduce the mouth to its final width (Fig. 4.2).

4.2.4 Formation of the palate (7–9 weeks i.u.)

At the beginning of the 7th week i.u., the floor of the nasal cavity is a posterior extension of the intermaxillary process known as the primary palate. During the 7th week, the medial walls of the maxillary swellings begin to produce a pair of thin medial extensions, 'palatine shelves', which grow inferiorly on either side of the tongue. The tongue moves downward and the palatine shelves rapidly rotate upwards towards the midline, growing horizontally during the 8th week i.u. The palatine shelves begin to fuse ventrodorsally with each other, the primary palate and the inferior border of the nasal septum in the 9th week (Fig. 4.3).

Any disturbance in the timing and/or process of palatal shelve elevation from a vertical to a horizontal orientation and their subsequent fusion is likely to cause clefting. The processes that bring about shelf elevation involve both an internal shelf-elevating force and developmental changes in the surrounding face. The internal shelf-elevating force results from progressive accumulation and hydration of glycosaminoglycans which creates a strongly hydrated space-filling gel resulting in swelling of the extracellular matrix. The developmental changes include unfolding of the embryo lowering the developing heart and allowing differential growth of the face – an increase in vertical dimension with constant transverse dimension. Also, sagittal growth of Meckel's cartilage displaces the tongue via the attachment of the genioglossus muscle. Once the shelves have elevated and the medial edges are in contact, disruption of the surface cells forming the epithelial seam is required to establish ectomesenchymal continuity. A number of methods are recognized: apoptosis (programmed cell death) of the epithelial cells; epithelial-mesenchymal transformation leading to the cells adopting a fibroblastic morphology and remaining within the palatal mesenchyme, and migration of the epithelial cells to the oral and nasal surface epithelia where they differentiate into keratinocytes.

Clefts of the lip and palate (CLP) are the most common craniofacial malformation in humans with an incidence of 1 in every 700 live births. The incidence varies with racial groups being much higher in Native Americans and much lower in black Africans. Clefts of the lip may be unilateral or bilateral with the majority of unilateral cases occurring on the left. Males are affected more frequently. Isolated clefts of the palate are a separate entity, occurring in 1 per 2000 live births and affecting females more than males.

The aetiology of CLP may be explained by a failure to merge of the maxillary and intermaxillary processes and the palatal shelves and may occur from inadequate migration of NC or excessive cell death. Research suggests that clefts of both lip and palate can be caused by deficiency of NC cells. Isolated cleft palate aetiology is usually considered to be of a physical nature

The role of the orthodontist in the treatment of individuals with clefts of the lip and palate is covered in Chapter 22.

4.3 Mechanisms of bone growth

The process by which new mineralised bone is formed is termed ossification. Ossification occurs in one of two ways: by membrane activity (intramembranous ossification), and by bony replacement of a cartilaginous model (endochondral ossification). The adult structure of osseous tissue formed by the two methods is indistinguishable, both methods can be utilised in the same bone and both processes need induction by interaction of the mesenchyme with overlying epithelium.

Intramembranous ossification is seen during embryonic development by direct transformation of mesenchymal cells into osteoblasts and occurs in sheet-like osteogenic membranes. Intramembranous

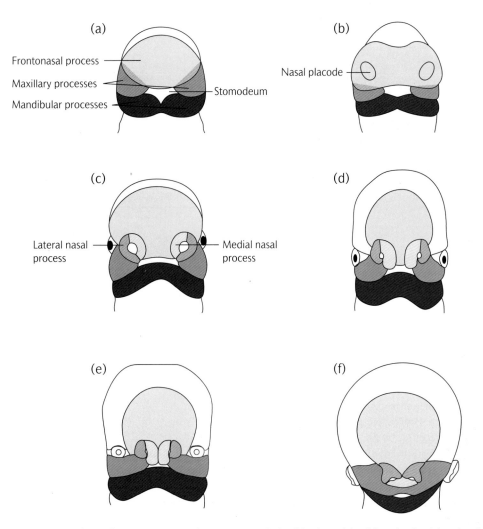

Fig. 4.2 Diagrammatic representation of early facial development from 4 to 10 weeks i.u. (a) 4th week i.u. (b) 28 days i.u. (c) 32 days i.u. (d) 35 days i.u. (e) 48 days i.u. (f) 10 weeks i.u. Further detail given in the text: Section 4.2.3. (Redrawn from a previously available electronic source: http://www.biomed2.man.ac.uk/ugrad/biomedical/calpage/sproject/rob/glossary.html).

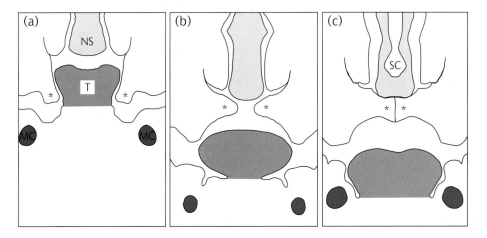

Fig. 4.3 Diagrammatic representation of palatal shelf elevation and subsequent fusion. (a) During the 7th week i.u. the palatal shelves begin to develop and lie on either side of the tongue. (b) During the 8th week i.u. the palatine shelves elevate rapidly due to the internal shelf-elevating force and developmental changes in the face. (c) During the 9th week i.u. the shelves fuse with each other, the primary palate and the nasal septum. NS = nasal septum, T = tongue, MC = Meckel's cartilage, SC = septal cartilage, * = palatal shelves.

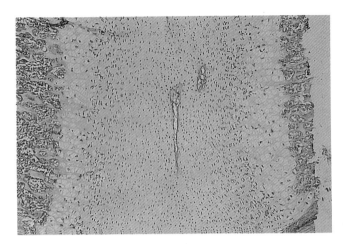

Fig. 4.4 Synchondrosis: ossification is taking place on both sides of the primary growth cartilage. (Photograph: D. J. Reid).

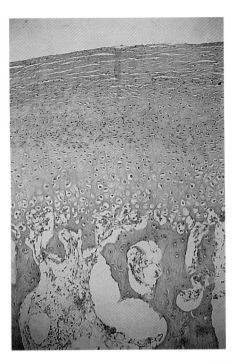

Fig. 4.5 Condylar cartilage of young adult. (Photograph: D. J. Reid).

ossification is seen in the bones of the calvaria, the facial bones, the mandible and the clavicle.

Endochondral ossification is seen in the long bones of the limbs, the axial skeleton and the bones of the cranial base. Ossification takes place in a hyaline cartilage framework and begins in a region known as the primary ossification centre. Ossification spreads from the primary ossification centre. At growth centres, the chrondroblasts are aligned in columns along the direction of growth, in which there are recognizable zones of cell division, cell hypertrophy, and calcification. This process is seen in both the epiphyseal plates of long bones and the synchondroses of the cranial base. Growth at these primary centres causes expansion, despite any opposing compressive forces such as the weight of the body on the long bones.

Structurally, **synchondroses** resemble two epiphyseal cartilages placed back to back and have a common central zone of resting cells. Therefore, they have two directions of linear growth in response to functional and non-functional stimuli and the bones on either side of the synchondrosis are moved apart as it grows (Fig. 4.4). Differential growth can occur. At birth, there are three synchondroses in the cranial base, the most important of which is the spheno-occipital synchondrosis.

Condylar cartilage also lays down bone, and for a long time this was thought to be a similar mechanism to epiphyseal growth, but developmentally it is a secondary cartilage and its structure is different. Proliferating condylar cartilage cells do not show the ordered columnar arrangement seen in epiphyseal cartilage, and the articular surface is covered by a layer of dense fibrous connective tissue (Fig. 4.5). The role of the condylar cartilage during growth is not yet fully understood, but it is clear that it is different from that of the primary cartilages and its growth seems to be a reactive process in response to the growth of other structures in the face.

Bone does not grow interstitially, i.e. it does not expand by cell division within its mass; rather, it grows by activity at the margins of the bone tissue. Overall bone growth is a function of two phenomena, **remodelling** and **displacement/transposition**. Growth does not consist simply of enlargement of a bone by deposition on its surface: periosteal (surface) remodelling is also needed to maintain the overall shape of the bone as it grows. Thus, as well as having areas where new bone is being laid down, a growing bone always undergoes resorption of some parts of its surface. At the same time, endosteal remodelling maintains the internal architecture of cortical plates and trabeculae. These processes of deposition and resorption together constitute remodelling. Remodelling is a very important mechanism of facial growth, and the complex patterns of surface remodelling brought about by the periosteum which invests the facial skeleton have been studied extensively. The change in position of a bony structure owing to remodelling of that structure is called **drift**, an example being where the palate moves downwards during growth as a result of bone being laid down on its inferior surface and resorbed on its superior surface.

The bones of the face and skull articulate together mostly at **sutures**, and growth at sutures can be regarded as a special kind of periosteal remodelling – an infilling of bone in response to tensional growth forces separating the bones on either side.

Growth which causes the mass of a bone to be moved relative to its neighbours is known as **displacement** of the bone and this is brought about by forces exerted by the soft tissues and by intrinsic growth of the bones themselves, e.g. epiphyseal plates and synchondroses; an example is forward and downward translation of the maxillary complex (Fig. 4.6).

Both remodelling and displacement can occur in the same bone in the same or different directions, but the relative contribution of each is difficult to determine.

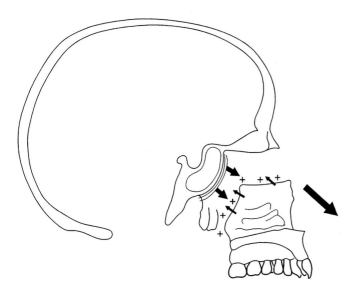

Fig. 4.6 Forward and downward displacement of the maxillary complex associated with deposition of bone at sutures. (After Enlow, D. H. (1990) *Facial Growth*, W. B. Saunders Co., Philadelphia).

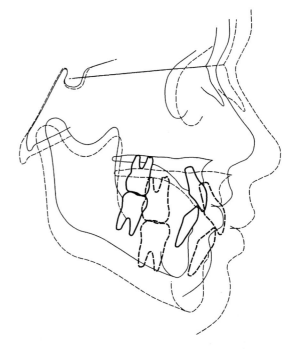

Fig. 4.7 Superimpositions on the cranial base showing overall downwards and forwards direction of facial growth. Solid line 8 years, broken line 18 years of age.

4.4 Postnatal craniofacial growth

Early cephalometric growth studies gave the impression that, overall, as the face enlarges it grows downwards and forwards away from the cranial base (Fig. 4.7). However, it is now known that growth of the craniofacial region is much more complex than this, with the calvaria, cranial base, maxilla and mandible experiencing differing rates of growth and differing mechanisms of growth at different stages of development, all of which are under the influence of a variety of factors. The overall pattern of facial growth results from the interplay between them and they must all harmonise with each other if a normal facial form is to result. Small deviations from a harmonious facial growth pattern will cause discrepancies of facial form and jaw relationships which are of major significance to the orthodontist.

4.4.1 Growth patterns

Different tissues have different growth patterns (curves) in terms of rate and timing, and four main types are recognized: neural, somatic, genital, and lymphoid (Fig. 4.8). The first two are the most relevant in terms of craniofacial growth.

Neural growth is essentially that which is determined by growth of the brain, with the calvarium following this pattern. There is rapid growth in the early years of life, but this slows until by about the age of 7 years growth is almost complete. The orbits also follow a neural growth pattern.

Somatic growth is that which is followed by most structures. It is seen in the long bones, amongst others, and is the pattern followed by increase in body height. Growth is fairly rapid in the early years, but slows in the prepubertal period. The pubertal growth spurt is a

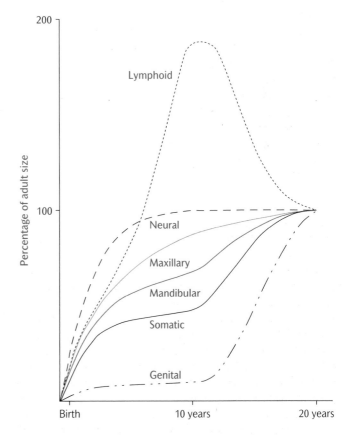

Fig. 4.8 Postnatal growth patterns for neural, lymphoid, somatic and genital tissues shown as percentages of total increase. The patterns for the maxilla and mandible are shown in blue (Redrawn from Proffit, W.R. (2000) *Contemporary Orthodontics*, 3rd edn, Mosby).

time of very rapid growth, which is followed by further slower growth. Traditionally, the pubertal growth spurt has been reported to occur on average at 12 years in girls, but there is evidence that the age of puberty is decreasing in girls. In boys the age of puberty is later at about 14 years.

The maxilla and mandible follow a pattern of growth that is intermediate between neural and somatic growth, with the mandible following the somatic growth curve more closely than the maxilla, which has a more neural growth pattern (Fig. 4.8).

Thus different parts of the skull follow different growth patterns, with much of the growth of the face occurring later than the growth of the cranial vault. As a result the proportions of the face to the cranium change during growth, and the face of the child represents a much smaller proportion of the skull than the face of the adult (Fig. 4.9).

4.4.2 Calvarium

The calvarium is that part of the skull which develops intramembranously to surround the brain and, therefore, it follows the neural growth pattern. Development of the calvaria is dependent upon the presence of the brain. It comprises the frontal bones, the parietal bones, and the squamous parts of the temporal and occipital bones. Ossification centres for each bone appear in the outer membrane surrounding the brain (ectomeninx) during the 8th week i.u. Bone formation spreads until the osteogenic fronts of adjacent bones meet and sutures are formed. Where more than two bones meet the intersections between the sutures are occupied by large membrane-covered fontanelles. Six fontanelles are present at birth which close by 18 months. By the age of 6 years the calvarium has developed inner and outer cortical tables which enclose the diploë. Its growth consists of a combination of displacement due to the expanding brain and osteogenesis at sutural margins, and remodelling to increase thickness and change shape. The intracranial aspects of the bones are resorbed while bone is laid down on the external surfaces. Growth of the calvaria corresponds closely to that of the brain and it ceases to grow in size by the age of 7 years. Eventually all sutures undergo varying degrees of fusion.

4.4.3 Cranial base

The cranial base develops by endochondral ossification. Cells within the ectomeninx differentiate into chondrocytes and form discrete condensations of cartilage from the 40th day i.u. These condensations of cartilage form three regional groups. A number of separate ossification centres appear in the cartilaginous model between 3 and 5 months i.u. Growth of the cranial base is influenced by both neural and somatic growth patterns, with 50 per cent of postnatal growth being complete by the age of 3 years. As in the calvarium, there is both remodelling and sutural infilling as the brain enlarges, but there are also primary cartilaginous growth sites in this region — the synchondroses. Of these, the spheno-occipital synchondrosis is of special interest as it makes an important contribution to growth of the cranial base during childhood, continuing to grow until 13–15 years in females and 15–17 years of age in males, fusing at approximately 20 years. Thus the middle cranial fossa follows a somatic growth pattern and enlarges both by anteroposterior growth at the spheno-occipital synchondrosis and by remodelling. The anterior cranial fossa follows a neural growth pattern and enlarges and increases in anteroposterior length by remodelling, with resorption intracranially and corresponding extracranial deposition. There is no further growth of the anterior cranial fossa between the sella turcica and foramen caecum after the age of 7 years. Therefore, after this age the anterior cranial base may be used as a stable reference structure upon which sequential lateral skull radiographs may be superimposed to analyse changes in facial form due to growth and orthodontic treatment. The Sella-Nasion line is not as accurate because Nasion can change position due to surface deposition and the development of the frontal sinuses (see Chapter 6).

The spheno-occipital synchondrosis is anterior to the temporomandibular joints, but posterior to the anterior cranial fossa, and, therefore, its growth is significant clinically as it influences the overall facial skeletal pattern (Fig. 4.10). Growth at the spheno-occipital synchondrosis increases the length of the cranial base, and since the maxillary complex lies beneath the anterior cranial fossa while the mandible articulates with the skull at the temporomandibular joints which lie beneath the

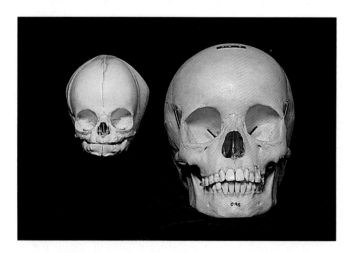

Fig. 4.9 The face in the neonate represents a much smaller proportion of the skull than the face of the adolescent (Photograph: B. Hill).

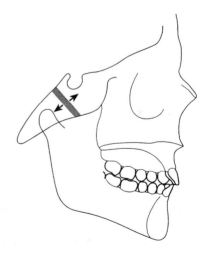

Fig. 4.10 Anteroposterior growth at the spheno-occipital synchondrosis affects the anteroposterior relationship of the jaws.

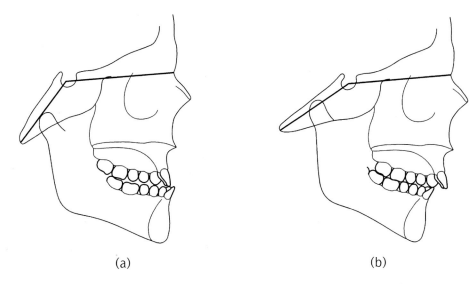

(a)   (b)

Fig. 4.11 View (a) Low cranial base angle associated with Class III skeletal pattern. View (b) Large cranial base angle associated with a Class II skeletal pattern.

middle cranial fossa, the cranial base plays an important part in determining how the mandible and maxilla relate to each other. For example, a Class II skeletal facial pattern is often associated with the presence of a long cranial base which causes the mandible to be set back relative to the maxilla.

In the same way, the overall shape of the cranial base affects the jaw relationship, with a smaller cranial base angle tending to cause a Class III skeletal pattern, and a larger cranial base angle being more likely to be associated with a Class II skeletal pattern (Fig. 4.11). The cranial base angle usually remains constant during the postnatal period, but can increase or decrease due to surface remodelling and differential growth at the spheno-occipital synchondrosis.

4.4.4 Maxillary complex

The maxilla derives from the first pharyngeal arch and ossification of the maxillary complex is intramembranous, beginning in the 6th week i.u. The maxilla is the third bone to ossify after the clavicle and the mandible. The main ossification centres appear bilaterally above the future deciduous canine close to where the infraorbital nerve gives off the anterior superior alveolar nerve. Ossification proceeds in several directions to produce the various maxillary processes. Postnatal growth of the maxilla follows a growth pattern that is thought to be intermediate between a neural and a somatic growth pattern (see Fig. 4.8).

Clinical orthodontic practice is primarily concerned with the dentition and its supporting alveolar bone which is part of the maxilla and premaxilla. However, the middle third of the facial skeleton is a complex structure and also includes, among others, the palatal, zygomatic, ethmoid, vomer, and nasal bones. These articulate with each other and with the anterior cranial base at sutures. Growth of the maxillary complex occurs in part by displacement with fill-in growth at sutures and in part by drift and periosteal remodelling. Passive forward displacement is important up to the age of 7 years, due to the effects of growth of the cranial base. When neural growth is completed, maxillary growth slows

and subsequently, approximately one-third of growth is due to displacement (0.2–1 mm per year) with the remainder due to sutural growth (1–2 mm per year). In total, up to 10 mm of bone is added by growth at the sutures.

Much of the anteroposterior growth of the maxilla is in a backward direction at the tuberosities which also lengthens the dental arch, allowing the permanent molar teeth to erupt. A forwards displacement of the maxilla gives room for the deposition of bone at the tuberosities (see Fig. 4.5). The zygomatic bones are also carried forwards, necessitating infilling at sutures, and at the same time they enlarge and remodel. In the upper part of the face, the ethmoids and nasal bones grow forwards by deposition on their anterior surfaces, with corresponding remodelling further back, including within the air sinuses, to maintain their anatomical form.

Downward growth occurs by vertical development of the alveolar process and eruption of the teeth, and also by inferior drift of the hard palate, i.e. the palate remodels downwards by deposition of bone on its inferior surface (the palatal vault) and resorption on its superior surface (the floor of the nose and maxillary sinuses) (see Fig. 4.6). These changes are also associated with some downward displacement of the bones as they enlarge, again necessitating infilling at sutures. Lateral growth in the mid-face occurs by displacement of the two halves of the maxilla, with deposition of bone at the midline suture. Internal remodelling leads to enlargement of the air sinuses and nasal cavity as the bones of the mid-face increase in size.

Therefore, growth is accompanied by complex patterns of surface remodelling on the anterior and lateral surfaces of the maxilla which maintain the overall shape of the bone as it enlarges. Despite being translated anteriorly, in fact much of the anterior surface of the maxilla is resorptive in order to maintain the concave contours beneath the pyriform fossa and zygomatic buttresses.

Growth of the nasal structures is variable but occurs at a more rapid rate than the rest of the maxilla. During the pubertal growth spurt, nasal dimensions increase 25 per cent faster than maxillary dimensions.

Maxillary growth slows to adult levels on average at about 15 years in girls and rather later, at about 17 years, in boys (see Section 4.6).

4.4.5 Mandible

The mandible derives from the first pharyngeal arch and ossifies intramembranously, beginning in the 6th week i.u. It is the second bone to ossify after the clavicle. It ossifies laterally to Meckel's cartilage with the ossification centres appearing bilaterally at the bifurcation of the inferior alveolar nerve into the mental and incisive branches. Ossification extends forwards, backwards and upwards to form the body, alveolar processes and ramus. Secondary cartilages appear, including the condylar cartilage during the 10th week i.u. Endochondral bone appears in the condylar cartilage by the 14th week i.u. Both inferior and superior joint spaces have appeared by the 11th week and by 22 weeks i.u. the glenoid fossa and articular eminence have formed. The role of the condylar cartilage in the growth of the mandible is not yet entirely clear. It is not a primary growth centre in its own right, but rather it grows in response to some other controlling factors. However, normal growth at the condylar cartilage is required for normal mandibular growth to take place.

Postnatal growth of the mandible follows a pattern intermediate between a neural and somatic pattern, although it follows the somatic pattern more closely than does the growth of the maxilla (Fig 4.8). Most mandibular growth occurs as a result of periosteal activity. Muscular processes develop at the angles of the mandible and the coronoid processes, and the alveolar processes develop vertically to keep pace with the eruption of the teeth. As the mandible is displaced forwards growth at the condylar cartilage fills in posteriorly while at the same time periosteal remodelling maintains its shape (Fig. 4.12). Bone is laid down on the posterior margin of the vertical ramus and resorbed on the anterior

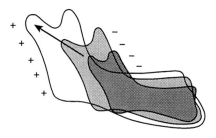

Fig. 4.12 Growth at the condylar cartilage 'fills in' for the mandible following anterior displacement, while its shape is maintained by remodelling, including posterior drift of the ramus. (After Enlow, D. H. (1990) *Facial Growth*, Saunders, Philadelphia).

margin, and this posterior drift of the ramus allows lengthening of the dental arch posteriorly. At the same time the vertical ramus becomes taller to accommodate the increase in height of the alveolar processes. Remodelling also brings about an increase in the width of the mandible, particularly posteriorly. Lengthening of the mandible and anterior remodelling together cause the chin to become more prominent, an obvious feature of facial maturation especially in males. Indeed, just as in the maxilla, the whole surface of the mandible undergoes many complex patterns of remodelling as it grows in order to maintain its proper anatomical form.

Before puberty growth occurs at steady rate with an increase of 1–2 mm per year in ramus height and 2–3 mm per year in body length. However, growth rates can double during puberty and the associated growth spurt.

Mandibular growth slows to adult levels rather later than maxillary growth, on average at about 17 years in girls and 19 years in boys, although it may continue for longer.

4.5 Growth rotations

Early studies of facial growth indicated that during childhood the face enlarges progressively and consistently, growing downwards and forwards away from the cranial base (see Fig. 4.7). These studies looked only at average trends and failed to demonstrate the huge variation which exists between the growth patterns of individual children. Later work by Björk has shown that the direction of facial growth is curved, giving a rotational effect (Fig. 4.13). The growth rotations were demonstrated by placing small titanium implants into the surface of the facial bones and subsequently taking cephalometric radiographs at intervals during growth. Since bone does not grow interstitially, the implants could be used as fixed reference points on the serial radiographs from which to measure the growth changes.

Growth rotations are most obvious and have their greatest impact on the mandible; their effects on the maxilla are small and are almost completely masked by surface remodelling. In the mandible, however, their effect is significant, particularly in the vertical dimension. Mandibular growth rotations result from the interplay of the growth of a number of structures which together determine the ratio of posterior to anterior facial heights (Fig. 4.14). The posterior face height is determined by factors including the direction of the growth at the condyles, vertical growth at the spheno-occipital synchondrosis and the influence of

the masticatory musculature on the ramus. The anterior facial height is affected by the eruption of teeth and vertical growth of the soft tissues, including the suprahyoid musculature and fasciae, which are in turn influenced by growth of the spinal column. The overall direction of growth rotation is thus the result of the growth of many structures.

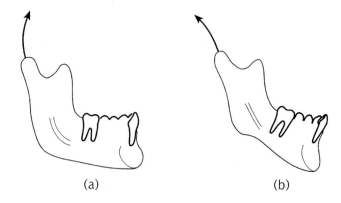

(a)   (b)

Fig. 4.13 Direction of condylar growth and mandibular growth rotations: (a) forward rotation; (b) backward rotation.

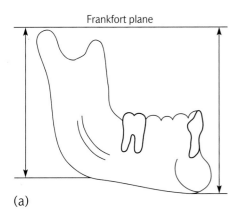

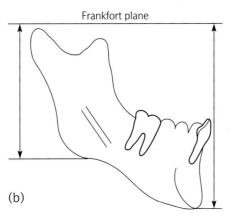

Frankfort plane

Frankfort plane

(a)

(b)

Fig. 4.14 Mandibular growth rotations reflect the ratio between the anterior and posterior face heights, here shown relative to the Frankfort horizontal plane: (a) forward rotation; (b) backward rotation.

Forward growth rotations are more common than backward rotations, with the average being a mild forward rotation which produces a well-balanced facial appearance. A marked forward growth rotation tends to result in reduced anterior vertical facial proportions and an increased overbite (Fig. 4.15), and the more severe the forward rotation the more difficult it will be to reduce the overbite. Similarly, a more backward rotation will tend to produce increased anterior vertical facial proportions and a reduced overbite or anterior open bite (Fig. 4.16).

Not only is the vertical dimension affected, but there are also important anteroposterior effects. For example, correction of a Class II malocclusion will be helped by a forward growth rotation, but made more difficult by a backward rotation. Growth rotations may also have an effect on the position of the lower labial segment. A forward growth rotation tends to cause retroclination of the lower labial segment which is often associated with shortening of the dental arch anteriorly and crowding of the lower incisors. A possible explanation for this is that, as the lower arch is carried forwards with mandibular growth, forward movement of the lower incisor crowns is limited by contact with the upper incisors, causing them to crowd. This is common in the very late stages of growth when mandibular growth continues after maxillary growth has finished, although facial growth is only one of a number of possible aetiological factors in late lower incisor crowding.

Thus growth rotations play an important part in the aetiology of certain malocclusions and must be taken into account in planning orthodontic treatment. It is necessary to try to assess the direction of mandibular growth rotation clinically. This is not entirely straightforward since the effect of growth rotation upon the mandible is masked to some extent by surface remodelling, particularly along the lower border of the mandible and at the angle. However, it is possible to make a useful assessment of a patient's facial growth pattern by examining the anterior facial proportions and mandibular plane angle

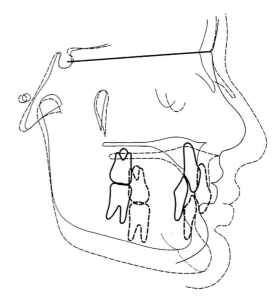

Fig. 4.15 Forward growth rotation. Solid line 11 years, broken line 18 years of age.

as described in Chapter 5. Increased facial proportions and a steep mandibular plane indicate that the direction of mandibular growth has a substantial downward component, while reduced facial proportions and a horizontal mandibular plane suggest that the direction of growth is more forwards. It is also helpful to examine the shape of the lower border of the mandible. A concave lower border with a marked antegonial notch is often associated with a backward rotation, while a convex lower border is associated with a forward growth rotation (see Figs 4.15 and 4.16).

4.6 Craniofacial growth in the adult

Analysis of longitudinal data from 163 cases aged 17–83 years of age from the Bolton growth study in the USA indicated that facial dimensions continued to increase throughout life.

Nearly all subjects (95 per cent) showed an increase in size for a particular measurement. An increase in size of between 2 and 10 per cent was the average. The cranial base altered the least; there was a moderate increase

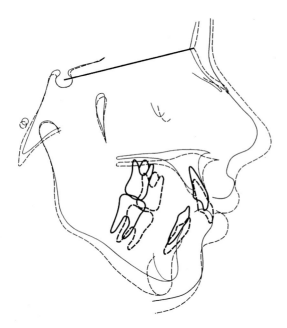

Fig. 4.16 Backward growth rotation. Solid line 12 years, broken line 19 years of age.

Table 4.2 Age of decline of growth to adult levels

Dimension	Female	Male
Transverse	12 years (maxilla)	12 years (maxilla)
(intercanine width)	9 years (mandible)	9 years (mandible)
Anteroposterior	2–3 years after first menstruation	4 years after sexual maturity
	14–15 years (maxilla)	17 years (maxilla)
	16–17 years (mandible)	19 years (mandible)
Vertical	17–18 years	Early 20s

in size of the facial bones; the frontal sinuses increased in size more than the facial bones, and the soft tissues increased the most. Vertical changes predominated later in adulthood with a forward rotation of the mandible more common in males and a backward rotation more common in females.

Facial growth is no longer referred to as being complete, rather it declines to adult levels of growth following the peak rate of growth seen during the pubertal growth spurt. The decline to adult levels of growth occurs in a predictable manner (Table 4.2).

4.7 Growth of the soft tissues

So far in this chapter we have concentrated on the growth of the facial skeleton. However, the bony facial form can be masked or accentuated by the form and function of the nasal and circumoral soft tissues. The circumoral soft tissues (musculature) are important also in relation to orthodontic treatment because they influence significantly the form of the dental arches, since the teeth are positioned in an area of relative stability between the tongue lingually, and the lips and cheeks labially and buccally. Therefore they are important factors in the aetiology of malocclusion, and affect the stability of the result after orthodontic treatment.

The facial musculature is well developed at birth, considerably in advance of the limbs, because of the need for the baby to suckle and maintain the airway. Other functions soon develop: mastication as teeth erupt, facial expressions, a mature swallowing pattern (as opposed to suckling), and speech.

The lips, tongue, and cheeks guide the erupting teeth towards each other to achieve a functional occlusion. This serves as a compensatory mechanism for a discrepancy in the skeletal pattern; for example, in a Class III subject the lower incisors may become retroclined and the upper incisors proclined to obtain incisor contact. Sometimes this compensatory mechanism fails, either because the skeletal problem is too severe or the soft tissue behaviour is abnormal. An example of this is where lower lip function worsens a Class II division 1 malocclusion by acting behind the upper incisors rather than anteriorly to them.

A knowledge of the likely changes in soft tissue form which occur because of growth is essential for the orthodontist, especially during the treatment planning phase. Significant changes occur during the adolescent growth spurt, some of which show sexual dimorphism. The timing of the greatest overall change in the soft tissues occurs between 10 and 15 years of age in girls, with the majority of the changes having occurred by the age of 12 years, but in boys the greatest overall change occurs between the ages of 15 and 25 years, although most changes are complete by the late teens.

The nasal structures undergo the most growth during adolescence and increase in size by 25 per cent more than the maxilla. Nasal growth in girls peaks at age 12 years and is complete, on average, by the age of 16 years. However, nasal growth in boys peaks between the ages of 13 and 14 years and continues for much longer. There is still significant growth of the nose in men during adulthood. The lips undergo increases in length and thickness in both sexes, although the growth in both is more for boys and continues for longer. Growth of the soft tissues covering the bony chin follow that of the bones closely and therefore, the chin becomes more prominent in males due to the upward and forward growth rotation of the mandible. In both sexes there is also a greater prominence of the brows, deepening of the eyes and flattening of the cheeks. However, in general the changes are greater in boys than girls and occur approximately 2 years later in boys than in girls.

The combination of the above growth patterns of the different structures has an important influence on facial appearance: the nose becomes more prominent in both sexes which leads to an apparent retrusion or flattening of the lips in both sexes, despite the increase in thickness of the lips; the chin becomes more prominent in males, but changes little, or may become more retrusive in girls, especially during adulthood. The 3D changes in soft-tissue pattern and in facial shape in non-treated inividuals and those subjects who have undergone various types of orthodontic treatment are an area of very active research.

The apparent retrusion of the lips during the pubertal growth of the soft tissues needs to be taken into consideration during treatment planning, especially in individuals with a Class II malocclusion. However, the increase in length of the lips is very beneficial during the treatment of patients with increased overjets as the increase in lip length is useful for stability of overjet correction.

4.8 Control of craniofacial growth

The mechanisms that control facial growth are poorly understood, but are the subject of considerable interest and research. As with all growth and development, there is an interaction between genetic and environmental factors, but if environmental factors can make a significant impact on facial growth then the possibility exists for clinicians to alter facial growth with appliances.

It is often difficult to distinguish the effects of heredity and environment, but it is helpful to consider how tightly the growth and development of a structure or tissue are under genetic control. Two simple examples illustrate this: gender is genetically determined and does not change no matter how extreme the environmental conditions, while obesity is strongly affected by environmental influences – the nature and amount of food consumed and exercise undertaken. Most structures, including the facial skeleton and soft tissues, are influenced by both genetic and environmental factors, and the effect that the latter can have depends upon how tightly growth is under genetic control.

Genetic control is undoubtedly significant in facial growth, as is clearly shown by facial similarities in members of a family. Twin studies, although methodologically flawed in many ways, have indicated that the genotype has more influence on anteroposterior facial form than vertical facial form. Class III malocclusions are good examples of genetic influences. In one study, 33 per cent of children of Class III parents were also Class III and 16 per cent had Class III siblings. Also Class III malocclusions are much more common in some racial groups and are very prevalent in South East Asia, whereas Class II malocclusions are more common in North West Europeans.

The extent to which the facial skeleton itself is under genetic control has been debated at length in recent decades, with the development of two opposing schools of thought. Growth at the primary cartilages is regarded as being under tight genetic control, with the cartilage itself containing the necessary genetic programming. Therefore, those who view growth of the whole facial skeleton as being directly and tightly genetically controlled have looked for primary cartilaginous growth centres in the facial bones. Originally, it was thought that the condylar cartilages fulfilled this role in the mandible, while the nasal septal cartilage served a similar function in the maxilla. However, the structure and behaviour of these cartilages is different from primary growth cartilages, and at present it is thought that, while their presence is necessary for normal growth to take place, they are not primary growth centres in their own right.

The opposing school of thought proposed that bone growth itself is only under loose genetic control and takes place in response to growth of the surrounding soft tissues – the **functional matrix** which invests the bone. A good example of a functional matrix is the neural growth pattern of the calvarium and orbits, which develop intramembranously and enlarge in response to growth of the brain and eyes. The functional matrix theory also works with respect to the mandible: the shape of the coronoid process and the angle of the mandible are affected by the function of the attached musculature (temporalis and masseter and medial pterygoid respectively). Also, the alveolar processes only develop if teeth are present. However, the functional matrix theory cannot easily explain the growth of the midface as there is no soft tissue growth to influence this region. The theory has attracted much attention as, if taken to its logical conclusion, it implies that orthodontic appliances can be used to alter facial growth.

Most current research activity in relation to the genetic control of facial development and growth is concentrating on the role of Hox genes and various growth factors and signalling molecules in influencing facial growth. However, three main theories of the possible environmental influences on vertical facial development exist: mouth breathing; soft tissue stretching and the structure/function of the muscles of mastication.

The theory that mouth breathing caused the teeth to be out of occlusion and, therefore, allowed an over-development of dento-alveolar structures pushing the mandible downwards and backwards (a posterior growth rotation) was devised in the 1970s. It was observed that children who required adenoidectomy were mouth breathers because the enlarged adenoids had reduced the ability to breathe through the nose. The study showed that 26 per cent of children who underwent the removal of their adenoids reverted to a more 'normal' pattern of vertical growth. Unfortunately, there were no controls in the study. More recent evidence has suggested that the reported increase in growth of the mandible following adenoidectomy is more likely due to normalisation of nocturnal growth hormone secretion, which is reduced in patients prior to adenoidectomy. These children also display an acceleration of somatic growth post-operatively and it has been postulated that growth at the mandiblular condyle is responsible for the change in direction of mandibular growth, rather than the change in breathing pattern.

It was noted, also in the 1970s that the angle that the anterior cranial base made with the cervical vertebrae differed between subjects with long faces and those with normal or short faces. It was proposed that an impairment to nasal breathing caused the subject to extend the head to open up the nasal airway. This led to stretching of the soft tissues of the neck which attach to the mandible and this, in turn, led to a posterior growth rotation of the mandible.

Interest in the role of the muscles of mastication (masseter) was generated in the late 1960s when it was shown that subjects with short faces have a much stronger bite force than subjects with long faces. These observations generated the theory that weak muscles allow the mandible to rotate backwards whereas strong muscles increase the anterior growth rotation. Whilst this theory does explain the development of short faces as well as long faces, recent research has shown that the occlusion has a significant effect on the structure/function of the masseter. Therefore, the muscles may influence facial form and, hence, the occlusion, but the occlusion (malocclusion) influences the function/structure of the muscles. Taking this argument to its logical conclusion suggests that any environmental influence on the occlusion, for example mouth breathing, thumb sucking, dental treatment, may, in genetically predisposed individuals, affect the structure and function of the masticatory musculature to an extent that influences future facial growth in the vertical dimension.

There is much yet to be understood about how growth of the face is controlled and whether orthodontic appliances can influence facial growth. Research into the effect of orthodontic appliances is difficult and, at present, the evidence is that the impact of current orthodontic treatment methods on facial growth is, on average, quite small. However, there is considerable variation in the response of individual patients.

4.9 Growth prediction

It would be extremely useful if we could predict the future growth of a child's face, particularly in cases which are at the limits of what orthodontic treatment can achieve. For growth prediction to be useful clinically it would need to be able to predict the amount, direction, and timing of growth of the various parts of the facial skeleton to a high level of accuracy.

At present there are no known predictors which can be measured, either clinically on the patient or from radiographs, which will enable future growth to be predicted with the necessary precision. Much work has been undertaken to try to find measurements which can be taken from cephalometric radiographs which will predict future facial growth to a useful level of precision, but so far with limited success. Assessment of stature (height) and secondary sex characteristics help to indicate whether the patient has entered the pubertal growth spurt, an important observation when functional appliances are being considered. Historically, growth of the jaws was thought to follow a somatic growth pattern, and the possibility has been investigated that observation of the developmental stage of other parts of the skeleton would give an indication of the stage of facial development. The stage of maturation of the metacarpal bones and the phalanges as seen on a hand–wrist radiograph and the stage of maturation of the cervical vertebrae as seen on lateral cephalometric radiographs are both used as an indication of the stage of puberty of an individual. However, the correlation of this with jaw growth has been found to be too poor to give clinically useful

information, perhaps because the growth of the maxilla and mandible follows a pattern intermediate between the neural and somatic patterns.

The best which can be done is to add average growth increments to the patient's existing facial pattern, but this has only limited value. This can be done manually using a grid superimposed on the patient's lateral cephalometric tracing, and average annual growth increments are read off to predict the change in position of the various cephalometric landmarks. Computer programs can be used for the same purpose, after the points and outlines from the lateral skull radiograph have been digitised. These programs can refine the prediction process further but they still have to make some assumptions about the rate and direction of facial growth. Unfortunately, the assumption that a patient's future growth pattern will be average is least appropriate in those individuals whose facial growth differs significantly from the average, and who are the very subjects where accurate prediction would be most useful. As growth proceeds, the rate and direction of growth in an individual vary enough that study of the past pattern of a patient's facial growth does not allow prediction of future growth to the level of precision required for it to be clinically useful. However, many clinicians find it helpful to assess the direction of mandibular growth rotation (see Section 4.8) on the assumption that this pattern is likely to continue.

Clinical experience has shown that for most patients, whose growth patterns are close to the average, it can be assumed for treatment-planning purposes that their growth will continue to be average.

4.10 Biology of tooth movement

The ability of the periodontium to respond to mechanical loading by remodelling of the alveolar bone and translocation of the tooth and periodontium is fundamental to the practice of orthodontics. It is the cells of the periodontal ligament which orchestrate, and are responsible for, the bony remodelling.

For many years, students of orthodontics have been taught that, when optimal force levels are applied to a tooth, bone is laid down where the periodontal ligament is under tension and resorbed from areas where the periodontal ligament is being compressed. This over-simplified statement, whilst true in essence, was based on evidence gained from histological studies and does not do justice to the complex molecular and cellular interactions which take place to bring about tooth movement. The rapid advances made in scientific knowledge and techniques over the last 20–25 years have enabled a greater understanding of these

complex interactions and the molecular biology of tooth movement attracts international research interest.

4.10.1 The periodontal ligament

The periodontal ligament (PDL) consists of a number of cell types embedded in an extracellular matrix composed mainly of type I collagen fibres with ground substance (proteoglycans and glycoproteins) and oxytalin fibres. There are four main cell types that are considered to be cells of the PDL: the fibroblast, responsible for producing and degrading the extracellular matrix; the cementoblast, responsible for the production of cementum; the osteoblast, responsible for bone production and the co-ordination of bone deposition and resorption, and the osteoclast, responsible for bone

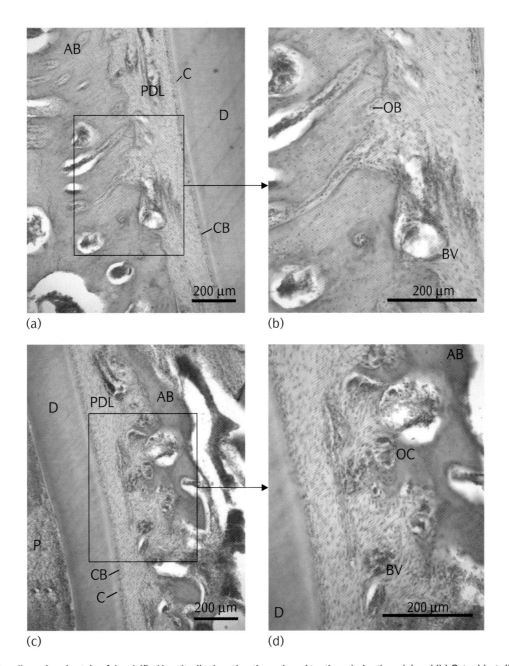

Fig. 4.17 Haematoxylin and eosin stain of decalcified longitudinal section through and tooth periodontium. (a) and (b) Osteoblasts lining the bone surface; (c) and (d) osteoclasts in Howship's lacunae. Note the vascularity of the periodontal ligament with the blood vessels forming a plexus more closely associated with the alveolar bone. AB = alveolar bone, BV = blood vessel, C = cementum, CB = cementoblast, D = dentine, OB = osteoblast, OC = osteoclast, PDL = periodontal ligament. Photomicrographs courtesy of Dr R. C. Shore, Visiting Fellow in Oral Biology, University of Leeds.

resorption. Also found are small 'islands' of cells, the cell rests of Malassez, and macrophages. Macrophages are found in the vicinity of the blood vessels and make up to 4 per cent of the cell population (Fig. 4.17).

The PDL has a number of structural and biochemical features reminiscent of immature connective tissue which it retains even in an adult: it contains a large number of cells, mainly fibroblasts, making up to 50 per cent of the connective tissue volume in some areas; it has a very high turnover rate and the fibroblasts are metabolically very active,

indicated by the large amounts of rough endoplasmic reticulum seen within these cells, and it is very vascular. The rich blood supply derives from the superior and inferior alveolar arteries and whilst some of the capillary bed in the ligament originates in the vessels entering the tooth apex, the majority of capillaries within the ligament originate in the intra bony spaces of the alveolus and from arterioles within the gingivae. The blood vessels within the ligament form a plexus around the tooth which is situated more towards the alveolus and may occupy up to 50 per cent of the periodontal space.

4.10.2 Cells involved in bone homeostasis

There are three main cell types involved in bone homeostasis: the osteoblast, the osteocyte and the osteoclast. The osteoblast derives from mesenchymal stromal cells and lies on the surface of the bone. Osteoblasts are responsible for the production of the bone organic matrix and its subsequent mineralisation. They are also responsible for the recruitment and activation of osteoclasts via the production of various cytokines and are the main regulators of bone homeostasis. When osteoblasts become surrounded by mineralised bone they become osteocytes.

Osteocytes continue to communicate with each other via cytoplasmic extensions which run though the canaliculi in the bone. They derive their nutrition from the blood vessels which run though the centre of the Haversion systems. They are thought to be responsible for detecting mechanical load on the bone.

The osteoclasts derive from blood monocytes and are recruited, when necessary, by signalling from the osteoblasts. They are responsible for resorption of bone. They are large multinucleated cells found on periosteal and endosteal bone surfaces in resorption pits called Howship's lacunae. They have a brush border adjacent to the bone surface which provides a large surface area over which active resorption takes place.

The organic matrix consists of collagen type I fibres, proteoglycans and a large number of growth factors. Bone contains more growth factors than any other tissue and this is thought to be why bone is so capable of regeneration, repair and remodelling. Numerous growth factors and signalling molecules have now been shown to be associated with bone homeostasis, many of which have been shown to play an active role in the bone remodelling associated with orthodontic tooth movement (Table 4.3).

4.10.3 Cellular events in response to mechanical loading

It is now well established that during normal everyday function there is a balance maintained between bone resorption and bone deposition, with the osteoblast controlling these processes. The exact cellular and molecular biological events that occur during orthodontic tooth movement are the subject of extensive research.

Mechanical load, for example force on a tooth from an orthodontic appliance, leads to deformation of the alveolar bone, possibly due to the effects of fluid movement within the viscoelastic PDL as the tooth is displaced, and stretching or compression of the collagen fibres and extracellular matrix. These distortions are detected by the cells (fibroblasts, osteoblasts, and osteocytes) because their cytoskeleton is connected to the extracellular matrix (ECM) by integrins embedded in their cell walls. Osteocytes communicate with each other via gap junctions. There is evidence that the shape of a cell can influence its activity; rounded cells tend to be catabolic where as flattened cells are anabolic and it is possible that the changes in shape of the cells in the PDL are at least partly responsible for the chain of events seen in areas where the PDL is compressed or under tension (Boxes 4.2 and 4.3 and Fig. 4.18). A recent review of the mechanobiology of tooth movement has suggested the following four stages may be described:

(1) Matrix strain and fluid flow in the alveolar bone and PDL

(2) Cell strain, as a result of matrix strain and fluid flow

(3) Cell activation and differentiation (osteoblasts, osteocytes, fibroblasts and osteoclast precursors)

(4) Remodelling of PDL and alveolar bone

Table 4.3 Factors involved in the regulation of bone remodelling during orthodontic tooth movement

Name	Function
RUNX-2	One of the most important bone-specific genes, vital for mesenchymal differentiation into osteoblasts
Interleukin-1 (IL-1)	Potent stimulator of bone resorption, acting both directly and by increasing prostaglandin synthesis. Also an inhibitor of bone formation. Produced by macrophages and osteoblasts
RANKL (Receptor activator of nuclear factor (NF-kB) ligand)	Secreted by osteoblasts and binds the RANK receptors found within the cell membrane of osteoclast precursors. It is an essential stimulatory factor for the differentiation, fusion, activation and survival of osteoclastic cells
OPG (osteoprotegerin)	Secreted by osteoblasts and blocks the effects of RANKL, thereby decreasing the activity of osteoclasts. Acts as a decoy receptor by binding RANKL extracellularly
M-CSF (macrophage-colony stimulating factor) aka CSF-1	Polypeptide growth factor found in bone matrix and produced by osteoblasts. Acts directly on osteoclast precursor cells to control proliferation and differentiation
PGE-2 (prostaglandin E2)	Potent mediator of bone resorption found in sites of inflammation. Produced by cells in response to mechanical loading. Elevates intracellular messengers
Leukotrienes	Actions on both bone destruction and bone formation, found in sites of inflammation. Produced by cells in response to mechanical loading. Elevates intracellular messengers
MMPs (matrix metalloproteinases)	Range of enzymes e.g. collagenase, gelatinase, produced by various cell types to break down unmineralised extracellular matrix
TIMPs (tissue inhibitors of metalloproteinases)	Produced by various cell types to bind to MMPs extracellularly to reduce/inhibit their activity
ERKs (extracellular signal-related kinases)	Members of the MAP kinase family of intracellular messengers that provide a key link between membrane bound receptors and changes in the pattern of gene expression

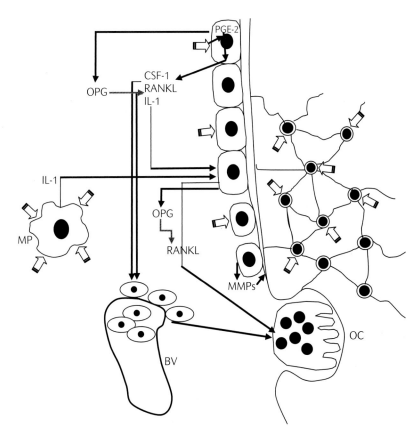

Fig. 4.18 Schematic diagram of cellular signalling involved in bone remodelling response to compressive load. BV = blood vessel, MP = macrophage, OC = osteoclast. All black arrows indicate up-regulation of expression of the particular factors. Red arrows indicate inhibition. Note the osteoblasts lining the bone surface (osteoid), the osteocytes within the bone detecting the mechanical load, and the monocytes exiting the blood vessel in response to RANKL and CSF-1.

Box 4.2 Possible chain of cellular events when the periodontal ligament is subjected to a compressive load

- The mechanical load causes strain in the extracellular matrix (ECM) of PDL and in alveolar bone causing fluid flow in both tissues

- The strain in the ECM is sensed by PDL cells due to the connection of their cytoskeleton to the ECM via integrins. Osteocytes sense the mechanical force by fluid flow through the canaliculi

- Osteocytes respond to mechanical deformation by producing bone morphogenic proteins (BMPs) and other cytokines which activate osteoblasts; fibroblasts respond by producing MMPs; osteoblasts respond by producing prostaglandins e.g. PGE-2 and leukotrienes

- Osteoblast production of PGE-2 and luekotrienes leads to an elevation of intracellular messengers. These induce IL-1 and CSF-1 production by the osteoblast and also increase the production of RANKL by the osteoblast

- Macrophages respond to mechanical deformation by increasing production of IL-1

- IL-1 produced by osteoblasts and macrophages increases the production of RANKL by the osteoblast

- RANKL and CSF-1 cause increased attraction and proliferation of blood monocytes to the area which fuse to form osteoclasts. RANKL also stimulates the osteoclasts to become active

- The osteoblasts round up to expose the underlying osteoid and produce MMPs to degrade this to give the osteoclasts access to the underlying mineralised bone. They also produce osteopontin (OPN) which causes the osteoclasts to attach to the exposed bone surface

- The osteoclasts resorb the bone by first softening the hydroxyapetite crystals by excreting hydrogen ions into the matrix and then using proteases such as cathepsin K to break down the extracellular matrix

- The osteoblasts also produce inhibitors of some of the enzymes and cytokines which they produce e.g. TIMPS and OPG in order that the bone resorption is tightly controlled

---

Box 4.3 Possible chain of cellular events when the periodontal ligament is subjected to tension

- In areas of tension the osteoblasts are flattened and the osteoid remains unexposed

- It has been shown recently that cells in the PDL increase the amount of a specific secondary messenger (ERK) in response to tension

- ERK signalling induces the expression of RUNX-2 which, in turn, causes an increase in osteoblast activity and bone production

- There is no increase in total cell number in areas of the PDL under tension, although there is an increase in number of osteoblasts. This indicates that RUNX-2 may be inducing fibroblasts of the PDL to differentiate into osteoblasts

---

4.11 Cellular events associated with loss of anchorage

Simply put, anchorage is the resistance to unwanted tooth movement. This unwanted tooth movement occurs as a result of Newton's Third Law – every action has an equal and opposite reaction. The accurate planning of anchorage requirements is fundamental to the success of orthodontic treatment and is discussed further in Chapter 15. Loss of anchorage – the term given to the situation when unwanted tooth movement does occur – may occur as a consequence of inadequate treatment planning, but may also occur due to excessive force levels being applied to the teeth. Loss of anchorage usually results in a poor treatment outcome.

If the force applied to a tooth exceeds the pressure in the capillaries (30 mmHg) then the capillaries will occlude and the provision of essential nutrients ceases. This causes cell death in the compressed periodontal ligament which undergoes a sterile necrosis and takes on a glassy appearance under the light microscope – the periodontal ligament is said to be **hyalinised**.

Under more physiological conditions, bone is resorbed by osteoclasts formed by the fusion of blood monocytes, under the control of the osteoblast. However, the cell death in the avascular periodontal ligament means that there are no osteoblasts and no osteoclasts can be recruited for frontal resorption of the alveolar bone to take place. Therefore, remodelling of the bone has to be performed by cells that have migrated from adjacent undamaged areas. It may take several days before these cells begin to invade the necrotic area. However, under these conditions, the resorption of the bone is mainly carried out by osteoclasts which appear within the adjacent marrow spaces and begin to resorb the bone, from cancellous bone out towards the periodontal ligament. This resorption process is termed **undermining resorption**. When hyalinisation and undermining resorption occur there is a delay in tooth movement because, firstly, there is a delay in stimulating the cells within the marrow spaces to differentiate and, secondly, a considerable amount of bone may need to be removed before tooth movement can take place. This causes a delay of 10–14 days before tooth movement can continue.

During this time, although movement of the tooth in question may not occur, the force is still being applied and is being dissipated around the other teeth included in the appliance. The forces to the anchor teeth may well be adequate to induce tooth movement in these teeth – anchorage will have been lost.

A recent (2009) systematic review of the literature related to hyalinisation following application of orthodontic forces concluded that, despite the fact that hyalinisation is considered to be an undesirable side-effect of orthodontic tooth movement, little attention has been paid to the phenomenon itself and its possible relationship with stress/strain levels in the PDL and alveolar bone or the rate of tooth movement. The authors comment that high quality studies on hyalinisation are urgently needed in order to better understand its role in orthodontic tooth movement and, as a consequence, improve the efficiency of tooth movement.

4.12 Cellular events during root resorption

External apical root resorption is a complex, sterile inflammatory process that occurs in virtually all patients undergoing treatment with fixed orthodontic appliances. The cells responsible for resorption of mineralised dental tissues are the odontoclasts which are multinucleated cells similar, but not identical, to osteoclasts. In the mildest cases only small areas of cementum are resorbed and these resorption craters are repaired with the deposition of cellular cementum once the force applied to the tooth has been removed. In more severe cases, the dentine is also resorbed and these defects are repaired also with cellular cementum. In severe cases the apical portion of the root is removed and the root length is decreased. Although the remaining dentine will become covered by cementum, the original length of the root is never re-established. Loss of root length is most commonly seen affecting the upper incisor teeth and

in the majority of cases up to 1 mm of root length is lost. However, in a small percentage of patients (1 or 2 per cent) up to half of the root length may be lost during a course of orthodontic treatment with fixed appliances and in these cases root resorption often affects all teeth that were included in the appliance. Root resorption is an iatrogenic event caused by orthodontic treatment and, as such, has generated much research interest. There is increasing evidence to suggest that the likelihood of root resorption is much more common where force levels are excessive, especially in areas under compression, and where forces are optimal, although small areas of root resorption may be seen, root resorption is less common. This is thought to be due to the association of root resorption with hyalinisation of the periodontal ligament. The exact reasons for this are unclear but a number of hypotheses have been proposed.

Firstly, *in vitro* work has indicated a possible protective effect of the periodontal ligament fibroblasts because they may be able to modulate the cascade of signals that results in root resorption. Furthermore, *in vivo* work suggests that root resorption continues, even after the force has been removed, until the periodontal ligament becomes re-attached to the root surface. During periodontal ligament hyalinisation, the protective effect of the fibroblasts would be lost. Secondly, the most severe root resorption is seen towards the root apex which is covered by cellular cementum and, hence, requires a patent blood supply for survival. Cellular cementum may be more prone to damage than acellular cementum if the blood vessels are occluded during orthodontic tooth movement, such as occurs in hyalinisation of the periodontal ligament, which may result in its subsequent removal by odontoclasts.

Recently, two separate pathways leading to odontoclast activation have been elucidated. The first causes odontoclast activation through an inflammation modulation pathway involving interleukin 1b (IL-1b). Local damage of tissue may result in release of cytokines including IL-1b. Such cytokines can recruit more monocytes and macrophages to eliminate apoptotic cells and prevent further necrosis. Studies involving genetically engineered mice that do not express IL-1b (IL-1b knockout mice) have shown significantly greater root resorption in the knockout mice than in wild type controls when undergoing experimental orthodontic treatments. Similarly, patients with IL-1b polymorphisms are more susceptible to external resorption associated with orthodontic treatment.

The second pathway involves the RANK/RANKL/OPG osteoclast program. Not surprisingly, excessive osteoclast activity induced by the inflammatory process will exacerbate root resorption. On the other hand, orthodontically induced root resorption may be associated with defective alveolar resorption and/or turnover along with tooth movement or force application, resulting in prolonged stress and strain i.e. hyalinisation, which links with the cellular hypotheses discussed above. Therefore, any risk factors that interfere with osteoclast function may actually contribute to more root resorption.

4.13 Summary

4.13.1 Facial Growth

- Facial development begins at the end of the 4th week i.u. with the development of five swellings (one frontonasal, two maxillary, two mandibular) around the stomodeum
- The maxilla and mandible derive from the first pharyngeal arch into which have migrated cranial neural crest cells
- Neural crest cells give rise to a number of pre-specified derivatives, the patterning of which is controlled by homeodomain transcription factors
- Bone formation occurs by either intramembranous ossification or endochondral ossification
- Bone growth occurs by remodelling and displacement
- The calvarium ossifies intramembranously, its growth closely follows that of the brain. Growth is complete by age 7 years
- The cranial base ossifies endochondrally. Growth at the spheno-occipital synchondrosis occurs in two directions until the mid teens
- The maxilla and mandible ossify intramembranously and both undergo complex patterns of remodelling during growth. They are displaced in a downward and forwards direction in relation to the cranial base and growth occurs posteriorly at the tuberosities (maxilla) and ramus (mandible)
- The mandible experiences rotational growth with most individuals having an upward and forward direction of rotation
- Facial growth continues at low levels in the adult. The decline to adult levels is seen first in the transverse dimension, followed by the anteroposterior dimension and finally the vertical dimension. Growth continues for longer in boys in the AP and vertical dimensions

- During puberty there is a large increase in nasal dimensions and the lips lengthen and thicken, especially in boys. Soft tissue growth continues throughout adulthood
- The control of facial growth is a combination of genetics and the environment. The environment may have a greater influence on growth in the vertical dimension
- Currently, it is not possible to accurately predict the timing, rate or amount of facial growth

4.13.2 Cellular basis of tooth movement

- Orthodontic treatment would not be possible without the ability of the alveolar bone to remodel
- The cells of the periodontal ligament are responsible for the bone remodelling and, hence, tooth movement
- The osteoblast is the bone forming cell and is responsible also for the recruitment and activation of osteoclasts (bone resorbing cells)
- A number of different growth factors and signalling molecules are now known to be intimately involved in bone removal and formation during orthodontic tooth movement with the RANK/RANKL/OPG osteoclast program being the most important

4.13.3 Anchorage

- Anchorage is the resistance to unwanted tooth movement
- Anchorage loss may occur when excessive force is applied because this causes hyalinisation of the periodontal ligament. This leads to a time delay (10–14 days) before the bone is removed by undermining resorption allowing tooth movement to continue

4.13.4 Root resorption

- Root resorption occurs in the majority of patients undergoing orthodontic treatment

- The cell responsible for the removal of cementum and dentine is the odontoclast

- Two distinct signalling pathways have been shown to be involved in root resorption, with defective bone removal leading to an increase in root resorption

Principal sources and further reading

Björk, A. and Skieller, V. (1983). Normal and abnormal growth of the mandible. A synthesis of longitudinal cephalometric implant studies over a period of 25 years. *European Journal of Orthodontics*, **5**, 1–46.

A summary of the implant work on mandibular growth rotations.

Cordero, D.R., Brugmann S., Chu, Y., Bajpai, R., Jame, M., and Helms, J.A. (2011) Cranial neural crest cells on the move: Their role in craniofacial development. *American Journal of Medical Genetics Part A*. **155**: 270–9.

A very interesting article for those wishing to further understand the role of cranial neural crest cells.

Enlow, D. H. and Hans M. G. (2008). *Essentials of facial growth*. 2nd edition. Saunders, Philadelphia.

The Bible of facial growth.

Henneman, S., Von den Hoff, J. W., and Maltha, J. C. (2008). Mechanobiology of tooth movement. *European Journal of Orthodontics*, **30**, 299–306.

An up-to-date and easy-to-understand review of the biology of orthodontic tooth movement.

Houston, W. J. B. (1979). The current status of facial growth prediction: a review. *British Journal of Orthodontics*, **6**, 11–17.

An authoritative assessment of the value of growth prediction.

Houston, W. J. B. (1988). Mandibular growth rotations – their mechanism and importance. *European Journal of Orthodontics*, **10**, 369–73.

A concise review of the aetiology and clinical importance of growth rotations.

Meikle, M. C. (2002). *Craniofacial development, growth and evolution*. Bateson Publishing, Norfolk, England.

A fascinating book. A little outdated now, but will serve as a useful 'first text' for the interested student.

Proffit, W. R. (2000). *Contemporary Orthodontics*, 3rd Edition. Mosby, St Louis, USA.

The standard text for postgraduate students in orthodontics.

Sandy, J. R., Farndale, R. W. and Meikle, M. C. (1993). Recent advances in understanding mechanically induced bone remodelling and their relevance to orthodontic theory and practice. *American Journal of Orthodontics and Dentofacial Orthopedics*, **103**, 212–22.

Still a key paper in understanding the cellular events behind orthodontic tooth movement.

Wang, Z. and McCauley, L. (2011) Osteoclasts and odontoclasts: signaling pathways to development and disease. *Oral Diseases*, **17**, 129–42.

An up-to-date account of the causes of orthodontists' worst nightmares.

References for this chapter can also be found at www.oxfordtextbooks.co.uk/orc/mitchell4e/. Where possible, these are presented as active links which direct you to the electronic version of the work, to help facilitate onward study. If you are a subscriber to that work (either individually or through an institution), and depending on your level of access, you may be able to peruse an abstract or the full article if available.

5

Orthodontic assessment

S. J. Littlewood

5.1 Introduction to orthodontic assessment

The purpose of an orthodontic assessment is to gather information about the patient to produce an accurate orthodontic diagnosis. This information is collected by:

- taking a full history
- undertaking a clinical examination
- collecting appropriate records

The assessment will produce a collection of data identifying a list of the patient's orthodontic problems, and it is this problem list that will form the basis of the orthodontic diagnosis (Fig. 5.1). Problems can be divided into pathological problems and developmental problems. Pathological problems are problems related to diseases, such as caries and periodontal disease, and need to be addressed before any orthodontic treatment is undertaken. Developmental problems are those factors related to the malocclusion and will be the focus of this chapter.

The management of the developing dentition has been discussed in Chapter 3, explaining how to recognize normal development and appreciate when to intercept any developing problems. Once in the mixed dentition a more detailed orthodontic assessment is required, and this should be systematic and comprehensive to ensure nothing is missed.

Orthodontic treatment is nearly always elective, and so it is important that the orthodontic assessment collects sufficient information not only to identify features that would benefit from treatment, but also

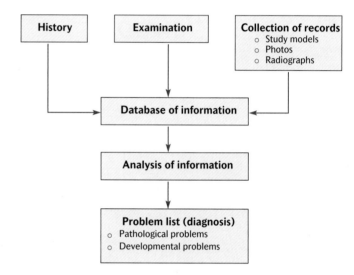

Fig. 5.1 The process of creating a problem list in orthodontics.

to identify any potential risks of proposed treatment (Chapter 1). By understanding both the risks and benefits of treatment the patient can make an informed decision as to whether they would like to proceed with treatment or not. (Informed consent is discussed in more detail in Section 7.8).

5.2 Taking an orthodontic history

The patient should be given the chance to describe their problem in their own words and the clinician can then guide them through a series of questions to address the areas summarized in Box 5.1.

When the patient is a child, the parent or guardian may lead this discussion, but it is important to get the child's input, as the child is the one who may undergo treatment and would therefore need to be willing and able to comply with the treatment plan.

5.2.1 Patient's perception of the problem

The patient should be given the opportunity to express, in their own words, what their problem is and what they would like corrected. They may perceive their problem as:

- functional (speech or mastication difficulties)
- related to dental health (like a traumatic overbite)
- aesthetics

It is important to recognize that the patient's perception of their problem may not always seem appropriate to the trained clinician. However, the patient is unlikely to be satisfied unless their problem is addressed as part of the treatment plan. Allowing the patient to describe their concerns will help to determine whether the patient's expectations are realistic and achievable (see Section 5.2.6).

5.2.2 Medical history

As with all aspects of dentistry, oral problems cannot be treated in isolation of the rest of the body. A clear understanding of a patient's medical problems and how this can affect potential orthodontic treatment is vital. Table 5.1 summarizes the key areas of the medical history of importance for orthodontic patients, and the section on further reading provides more details.

5.2.3 Dental history

The patient should be asked about their previous dental experience. This will provide an idea of their attitude towards dental health, what treatment they have had experienced previously and how this may affect their compliance with orthodontic treatment. In particular it is important to determine any ongoing dental problems, history of jaw joint problems, and any history of trauma to the teeth. There may also be a history of relevant inherited disorders affecting the dentition (e.g. hypodontia) and previous orthodontic treatment.

> **Box 5.1 Information to be gathered during the history-taking process**
>
> - Patient's complaint
> - Medical history – identifying any aspects that may affect orthodontic treatment
> - Dental history – any trauma, any previous or ongoing dental treatment, TMJ problems, any known inherited dental problems (e.g. hypodontia), any previous orthodontic treatment
> - Habits – details of any digit-sucking habits or other habits involving the dentition
> - Physical growth status (identifying whether growth is complete or still ongoing may affect the timing and nature of future treatment)
> - Patient (or parent's) motivation
> - Socio-behavioural factors – these may affect the patient's ability to complete the treatment

Table 5.1 Orthodontic relevance of some medical conditions

Medical condition	Relevance to orthodontics
Epilepsy	• Epilepsy needs to be under control before starting treatment
	• Extra-oral headgear may present an unacceptably high risk
	• Stress may induce a seizure
	• The anti-epileptic Phenytoin may cause gingival hyperplasia
Latex allergy	• Confirm allergy with the patient's doctor
	• Use latex-free gloves and orthodontic products
Nickel allergy	• Intra-oral reactions are very rare
	• Use plastic-coated headgear to avoid contact with skin
	• If intra-oral allergy is confirmed then use nickel-free orthodontic products
Diabetes	• Patient may be more prone to intra-oral infections and periodontal problems
	• Be aware of risk of hypoglycaemia if snacks or meals are missed, so schedule appointments appropriately
	• Treatment should be avoided in poorly controlled diabetics
Heart defects with a risk of infective endocarditis	• Antibiotic cover used to be prescribed routinely for patients with structural heart defects who were undergoing any form of dentogingival manipulation that could produce a bacteraemia
	• The guidelines have now changed as in many cases the risk of anaphylaxis caused by the antibiotic is greater than the risk of infective endocarditis
	• The clinician should refer to contemporary guidelines and contact the patient's doctor or cardiologist if in doubt
Bleeding disorders	• Generally orthodontic treatment is not contra-indicated
	• Precautions and medical advice are required for dental extractions
	• Avoiding trauma to soft tissues from wires or sharp edges is even more important for these patients
Asthma	• The regular use of steroid-based inhalers may predispose to intra-oral candidal infections, so excellent oral hygiene, particularly when using appliances that cover the palate, is important
Bisphosphonates	• These may predispose to osteonecrosis and affect bone turnover
	• The patient's physician should be contacted for advice about any proposed treatment plan, particularly if extractions may be required

The reader is referred to the section on further reading for more comprehensive information on this topic.

5.2.4 Habits

The patient should be asked about any previous or ongoing habits that involve the dentition. The most important are digit-sucking habits and the clinician needs to know the duration and nature of the habit. Other habits such as nail biting may predispose to an increased risk of root resorption.

5.2.5 Physical growth status

For some orthodontic treatment the patient's growth status is important. In some cases orthodontic treatment is more successful if they are still growing – for example when a patient has an underlying skeletal problem that could be improved using a process known as growth modification (see Chapters 7 and 19). In others, treatment planning is best undertaken when growth is complete (for example an adolescent with a Class III malocclusion). The patient, or their parents, can be asked questions to determine if they are still growing.

5.2.6 Motivation and expectation

Undergoing orthodontic treatment requires a great deal of active participation and co-operation from the patient. No matter how skilful the orthodontist, treatment will not be successful unless the patient is sufficiently motivated to comply will all aspects of their care. If a patient is not sufficiently motivated, then treatment should not be undertaken.

We have already explained the importance of finding out which features of their malocclusion a patient is unhappy with, and importantly, the result they are hoping for, or expect at the end of treatment. Where possible the clinician should formulate a plan that addresses the patient's area of concern. However, occasionally the patient's perception of their problem or their expectations may be unrealistic. The role of the orthodontist is then to counsel the patient carefully to explain what can or cannot be achieved. If a patient's expectations are unrealistic, then treatment should not be undertaken.

5.2.7 Socio-behavioural factors

Compliance for treatment is also affected by the patient's ability to attend regularly for appointments and any potential practical or social reasons that may make this impossible should be identified. Orthodontic treatment often requires long-term treatment with multiple appointments, and it is important to determine if the patient, and in the case of a child, their family or carer, are able to commit to the whole treatment. In addition, the patient's ability to comply with treatment may be affected by some behavioural problems.

5.3 Clinical examination in three dimensions

The purpose of the clinical examination is to identify pathological and developmental problems and determine which (if any) diagnostic records are required. It is important to remember that the face and dentition should be examined in all three planes (anteroposteriorly, vertically, and transversely). Box 5.2 summarizes how the different aspects of orthodontic assessment relate to the three planes.

5.4 Extra-oral examination

An appreciation of a patient's underlying skeletal pattern and overlying soft tissues will help to identify the aetiology of a malocclusion. This will help the clinician appreciate the anatomical limitations of any proposed treatment. In addition, a key aim of all orthodontic treatment should be to produce an aesthetic smile. Simply aligning teeth and producing a good occlusion does not necessarily guarantee a great smile. An understanding of the relationship between the teeth and the lips is vital and an assessment of the smile aesthetics should form part of any orthodontic assessment.

The patient needs to be examined in a frontal view and in profile. To ensure an accurate assessment representing the true skeletal relationships, it is important to ensure that the patient is in the 'Natural Head Position', which is the position the patient carries their head naturally. The patient should sit upright in the chair and be asked to focus on something in the distance. This same natural head position should also be used for any cephalometric radiographs to ensure consistency between all patient records (Section 6.1).

The key to the extra-oral assessment is an understanding of the normal proportions of the face and recognizing when patients deviate from these normal relationships. The patient is assessed extra-orally in the:

- frontal view (assessing in the vertical and transverse planes)
- profile view (assessing in the anteroposterior and vertical planes)

An assessment of the smile aesthetics, soft tissues (lips and tongue) and an examination of the temporomandibular joint should also be undertaken.

5.4.1 Anteroposterior assessment

This aims to assess the relationship between the tooth-bearing portions of the maxilla and mandible to each other, and also their relationships to the cranial base. The anteroposterior relationship can be assessed in three ways:

- assessing the relationship of the lips to a vertical line, known as zero meridian, dropped from soft tissue nasion (Fig. 5.2)
- palpating the anterior portion of the maxilla at A point and the mandible at B point (Fig. 5.3).
- assessing the convexity of the face by determining the angle between the middle and lower thirds of the face in profile (Fig. 5.4).

5.4.2 Vertical assessment

The face can be assessed vertically in two ways:

- using the rule of thirds
- measuring the angle of the lower border of the mandible to the maxilla

The face can be split into thirds (Fig. 5.5). In a face with normal proportions each third is approximately equal in size. Any discrepancy in these thirds may suggest a facial disharmony in the vertical plane. In particular orthodontists are interested in any increase or decrease in the proportion of the lower third of the face. The lower third of the face can also be split into thirds, with the upper lip lying in the upper third, and the lower lip lying in the lower two-thirds (Fig. 5.5).

Another clinical assessment that can be used to determine the vertical relationships is to assess the angle between the lower border of the mandible and the maxilla (Fig. 5.6). Placing a finger, or the handle of a dental instrument, along the lower border of the mandible gives an indication of the clinical mandibular plane angle.

5.4.3 Transverse Assessment

The transverse proportions of the face are best examined from the frontal view, but also by looking down on the face, by standing behind and above the patient (Fig. 5.7). No face is truly symmetrical, but any significant asymmetry should be noted. The soft tissue nasion, middle part of the upper lip at the vermillion border and the chin point should all be aligned. The face can also be divided into fifths, with each section being approximately equal to the width of an eye (Fig. 5.8).

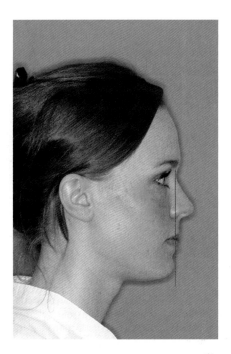

Fig. 5.2 Using zero meridian to estimate anteroposterior relationship. Zero meridian is the true vertical line dropped from the soft tissue nasion. In a Class I relationship (as shown here) the upper lip lies on or slightly anterior to this line and the chin point lies slightly behind it.

Box 5.2 The three dimensions of clinical examination

Anteroposterior

Extra-oral

Maxilla to mandible relationship (Class I, II or III)

Intra-oral

Incisor classification
Overjet
Canine relationship
Molar relationship
Anterior crossbite

Vertical

Extra-oral

Facial thirds
Angle of lower border of mandible to the maxilla

Intra-oral

Overbite, anterior open bite or lateral open bite

Transverse

Extra-oral

Facial asymmetry

Intra-oral

Centrelines
Posterior crossbites

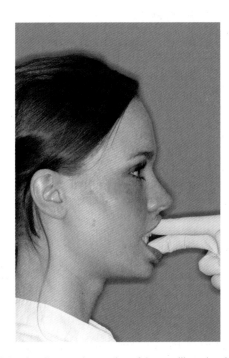

Fig. 5.3 Palpating the anterior portion of the maxilla at A point and the mandible at B point to determine the underlying skeletal anteroposterior relationship. In a normal (Class I) skeletal relationship, as shown here, the upper jaw lies 2–4 mm in front of the lower. In a Class II the lower jaw would be > 4 mm behind the upper jaw. In a Class III the lower jaw is < 2 mm behind the upper (in more severe Class III cases the lower jaw may be in front of the upper).

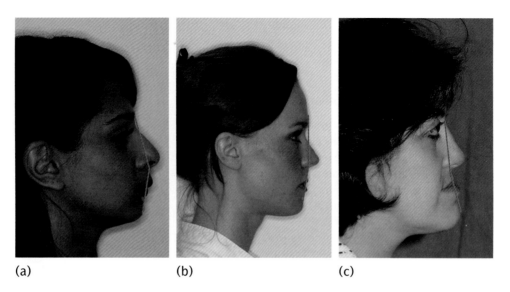

(a)   (b)   (c)

Fig. 5.4 The anteroposterior relationship of the jaws can also be assessed using the convexity of the face. This is assessed by the angle between the upper face (glabella to subnasale) and the lower face (subnasale to pogonion). The mean value is 12° ± 4°. (a) A patient with a convex profile with an increased angle of facial convexity indicating a Class II skeletal pattern. (b) A patient with a straighter profile with a normal angle of facial convexity indicating a Class I skeletal pattern. (c) A patient with a concave profile indicating a Class III skeletal pattern.

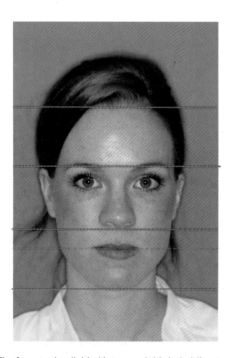

Fig. 5.5 The face can be divided into equal thirds: hairline to glabella between the eyebrows (forehead), glabella to subnasale (middle third), and subnasale to lowest part of the chin (lower third). The lower third can be further divided into the thirds, with the upper lip lying in the upper third and the lower lip lying at the top of the lower two-thirds.

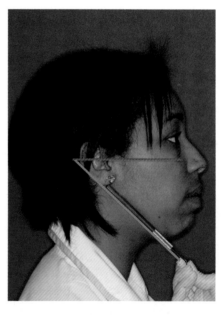

Fig. 5.6 The mandibular plane angle can be estimated clinically by looking at the point of contact of intersecting lines made up by the lower border of the mandible (in blue) and the Frankfort Horizontal Plane (in red). The Frankfort Plane is actually measured on a lateral cephalogram (between porion and orbital), but can be estimated clinically by palpation of the lower border of the orbit. The angle is considered normal if the two lines intersect at the occiput. In this case the lines intersect anterior to the occiput, which is consistent with an increased angle, suggesting increased vertical proportions. If the lines intersect posterior to the occiput, then the angle would be decreased, indicating reduced vertical proportions.

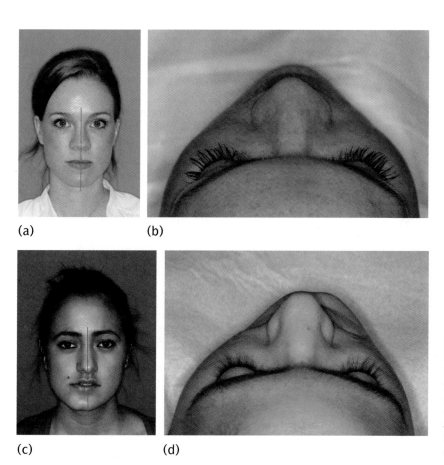

(a)　　　　　(b)

(c)　　　　　(d)

Fig. 5.7 The transverse examination of the face should be done from the front, and from above the patient (by standing behind and above the patient). (a) The patient has a symmetrical face, with the facial midline showing alignment of the soft tissue nasion, middle part of the upper lip at the vermillion border and the chin point. (b) The same patient viewed from behind, confirming the symmetry. (c, d) A patient with marked mandibular asymmetry to the right.

5.4.4 Smile aesthetics

Most patients seek orthodontic treatment to improve their smile, so it is important to recognize the various components of a smile that will improve the aesthetics (see section on Further reading).

A normal smile should show the following (Fig. 5.9):

- The whole height of the upper incisors should be visible on full smiling, with only the interproximal gingivae visible. This smile line is usually 1–2 mm higher in females.

- The upper incisor edges should run parallel to the lower lip (smile arc)

- The upper incisors should be close to, but not touching, the lower lip

- The gingival margins of the anterior teeth are important if they are visible in the smile. The margins of the central incisors and canines should be approximately level, with the lateral incisors lying 1 mm more incisally than the canines and central incisors

- The width of the smile should be such that buccal corridors should be visible, but minimal. The buccal corridor is the space between the angle of the mouth and the buccal surfaces of the most distal visible tooth.

- There should be a symmetrical dental arrangement

- The upper dental midline should be coincident to the middle of the face.

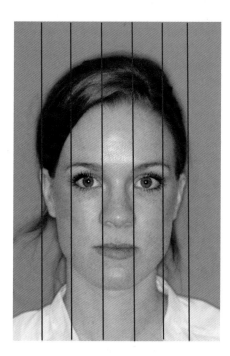

Fig. 5.8 In a face with normal transverse proportions, the face can divided into approximately five equal sections – each the width of an eye.

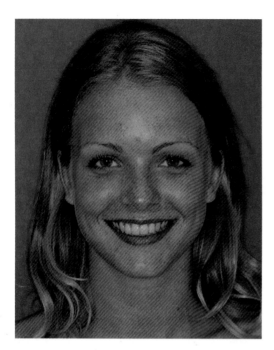

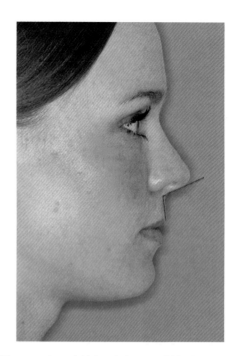

Fig. 5.9 The patient demonstrates many of the features of the normal smile: (1) the whole of the upper incisors is visible with only the interproximal gingivae visible; (2) the upper incisor edges are parallel to the lower lip – indicating a 'consonant' smile arc; (3) the upper incisors do not touch the lower lip; (4) the gingival margins of the central incisors and canines should be approximately level, with the lateral incisors lying 1 mm incisally; (5) the buccal corridors are visible, but minimal and (6) symmetrical dental arrangement. In this case the only aspect where the smile aesthetics deviate slightly from the normal, is that the upper dental centreline is slightly to the right of the facial midline.

Fig. 5.10 The normal nasolabial angle is 90–110°. This is important to note as the angle can be affected by orthodontic movement of the upper incisors.

Many aspects of facial or smile aesthetics cannot be influenced by orthodontics alone, or indeed cannot be influenced at all. This needs to be discussed with the patient, and if appropriate, surgical and restorative options may need to be considered.

5.4.5 Soft tissue examination

In addition to assessing the smile aesthetics, a soft tissue examination will also assess:

- Lips (see Box 5.3)
- Tongue

> **Box 5.3 Features of the lips to assess**
> - Lip competence
> - Lip fullness
> - Nasolabial angle
> - Method of achieving an anterior seal

Lips can be competent (that is meet together at rest), potentially competent (position of incisors prevents comfortable lip seal to be obtained) or incompetent (require considerable muscular activity to obtain a lip seal). Lip incompetence is common in preadolescent children, but increases with age due to vertical growth of the soft tissues. The ability to achieve lip competence is particularly important when reducing overjets in Class II division 1 cases, as the stability of the case is improved if the upper incisor position is under the control of competent lips at the end of treatment.

Lips should be everted at their base, with some vermillion border seen at rest. Protrusion of the lips does differ between different ethnic groups with patients of Afro-Caribbean origin being more protrusive than those of Caucasian origin (see Fig. 5.6). The use of Rickett's Esthetic line (E-line) provides a guide to the appropriate prominence of the lips within the face (see Section 6.9.2).

The nasolabial angle is formed between the base of the nose and the upper lip and should be 90–110° (Fig. 5.10). It can be affected by the shape of the nose, but also the drape of the upper lip. The drape of the upper lip can be affected by the support of the upper incisor. If the shape of the nose is normal, a high nasolabial angle could therefore indicate a retrusive lip, whereas a low nasolabial angle could indicate lip protrusion.

The reason why an assessment of the tongue is performed during the extra-oral examination, is to determine the method by which patients achieve an anterior seal during swallowing, and the position of the tongue at rest. In some patients with incompetent lips the tongue thrusts forward to contact with the lips to form an anterior seal. This is usually adaptive to the underlying malocclusion, so when the treatment is complete and normal lip competence can be achieved, the tongue thrust ceases. In some patients there is a so-called endogenous tongue thrust, which will re-establish itself after treatment, leading to relapse. Being able to identify cases that may have this strong relapse potential would be helpful. It is however very difficult to confidently distinguish between an adaptive tongue thrust and an endogenous tongue thrust. Patients with an endogenous tongue thrusts tend to show proclination of both the upper and lower incisors, an anterior openbite, an associated lisp, and the tongue tends to sit between the incisors at rest.

5.4.6 Temporomandibular (TMJ) examination

It is important to note the presence of any signs of pathology in the TMJ and muscles of mastication during the orthodontic assessment.

Any tenderness, clicks, crepitus and locking should be noted, as well as recording the range of movement and maximum opening. As mentioned in Chapter 1 (see Section 1.7), there is no strong evidence to suggest that TMJ disorders are either associated with malocclusions or cured by orthodontic treatment. However, if signs or symptoms are detected then they must be recorded and it may be worth referring the patient to a specialist before commencing orthodontic treatment.

5.5 Intra-oral examination

The intra-oral examination allows the clinician to assess the:

- stage of dental development (by charting the teeth present)
- soft tissues and periodontium for pathology
- oral hygiene
- overall dental health, including identifying any caries and restorations
- tooth position within each arch and between arches

5.5.1 Assessment of oral health

It is key that any pathology is identified in the mucosal surfaces, periodontally or in the teeth themselves. Generally any pathology needs to be treated and stabilised before any orthodontic treatment can be undertaken.

Periodontal disease is fortunately unusual in child patients, but is relatively common in adults. Any mucogingival or periodontal problems needs to be carefully noted. Section 20.3 discusses the importance of identifying and stabilising periodontal disease, allowing us to modify treatment planning and mechanics for these patients.

Excellent oral hygiene is essential for orthodontic treatment otherwise there is a high risk of decalcification. Treatment should not begin until a patient can demonstrate they can consistently maintain high levels of oral hygiene.

Dental pathology can have a significant influence on the treatment plan, and additional radiographs and special tests (such as vitality tests) may be required. We are particularly interested in detecting:

- caries
- areas of hypomineralisation
- effects of previous trauma
- tooth wear
- teeth of abnormal size or shape
- existing restorations which may change the way we bond to the tooth, as well determine our choice of extractions if space is required

---

Box 5.4 Describing the amount of crowding present

0–4 mm = Mild crowding

4–8 mm = Moderate crowding

>8 mm = Severe crowding

5.5.2 Assessment of each dental arch

Each arch is assessed individually for:

- crowding (see Box 5.4) or spacing
- alignment of teeth, including displacements or rotations of teeth
- inclination of the labial segments (proclined, upright or retroclined)
- angulation of the canines (mesial, upright or distal) as this affects anchorage assessment later
- arch shape and symmetry
- depth of Curve of Spee (see Section 7.7)

5.5.3 Assessment of arches in occlusion

The arches are now assessed in occlusion. The incisor relationships are assessed first: incisor classification, overjet or anterior crossbites (anteroposterior), overbite or openbite (vertical) and centrelines (transverse). Then the buccal relationships are assessed: canine and molar relationships (anteroposterior), any lateral openbites (vertical) and buccal crossbites (transverse).

Incisor classification

This is discussed in Section 2.3.

Overjet

This is measured from the labial surface of the most prominent incisor to the labial surface of the mandibular incisor (Fig. 5.11). This would normally be 2–4 mm. If the lower incisor lies anterior to the upper incisors, then overjet is given a negative value.

Overbite

This measures how much the maxillary incisors overlap the mandibular incisors vertically (Fig. 5.11). There are three features to note when assessing the overbite:

- amount of overlap
- whether the lower teeth are in contact with the opposing teeth or soft tissues (complete overbite) or if they are not touching anything (incomplete overbite)
- whether any soft tissue damage is being caused (when it is described as traumatic)

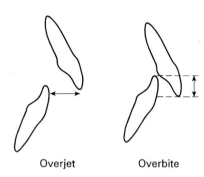

Fig. 5.11 Measurement of overjet and overbite.

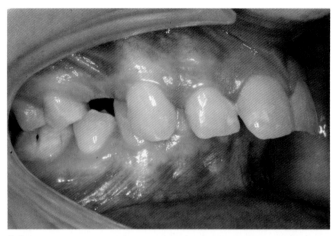

(a)

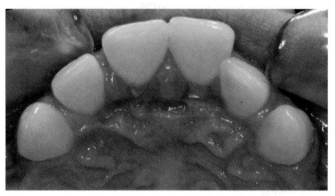

(b)

Fig. 5.12 Traumatic overbite. (a) A case with a very deep overbite; (b) demonstrates that the overbite is complete and traumatic (note damage associated with gingival stripping palatally of the upper central incisors).

A normal value would be 1/3 coverage of the crown of the lower incisor. If the overlap is greater than this the overbite is described as increased, and if it is less than this it is decreased. If there is no overlap at all it is an anterior open bite.

Occasionally an overbite can be traumatic. This usually happens when the teeth occlude with the junction between the tooth and cervical gingivae. This could be labial to the lower incisors, or palatal to the upper incisors (Fig. 5.12)

Centrelines

The centrelines should ideally be coincident with each other and to the facial midline.

Canine relationship

This is discussed in Section 2.3.

Molar relationship

This is discussed in Section 2.3.

Crossbites

A crossbite is a discrepancy in the buccolingual relationship of the upper and lower teeth. These relationships are described in more detail in Chapter 13. They can be described by:

- Location (anterior or posterior)
- Nature of the crossbite (see Box 5.5)

It is very important to note whether there is a displacement of the mandible on closure when any crossbite is present. This means that, due to the crossbite when the patient tries to close together there may be premature contact on a tooth or teeth that are in crossbite. This causes the mandible to move either left or right, and/or anteriorly into a new position to allow maximum intercuspation of the teeth. As a result there will be a discrepancy between the retruded contact position and intercuspal position (Fig. 5.13). It is vital that this displacement of the mandible is identified, because the crossbite is artificially holding the jaw in a different position, and as a result all the other measures of

---

Box 5.5 Description of crossbites

Buccal crossbite

The buccal cusps of the lower teeth occlude buccal to the buccal cusps of the upper teeth.

Lingual crossbite (or scissor bite)

The buccal cusps of the lower teeth occlude lingual to the lingual cusps of the upper teeth

---

occlusion will be inaccurate. The orthodontic treatment plan should be based on the retruded contact position, as this is the position the jaw will return to when the displacement is removed when the crossbite is corrected.

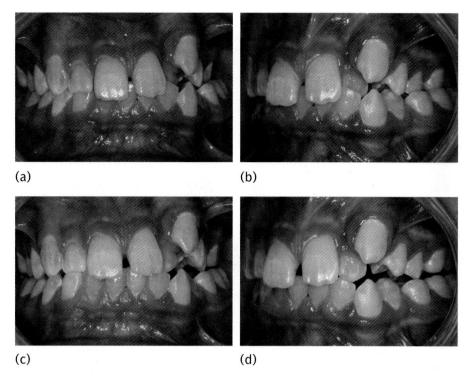

(a)

(b)

(c)

(d)

Fig. 5.13 This patient has an anterior crossbite on the upper left lateral incisor, and posterior crossbite affecting the upper left second premolar and upper left first molar. When examined carefully it is clear that the patient has a mandibular displacement forwards and to the left on closure, and this is caused by a premature contact on the upper left lateral incisor. (a, b) The patient with the teeth in maximum intercuspation (intercuspal position); (c, d) the patient before he displaces off the lateral incisor. Note the difference in the occlusal relationships, particularly the centrelines, as a result of the displacement of the mandible.

5.6 Diagnostic records

Orthodontic records may be required for a number of possible purposes:

- Diagnosis and treatment planning
- Monitoring growth
- Monitoring treatment
- Medico-legal record
- Patient communication and education
- Audit and research

5.6.1 Study models

Study models should show all the erupted teeth and be extended into the buccal sulcus. They are poured in dental stone and typically produced from alginate impressions. They should be mounted in occlusion, using a wax or polysiloxane bite. They are produced using a technique known as Angle trimming, which allows models to be placed on a flat surface and viewed in the correct occlusion from varying angles (Fig. 5.14).

Digital versions of study models, which should not deteriorate with time and do not take up physical space, are gradually replacing stone models.

5.6.2 Photographs

These provide a key colour record. The usual views taken are:

Four extra-oral (in natural head position):
- Full facial frontal at rest
- Full facial frontal smiling
- Facial three-quarters view
- Facial profile

Five intra-oral:
- Frontal occlusion
- Buccal occlusion (left and right)
- Occlusal views of upper and lower arch

Some operators are beginning to take short video clips of the patient talking and smiling, as this may provide additional useful information about the dentition and smile in function.

5.6.3 Radiographs

Any radiograph carries a low but identifiable risk, so each radiograph must be clinically justified. A radiograph is only prescribed after a full clinical

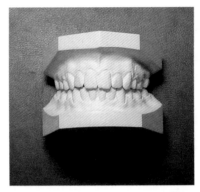

(a)

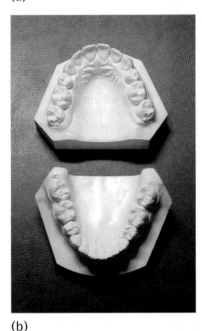

(b)

Fig. 5.14 Study models should be produced using a technique known as Angle's trimming. This means the models can be placed on a flat surface on different edges, so the correct occlusion can be viewed from different angles. (a) The teeth are shown in occlusion, on this occasion stood on their posterior trimmed base; (b) the two arches viewed independently.

examination to ensure that information cannot be gained by a less invasive method (see Box 5.6). When considering interceptive or active orthodontic treatment a radiograph may provide additional information on:

- Presence or absence of teeth
- Stage of development of adult dentition
- Root morphology of teeth
- Presence of ectopic or supernumerary teeth
- Presence of dental disease
- Relationship of the teeth to the skeletal dental bases, and their relationship to the cranial base

Dental Panoramic Tomograph (Fig. 5.15)

This is useful for confirming the presence, position and morphology of unerupted teeth, and a general overview of the teeth and their supporting structures. The focal trough is narrow in the incisor region, so additional views may be required for some patients in this region.

DPT should only be taken in the presence of specific signs and symptoms, so they should not be used as a method of screening clinically asymptomatic patients.

> **Box 5.6 Radiographs commonly used in orthodontic assessment**
>
> - Dental panoramic tomograph (DPT)
> - Cephalometric lateral skull radiograph
> - Upper standard occlusal radiograph
> - Periapical radiographs
> - Bitewing radiographs

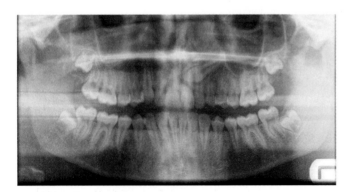

Fig. 5.15 Dental panoramic tomograph (DPT) showing an unerupted upper left canine and unerupted third permanent molars.

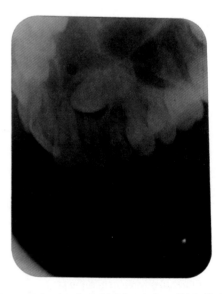

Fig. 5.16 Upper occlusal radiograph taken to investigate the impacted canine shown in Fig. 5.15. There is a suggestion of possible resorption of the root of the upper lateral incisor, associated with the crown of the palatally impacted upper left canine.

Cephalometric lateral skull radiograph

Sometimes referred to as a 'lateral ceph', this is discussed in more detail in Chapter 6.

Upper occlusal radiograph (Fig. 5.16)

This gives a view of the maxillary incisor region and is used to assess the root form of incisors, detect the presence of supernumerary teeth and to locate ectopic canine teeth. The location of teeth on radiographs often requires views to be taken at different angles using a technique known as parallax (see Section 14.5).

Periapical radiographs

These can be used in any part of the mouth and are useful for assessing root form and local pathology, and locating unerupted teeth (like the upper occlusal, they can be used with other radiographic views to identify the position of these teeth using parallax).

Bitewing radiographs

They may be useful in assessing caries and the condition of existing restorations.

5.6.4 Cone beam computed tomography (CBCT) and 3D imaging

Conventional computed tomography (CT) imaging involves the use of rotating X-ray equipment, combined with a digital computer, to obtain images of the body. Using CT imaging, cross-sectional images of body organs and tissues can be produced. CBCT is a faster, more compact version of traditional CT with a lower dose of radiation. Through the use of a cone-shaped X-ray beam, the size of the scanner, radiation dosage and time needed for scanning are all dramatically reduced. The three-dimensional views produced may be useful in certain orthodontic cases:

- Accurate location of impacted teeth and a more accurate assessment of any associated pathology, particularly resorption of adjacent teeth (Fig. 5.17)
- Assessment of alveolar bone coverage
- Assessment of alveolar bone height and volume (which may be relevant in potential implant cases)
- TMJ or airway analysis

Although the radiation dose is considerably smaller than conventional CT scanning, the dose is still higher than for the conventional radiographs discussed in Section 5.6.3 (see Section 6.1.1). At the present time CBCT should therefore only be used when conventional radiography has failed to give, or is very unlikely to give, the necessary diagnostic information.

Other 3D imaging techniques are also being developed for use in orthodontics, such as optical laser scanning and stereo photogrammetry. The use of 3D imaging in combined orthodontic and orthognathic surgery is covered in Section 21.10.1.

The use of 3D imaging is one of the most rapidly developing fields in orthodontics and the reader is directed to the section on Further reading for more details.

5.7 Forming a problem list

The information collected from the history, examination and records, produces a database identifying a list of problems. It is this list of problems that allows the clinician to form a diagnosis (Fig. 5.1). An example of an orthodontic patient assessment is given in Fig.5. 17.

Chapter 7 will discuss the process by which the problem list produces a list of aims of treatment. Once the aims of treatment are clear, various options for treatment can be discussed with the patient, considering the risks and benefits of each of the options. When the patient understands all the options a definitive treatment plan can be agreed.

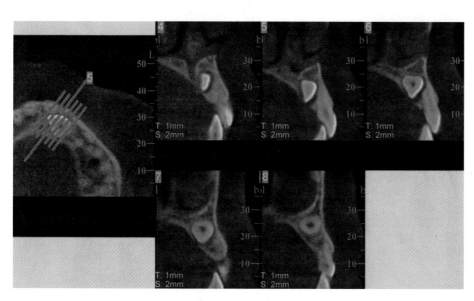

Fig. 5.17 Cone-beam computed tomography (CBCT) of the patient with the impacted canine shown in Figs 5.15 and 5.16, confirming that there is a small amount of root resorption occuring on the palatal aspect of the upper left lateral incisor, close to the apex of the tooth.

5.8 Case study: example case to demonstrate orthodontic assessment (case treated by Dr Taiyab Raja under the supervision of Simon Littlewood)

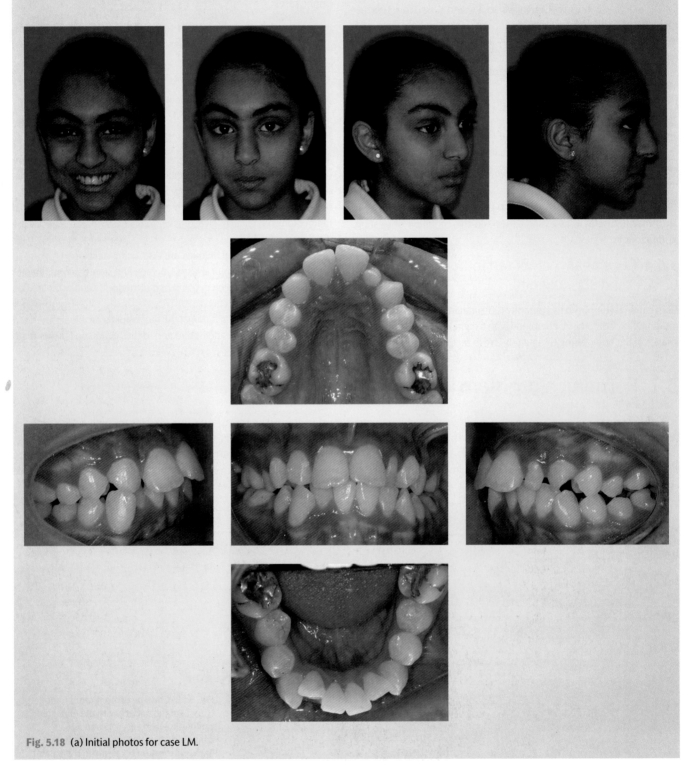

Fig. 5.18 (a) Initial photos for case LM.

Orthodontic Assessment Form

Patient Details

Name ▓▓▓▓▓ ▓▓▓▓▓	Referrer: ▓▓▓▓▓
Address ▓▓▓▓▓	Reason for referral
Tel Contact: ▓▓▓▓▓	*Missing lateral incisor*
Date of birth: ▓▓▓▓▓ Age 12 years 11 months	

History

Patient's complaint	Habits
Upper teeth stick out & are crooked	*None noted*
	Growth status
	Still growing
Medical history	**Motivation**
Medically fit & well	*Very keen for treatment with realistic expectations for treatment*
Dental History (including trauma & previous treatments)	
No trauma history. Regular dental attender, with experience of restorations in adult teeth	**Socio-behaviour factors** *Supportive family able to attend appointments. No apparent behavioral problems*

Extra-oral examination

Anteroposterior	Smile Aesthetics
Mild Class II	*Smile aesthetic compromised by missing upper right lateral incisor - creating unusual gingival margin relationships and asymmetrical dental arrangement*
Vertical	
Average vertical proportions	
	Soft tissues
	Lips incompetent at rest with lower lip behind upper incisors at rest. Normal swallowing pattern
Transverse	**TMJ**
Symmetrical	*No signs or symptoms reported*

Intra-oral examination

Teeth present:

7 6 5 4 3	1	1 2 3 4 5 6 7
7 6 5 4 3 2 1		1 2 3 4 5 6 7

Oral hygiene	Lower arch
Unsatisfactory – needs to improve	*Moderate crowding (approximately 7mm) Slightly mesially inclined lower canines*
Periondontal health	
Bleeding on probing in labial segments	**Upper arch**
Tooth quality	*Absent upper right lateral and peg-shaped upper left lateral incisor. Very mild crowding with upper right canine rotated mesio-palatally by 90°*
Heavily restored first permanent molars	

Teeth in occlusion

Incisor relationship	Molars
Class II division 1	Right ¾ unit Class II Left ¾ unit Class II
Overjet = 8 mm	**Canines**
	Right ¾ unit Class II Left ¾ unit Class II
Overbite	
Increased & incomplete	**Crossbites**
Centre-lines	*Crossbite tendency upper left second premolar*
Upper centre-line 2mm to right of facial midline	**Displacements**
Lower centre-line correct to facial midline	*None detected*

Fig. 5.18 (b) Completed orthodontic assessment sheet for case LM. A blank version of this form is available in the Appendix.

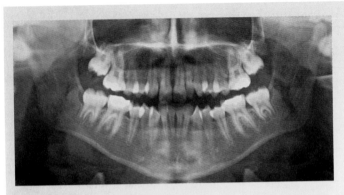

Fig. 5.18 (c) DPT for case LM. The DPT demonstrates the absence of the upper right lateral incisor and all third permanent molars. There is also large restorations in all first permanent molars, particularly the upper left and the lower right first permant molars.

Problem list for LM

Pathological problems

Oral hygiene is poor. The first permanent molars have large restorations and may therefore have a limited long-term prognosis.

Developmental (Orthodontic) problems

Patient's concerns: LM is concerned about her prominent and crooked upper teeth. She has good motivation for treatment and realistic expectations.

Facial and smile asthetics: The missing upper right lateral incisor is compromising her smile. This has caused an unusual gingival margin relationship and an asymmetric dental arrangement. Her mandible is slightly retrognathic, but acceptable. Her lips are incompetent at rest – competence can only be achieved by straining the lips.

Alignment and symmetry in each arch: The lower arch is symmetrical and U-shaped, with 7 mm of crowding. The upper arch is symmetrical and V-shaped with 1 mm of crowding. The upper right lateral incisor is developmentally absent and the upper left lateral incisor is peg-shaped. The upper incisors are proclined at 120° and the upper left canine is severely rotated.

Skeletal and dental problems in the transverse plane: There is no skeletal asymmetry. The upper centreline is 2 mm to the right of the facial midline, and the lower centreline is correct. There is a crossbite tendency on the upper left second premolar.

Skeletal and dental problems in anteroposterior plane: The mandible is slightly retrognathic, but clinically acceptable. There is an increased overjet of 8 mm. The molars and canines are ¾ unit Class II bilaterally.

Skeletal and dental problems in the vertical plane: The patient presents with normal vertical skeletal proportions. There is an average overbite, with an increased curve of Spee in the lower arch of 3 mm.

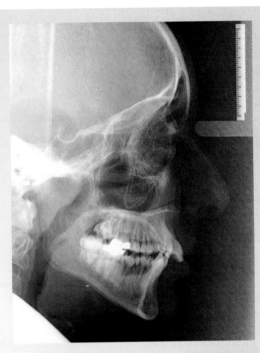

Fig. 5.18 (d) Lateral ceph radiograph of LM. Analysis of this radiograph shows the following values: SNA = 75°, SNB = 73°, ANB = 2°, upper incisor to maxilla = 120°, lower incisor to mandible = 90° and maxillary–mandibular planes angle = 28°. An Eastman correction on the ANB produces an ANB = 5°. Lateral ceph analysis will be explained further in Chapter 6. This radiograph confirms the clinical findings of a mild Class II skeletal pattern, with normal vertical proportions and proclined upper incisors.

Aims of treatment for LM

The **aims** of treatment are directly related to the problem list.

Patient's concerns: Address the patient's concerns by reducing slightly the prominent upper incisors and aligning the teeth.

Facial and smile aesthetics: Improve her smile by creating more normal gingival margin relationships, with the central incisors being higher than the adjacent tooth. Improve the symmetry of the smile by balancing the tooth proportions on the right and left in the upper labial segment. Allow her to obtain lip competence at rest by minimal retraction of the upper dentition.

Alignment and symmetry in each arch: Relieve the crowding in both arches. Maintain the lower archform and make the upper arch compatible with this. Improve the symmetry in the upper arch, reduce the prominence and proclination of the upper incisors, and align the teeth, including the rotated upper left canine.

Skeletal and dental problems in the transverse plane: Correct the upper centreline to the facial midline, and expand the upper arch to remove the crossbite tendency on the upper left second premolar.

Skeletal and dental problems in the anteroposterior plane: Reduce the overjet principally by retraction of the upper incisors. Some minimal proclination of the lower labial segment could be accepted. The canines should be treated to a Class I relationship. The mandible is slightly retrognathic so the case can be treated by othodontic camouflage.

Skeletal and dental problems in the vertical plane: Flatten the curve of Spee in the lower arch.

Treatment plan for LM

(The treatment planning process is discussed in Chapter 7.)

- Improve oral hygiene to level suitable for orthodontic treatment
- Extract peg-shaped upper left lateral incisor and all first permanent molars

- Transpalatal arch connecting upper second permanent molars (see Chapter 15)
- Upper and lower fixed appliances – aiming to close spaces anteriorly and camouflaging upper canines as upper lateral incisors, and camouflaging upper first premolars as upper canines. This should give a more symmetrical and aesthetic smile.
- Pericision to upper left canine to reduce relapse (see Section 16.7.1)
- Upper bonded retainer and upper and lower vacuum-formed retainers (see Chapter 16)

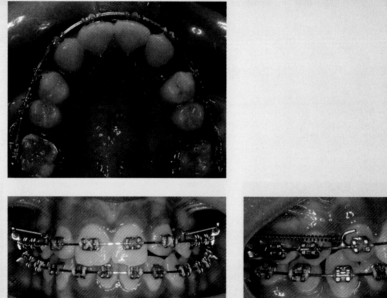

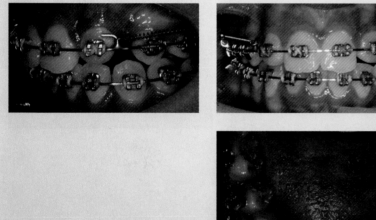

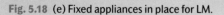

Fig. 5.18 (e) Fixed appliances in place for LM.

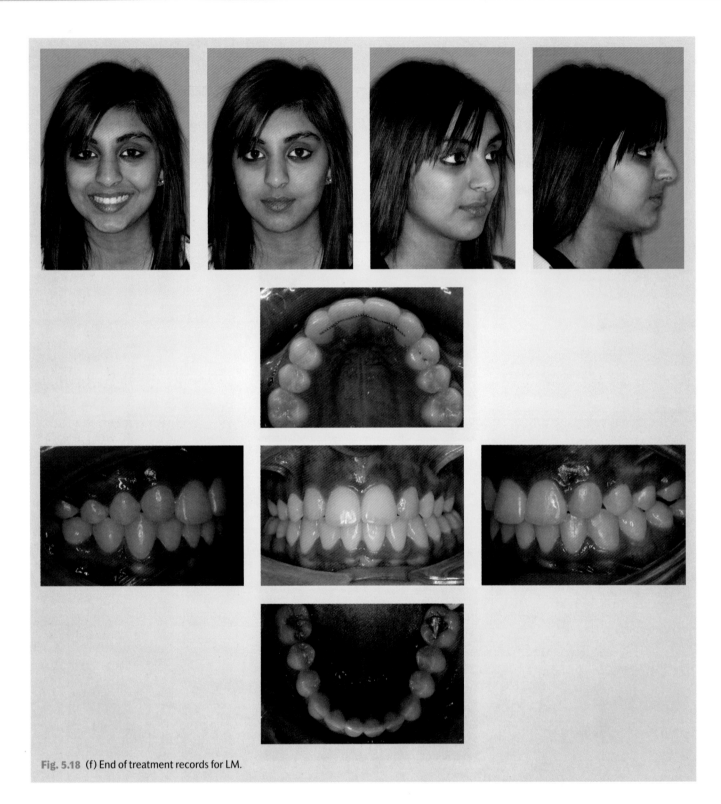

Fig. 5.18 (f) End of treatment records for LM.

Key points about orthodontic assessment

- Orthodontic assessment involves taking a history, undertaking a clinical examination and collecting appropriate diagnostic records
- The history should include the patient's presenting complaint, medical history, dental history (including any history of trauma and previous treatment), habits, physical growth status, patient motivation and any relevant socio-behavioural factors
- The clinical examination should be a systematic assessment of the face and dentition in three dimensions
- As well as assessing the patient extra-orally in three dimensions it is important to assess the smile aesthetics and soft tissues
- The intra-oral examination should assess the overall dental health, each arch individually, the arches in occlusion
- The history and examination should determine which diagnostic records are required. This may include study models, photographs and appropriate radiographs and possibly 3D imaging

Principal sources and further reading

Patel, A, Burden D.J., and Sandler J. (2009). Medical disorders and orthodontics. *Journal of Orthodontics*, **36**, 1–21.

This comprehensive article provides an excellent in-depth review of medical disorders that could affect orthodontic treatment.

Gill, D.S., Naini, F.B., and Tredwin, C.J. (2007). Smile aesthetics. *Dental Update*, **34**, 152–8.

Sarver, D.M. (2001). The importance of incisor positioning in the esthetic smile: the smile arc. *American Journal of Orthodontics and Dentofacial Orthopedics*, **120**, 98–111.

These two papers provide an overview of the important topic of smile aesthetics.

Isaacson, K.G., Thom, A.R., Horner, K., and Waites, E. (2008). *Orthodontic Radiographs: Guidelines* (3rd edn). British Orthodontic Society.

These radiographic guidelines have been specifically written for orthodontics.

Merrett, S.J., Drage, N.A., and Durning, P. (2009). Cone beam computed tomography: a useful tool in orthodontic diagnosis and treatment planning. *Journal of Orthodontics*, **36**, 202–10.

Benington, P.C.M., Khambay, B.S., and Ayoub, A.F. (2010). An overview of three-dimensional imaging in dentistry. *Dental Update*, **37**, 494–508.

These papers provide an introduction to the rapidly evolving field of 3D imaging

References for this chapter can also be found at www.oxfordtextbooks.co.uk/orc/mitchell4e/. Where possible, these are presented as active links which direct you to the electronic version of the work, to help facilitate onward study. If you are a subscriber to that work (either individually or through an institution), and depending on your level of access, you may be able to peruse an abstract or the full article if available.

Please note figure (5.18b) orthodontic assessment form can be downloaded from the OUP website www.oxfordtextbooks.co.uk/orc/mitchell4e/

6

Cephalometrics

Chapter contents

Cephalometry is the analysis and interpretation of standardized radiographs of the facial bones. In practice, cephalometrics has come to be associated with a true lateral view (Fig. 6.1). An anteroposterior radiograph can also be taken in the cephalostat, but this view is difficult to interpret and is usually only employed in cases with a skeletal asymmetry.

6.1 The cephalostat

In order to be able to compare the cephalometric radiographs of one patient taken on different occasions, or those of different individuals, some standardization is necessary. To achieve this aim the cephalostat was developed by B. Holly Broadbent in the period after the First World War (Fig. 6.2). The cephalostat consists of an X-ray machine which is at a fixed distance from a set of ear posts designed to fit into the patient's external auditory meatus. Thus the central beam of the machine is directed towards the ear posts, which also serve to stabilize the patient's head. The position of the head in the vertical axis is standardized by ensuring that the patient's Frankfort plane (for definition see below) is horizontal. This can be done by manually positioning the subject or, alternatively, by placing a mirror some distance away level with the patient's head and asking him or her to look into their own eyes. This is termed the natural head position, and some orthodontists claim that it is more consistent than a manual approach. It is normal practice to cone down the area exposed so that the skull vault is not routinely included in the X-ray beam.

Unfortunately, attempts to standardize the distances from the tube to the patient (usually between 5 and 6 feet (1.5 to 1.8 m)) and from the patient to the film (usually around 1 foot (around 30 cm)) have not been entirely successful as the values in parentheses would suggest. Some magnification, usually of the order of 7–8 per cent, is inevitable with a lateral cephalometric film. In order to be able to check the magnification and thus the comparability of different films, it is helpful if a scale is included in the view. In order to allow comparisons between radiographs of the same patient it is essential that the magnification for a particular cephalostat is standardized.

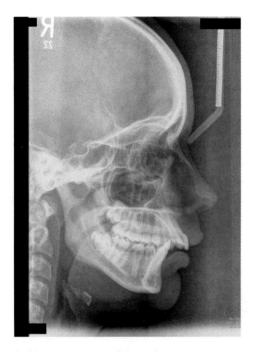

Fig. 6.1 A lateral cephalometric radiograph. An aluminium wedge has been positioned to attenuate the beam thereby enhancing the view of the soft tissues.

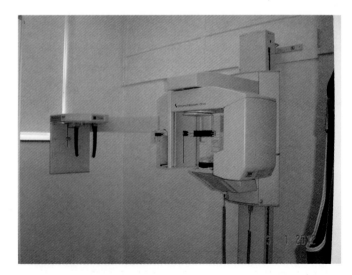

Fig. 6.2 A cephalostat.

Box 6.1 Types of digital radiographs

Charged Couple Device (CCD)

- CCD converts energy into electrical charge
- Sensor is placed in mouth for IO X-rays
- For EO X-rays sensor replaces film
- Sensor is connected by a cable to computer
- Information is displayed 'real-time' on computer screen

Photo-Stimuable Phosphor Imaging (PSP)

- Phosphor plate is placed in cassette
- After imaging, plate is read by a laser
- Therefore there is a delay in image appearing on screen

To give a better definition of the soft tissue outline of the face an aluminium wedge is positioned so as to attenuate the beam in that area

(see Fig 6.1). This step is however required less frequently with newer digital systems.

6.1.1 Digital radiographs

Conventionally, following the exposure of the X-ray beam onto the radiographic film, it is processed to give an individual radiograph. With digital radiographs the image is stored electronically and viewed directly on a computer screen. This approach has the advantage that processing faults are eliminated and the storage and transfer of images is facilitated.

There are currently two main approaches used to produce digital radiographs (see Box 6.1).

The resultant view can be digitized directly and the values noted or alternatively a proprietary software package can be used for digitization and analysis of the computer image.

6.2 Indications for cephalometric evaluation

An increasing awareness of the risks associated with X-rays has led clinicians to re-evaluate the indications for taking a cephalometric radiograph (Table 6.1). The following are considered valid.

6.2.1 An aid to diagnosis

It is possible to carry out successful orthodontic treatment without taking a cephalometric radiograph, particularly in Class I malocclusions. However, the information that cephalometric analysis yields is helpful in assessing the probable aetiology of a malocclusion and in planning treatment. The benefit to the patient in terms of the additional information gained must be weighed against the X-ray dosage. Therefore a lateral cephalometric radiograph is best limited to patients with a skeletal discrepancy and/or where anteroposterior movement of the incisors is planned. In a small proportion of patients it may be helpful to monitor growth to aid the planning and timing of treatment by taking serial cephalometric radiographs, although again the dosage to the patient must be justifiable.

In addition, a lateral view is often helpful in the accurate localization of unerupted displaced teeth and other pathology.

6.2.2 A pre-treatment record

A lateral cephalometric radiograph is useful in providing a baseline record prior to the placement of appliances, particularly where movement of the upper and lower incisors is planned.

6.2.3 Monitoring the progress of treatment

In the management of severe malocclusions, where tooth movement is occurring in all three planes of space (for example treatments involving functional appliances, or upper and lower fixed appliances), it may be helpful to take a lateral cephalometric radiograph during treatment to monitor incisor inclinations and anchorage requirements. A lateral cephalometric radiograph may also be useful in monitoring the movement of unerupted teeth and for assessing upper incisor root resorption if this is felt to be a potential risk during treatment.

6.2.4 Research purposes

A great deal of information has been obtained about growth and development by longitudinal studies which involved taking serial cephalometric radiographs from birth to the late teens or beyond. While the data provided by previous investigations are still used for reference purposes, it is no longer ethically possible to repeat this type of study. However, those views taken routinely during the course of orthodontic diagnosis and treatment can be used to study the effects of growth and treatment.

Table 6.1 Approximate effective dosages of different types of radiographs

Radiograph	Approximate effective dose (µSv)
Upper anterior occlusal	8
OPT	3–24
Lateral cephalogram	<6
Cone Beam CT	11–1025 (usually 50 to 500)

6.3 Evaluating a cephalometric radiograph

Before starting a tracing it is important to examine the radiograph for any abnormalities or pathology. For example, a pituitary tumour could result in an increase in the size of the sella turcica. A lateral cephalometric view is also helpful in assessing the patency of the airway, as enlarged adenoids can be easily seen.

6.3.1 Hand tracing

In order to be able to derive meaningful information, an accurate and systematic approach is required which also involves selecting the right conditions and equipment for the task.

- The tracing should be carried out in a darkened room on a light viewing box. All but the area being traced should be shielded to block out any extraneous light.
- Proprietary acetate sheets are the best medium as their transparency facilitates landmark identification.

- A sharp pencil should be used. The author recommends a 0.3-mm leaded propelling pencil (as this saves hours searching for pencil sharpeners).
- The acetate sheet should be secured onto the film with masking tape, which does not leave a sticky residue when removed. The tracing should be oriented in the same position as the patient was when the radiograph was taken, i.e. with the Frankfort plane horizontal.
- Some orthodontists use stencils to obtain a neat outline of the incisor and molar teeth. However, too much artistic licence can lead to inaccuracies, particularly if the crown root angle of a tooth is not 'average'.
- For landmarks which are bilateral (unless they are directly superimposed) an average of the two should be taken.
- With a careful technique tracing errors should be of the order of ±0.5 mm for linear measurements and ±0.5° for angular measurements.
- It is a valuable 'learning experience' to trace the same radiograph on two separate occasions and compare the tracings. This helps to reduce the temptation to place undue emphasis upon small variations from normal cephalometric values.

An example of a tracing is shown in Fig. 6.3 (see also Fig. 6.4). Definitions of the various points and reference planes are given in Section 6.5.

6.3.2 Digitizing

Information from a conventional hard copy lateral cephalometric film can be entered into a computer by means of a digitizer which comprises an illuminated radiographic viewing screen which is connected to the computer and a cursor used to record the horizontal and vertical (x, y) co-ordinates of cephalometric points and bony and soft tissue outlines. For digital radiographs the points can be entered directly by a

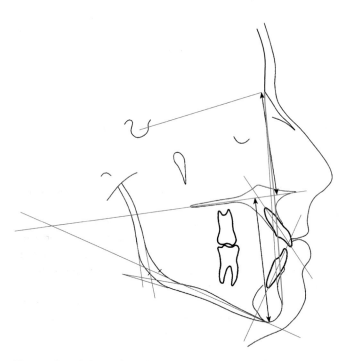

Fig. 6.3 A cephalometric tracing: patient LH (male) aged 14 years.

	LH	Mean
SNA	78.5°	81° ± 3°
SNB	77°	78° ± 3°
ANB	1.5°	3° ± 2°
UInc-MxPl	117.5°	109° ± 6°
LInc-MnPl	91.5°	93° ± 6°
MMPA	31°	27° ± 4°
LInc to APog	4 mm	1 mm ± 2 mm
FP	55%	55% ± 2%

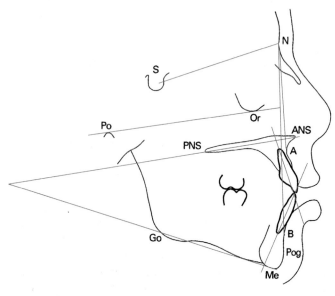

Fig. 6.4 Commonly used cephalometric points and planes.

mouse click. Specialized software can then be employed to utilize the information entered to produce a tracing and/or the analysis of choice. Studies have shown digitizing to be as accurate as tracing a radiograph by hand and with the increasing use of digital radiographs this now becoming the norm.

Clearly, this approach is particularly useful for research as any number of radiographs can be entered, superimposed, and/or compared statistically.

6.4 Cephalometric analysis: general points

The orthodontic literature is replete with different cephalometric analyses, which in itself suggests that no single method is sufficient for all purposes and that all have their drawbacks. In a book of this size it is more appropriate to consider one analysis in depth. Therefore one of the approaches used commonly in the UK will be considered (Table 6.2). For details of other analyses the reader is referred to the publications cited in the section on Further reading.

Cephalometric analyses are often based upon comparison of the values obtained for certain measurements for a particular individual (or group of individuals) with the average values for their population (e.g. Caucasians). An indication of the significance of any difference between the actual measurement for an individual and the 'average' value can be obtained from the standard deviation. The range given by one standard deviation around the mean will include 66 per cent of the population and two standard deviations will include 95 per cent.

Cephalometric analysis is also of value in identifying the component parts of a malocclusion and probable aetiological factors – it is useful when a tracing is finished to reflect why that individual has that particular malocclusion. However, it is important not to fall into the trap of giving more credence to cephalometric analysis than it actually merits; it should always be remembered that it is an adjunctive tool to clinical diagnosis, and differences of cephalometric values from the average are not in themselves an indication for treatment, particularly as variations from normal in a specific value may be compensated for elsewhere in the facial skeleton or cranial base. In addition, cephalometric errors can occur owing to incorrect positioning of the patient and incorrect identification of landmarks (see Section 6.11).

6.5 Commonly used cephalometric points and reference lines

The points and reference lines are shown in Fig. 6.4.

A point (A): this is the point of deepest concavity on the anterior profile of the maxilla. It is also called subspinale. This point is taken to represent the anterior limit of the maxilla and is often tricky to locate accurately. However, tracing the outline of the root of the upper central incisor first and shielding all extraneous light often aids identification. A point is located on alveolar bone and is liable to changes in position with tooth movement and growth.

Anterior nasal spine (ANS): this is the tip of the anterior process of the maxilla and is situated at the lower margin of the nasal aperture.

B point (B): the point of deepest concavity on the anterior surface of the mandibular symphysis. B point is also sited on alveolar bone and can alter with tooth movement and growth.

Gonion (Go): the most posterior inferior point on the angle of the mandible. This point can be 'guesstimated', or determined more accurately by bisecting the angle formed by the tangents from the posterior border of the ramus and the inferior border of the mandible (Fig. 6.5).

Menton (Me): the lowest point on the mandibular symphysis.

Nasion (N): the most anterior point on the frontonasal suture. When difficulty is experienced locating nasion, the point of deepest concavity at the intersection of the frontal and nasal bones can be used instead.

Orbitale (Or): the most inferior anterior point on the margin of the orbit. By definition, the left orbital margin should be used to locate this point. However, this can be a little tricky to determine radiographically, and so an average of the two images of left and right is usually taken.

Pogonion (Pog): the most anterior point on the mandibular symphysis.

Porion (Po): the uppermost outermost point on the bony external auditory meatus. This landmark can be obscured by the ear posts of the cephalostat, and some advocate tracing these instead. However, this is not recommended as they do not approximate to the position of the external auditory meatus. The uppermost surface of the condylar head is at the same level, and this can be used as a guide where difficulty is experienced in determining porion.

Posterior nasal spine (PNS): this is the tip of the posterior nasal spine of the maxilla. This point is often obscured by the developing third molars, but lies directly below the pterygomaxillary fissure.

Sella (S): the midpoint of the sella turcica.

SN line: this line, connecting the midpoint of sella turcica with nasion, is taken to represent the cranial base.

Frankfort plane: this is the line joining porion and orbitale. This plane is difficult to define accurately because of the problems inherent in determining orbitale and porion.

Mandibular plane: The line joining gonion and menton. This is only one of several definitions of the mandibular plane, but is probably the most widely used. Other definitions can be found in the publications listed in the section on Further reading.

Maxillary plane: the line joining anterior nasal spine with posterior nasal spine. Where it is difficult to determine ANS and PNS accurately, a line parallel to the nasal floor can be used instead.

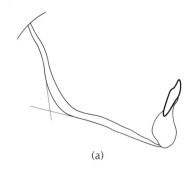

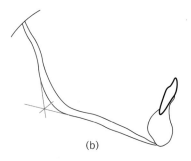

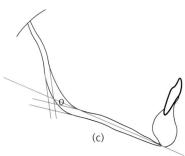

Fig. 6.5 Construction of Gonion (Go): (a) draw tangents to posterior and inferior borders; (b) bisect the angle formed by the tangents and mark where it crosses the angle of the mandible; (c) repeat for the other outline (if one is visible). Gonion is located midway between the two points.

Table 6.2 Cephalometric norms for Caucasians (Eastman Standard)

Measurement	Mean value	Standard deviation	Measurement	Mean value	Standard deviation
SNA	81°	3°	Inter-incisal angle	135°	10°
SNB	78°	3°	MMPA	27°	4°
ANB	3°	2°	Facial proportion	55%	2%
UInc to MxPl	109°	6°	LInc to APog line	+1 mm	2 mm
LInc to MnPl	93°*	6°	SN to MxPl	8°	3°

For definitions see Section 6.5.
*Or 120° – MMPA (see Section 6.8).

Functional occlusal plane: a line drawn between the cusp tips of the permanent molars and premolars (or deciduous molars in mixed dentition). It can be difficult to decide where to draw this line, particularly if there is an increased curve of Spee, or only the first permanent molars are in occlusion during the transition from mixed to permanent dentition. The functional plane can change orientation with growth and/or treatment, and so is not particularly reliable for longitudinal comparisons.

6.6 Anteroposterior skeletal pattern

6.6.1 Angle ANB

In order to be able to compare the position of the maxilla and mandible, it is necessary to have a fixed point or plane. The skeletal pattern is often determined cephalometrically by comparing the relationship of the maxilla and mandible with the cranial base by means of angles SNA and SNB. The difference between these two measurements, angle ANB, is classified broadly as follows:

ANB < 2°	Class III
2° ≤ ANB ≥ 4°	Class I
ANB > 4°	Class II

However, this approach assumes (incorrectly in some cases) that the cranial base, as indicated by the line SN, is a reliable basis for comparison and that points A and B are indicative of maxillary and mandibular basal bone. Variations in the position of nasion can also affect angles SNA and SNB and thus the difference ANB (Fig. 6.7); however, variations in the position of sella do not. If SNA is increased or reduced from the average value, this could be due to either a discrepancy in the position of the maxilla (as indicated by point A) or nasion. The following (rather crude) modification is often used in order to make allowance for this:

Provided the angle between the maxillary plane and the sella–nasion line is within 5–11°:

- if SNA is increased, for every degree that SNA is greater than 81°, subtract 0.5° from ANB;

- if SNA is reduced, for every degree that SNA is less than 81°, add 0.5° to ANB.

If the angle between the maxillary plane and the sella–nasion line is not within 5–11°, this correction is not applicable.

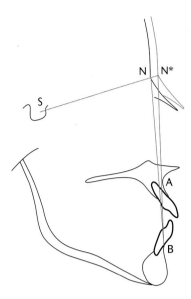

Fig. 6.7 Effect of variations in the position of nasion on angles SNA, SNB and ANB:

SNA = 78.5° SN*A = 81°
SNB = 77° SN*B = 81°
ANB = 1.5° AN*B = 0°

Alternatively, an approach which avoids the cranial base (e.g. the Ballard conversion or the Wits analysis) can be used to supplement the above analysis, particularly where the cephalometric findings are at variance with the clinical assessment.

6.6.2 Ballard conversion

This analysis uses the incisors as indicators of the relative position of the maxilla and mandible. It is easy to confuse a Ballard conversion and a prognosis tracing (see Fig. 6.12), but in the former the aim is to tilt the teeth to their normal angles (thus eliminating any dento-alveolar compensation) with the result that the residual overjet will indicate the relationship of the maxilla to the mandible.

6.6.3 Wits analysis

This analysis compares the relationship of the maxilla and mandible with the occlusal plane. There are several definitions of the occlusal plane, but for the purposes of the Wits analysis it is taken to be a line drawn between the cusp tips of the molars and premolars (or deciduous molars), which is known as the functional occlusal plane. Perpendicular lines from both point A and point B are dropped to the functional occlusal plane to give points AO and BO. The distance between AO and BO is then measured. The mean values are 1 mm (SD ±1.9 mm) for males and 0 mm (SD ±1.77 mm) for females.

The main drawback to the Wits analysis is that the functional occlusal plane is not easy to locate, which obviously affects the accuracy and reproducibility of the Wits analysis. A slight difference in the angulation of the functional occlusal plane can have a marked effect on the relative positions of AO and BO.

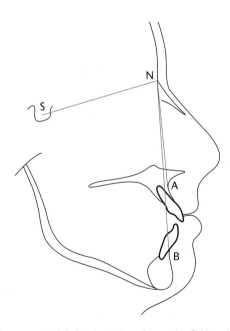

Fig. 6.6 Assessment of skeletal pattern using angles SNA and SNB: patient LH (male) aged 14 years.

	LH	**Mean**
SNA	78.5°	81° ± 3°
SNB	77°	78° ± 3°
ANB	1.5°	3° ± 2°

Corrected ANB $= 1.5° + \dfrac{81° - 78.5°}{2} = 2.75°$

This would normally be rounded to the nearest 0.5° giving a corrected value of 3°. The ANB difference suggests a mild Class III skeletal pattern. However, if the ANB difference is corrected for the low value of SNA, this suggests a Class I skeletal pattern.

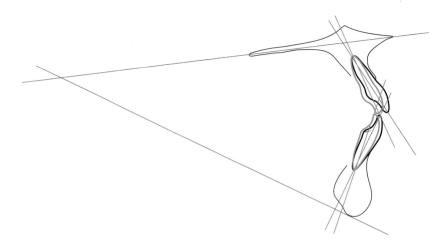

Fig. 6.8 Ballard conversion LH (male) aged 14 years: average upper incisor angle to maxillary plane, 109°; lower incisor angle to mandibular plane, 120° − 31° = 88°.

The method is as follows.

(1) Trace on a separate piece of tracing paper the outline of the maxilla, the mandibular symphysis, the incisors, and the maxillary and mandibular planes.

(2) Mark the 'rotation points' of the incisors one-third of the root length away from the root apex.

(3) By rotating around the point marked, reposition the upper incisor at an angle of 109° to the maxillary plane. Repeat for the lower incisor (allowing for the maxillary mandibular planes angle of 31° in this case).

(4) The residual overjet reflects the underlying skeletal pattern. In this case the Ballard conversion indicates a mild Class III skeletal pattern as the repositioned incisors are nearly edge to edge.

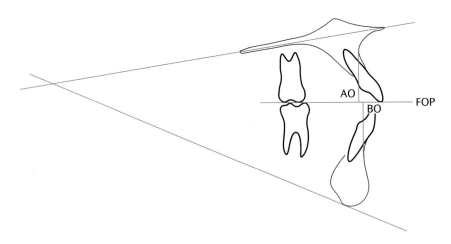

Fig. 6.9 Wits analysis: LH (male) aged 14 years. The method is as follows.

(1) Draw in the functional occlusal plane (FOP).

(2) Drop perpendiculars from point A and point B to the FOP to give points AO and BO.

(3) Measure the distance between AO and BO.

The average value is 1 mm (± 1.9 mm) for males and 0 mm (± 1.77 mm) for females. The distance from AO to BO for LH (male) is 2 mm, suggesting a mild Class III skeletal pattern.

6.7 Vertical skeletal pattern

Again there are many different ways of assessing vertical skeletal proportions. The more commonly used include the following.

- The Maxillary–Mandibular Planes Angle (Fig. 6.10). The average angle between the maxillary plane and the mandibular plane (MMPA) is 27 ±4°.
- Frankfort Mandibular Planes Angle (FMPA) Fig. 6.10). The average angle is 28 ±4°. However, the maxillary plane is easier to locate accurately and is therefore more widely used.
- The Facial Proportion (Fig. 6.11). This is the ratio of the lower facial height to the total anterior facial height measured perpendicularly from the maxillary plane, calculated as a percentage:

$$\text{Facial proportion (FP)} = \frac{\text{MxPl to Me}}{\text{MxPl to Me} + \text{MxPl to N}} \times 100.$$

If there appears to be a discrepancy between the results for the maxillary–mandibular planes angle and the facial proportion, it should be remembered that the MMPA reflects both posterior lower facial height and anterior lower facial height. Therefore in the case of patient LH who has an increased maxillary–mandibular planes angle but an average facial proportion it would appear that the posterior lower facial height is reduced (as opposed to an increased anterior lower facial height).

6.8 Incisor position

The average value for the angle formed between the upper incisor and the maxillary plane is 109°. The 'normal' value for lower incisor angle given in Table 6.1 is for an individual with an average MMPA of 27°. However, there is a relationship between the MMPA and the lower incisor angle: as the MMPA increases, the lower incisors become more retroclined. As the sum of the average MMPA (27°) and the average lower incisor angle (93°) equals 120°, an alternative way of deriving the 'average' lower incisor angulation for an individual is to subtract the MMPA from 120°: Lower incisor angle = 120° – MMPA

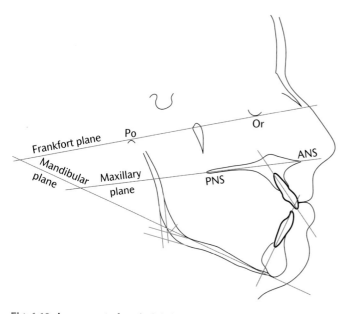

Fig. 6.10 Assessment of vertical skeletal pattern using the MMPA and FMPA: LH (male) aged 14 years.

	LH	**Mean**
MMPA	31.5°	27° ± 4°
FMPA	34.5°	28° ± 4°

Both the MMPA and the Frankfort mandibular planes angle are increased. This may be due to either an increased lower anterior face height or a reduced lower posterior face height.

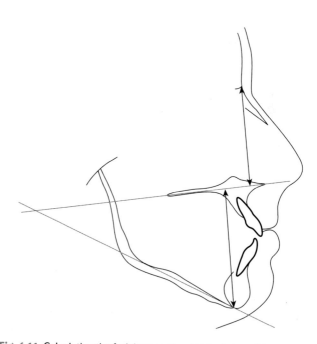

Fig. 6.11 Calculating the facial proportion: LH (male) aged 14 years.

$$\text{Facial proportion} = \frac{\text{MxPl to Me}}{\text{MxPl to Me} + \text{MxPl to N}} \times 100$$

$$= \frac{70\,\text{mm}}{57.5\,\text{mm} + 70\,\text{mm}} = \frac{70\,\text{mm}}{127.5\,\text{mm}}$$

$$= 55\% \text{ (average value)}.$$

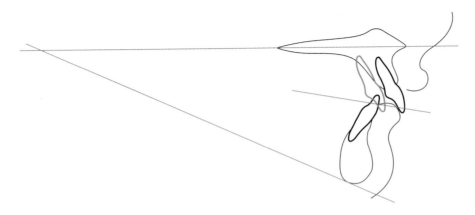

Fig. 6.12 Prognosis tracing: CP (female) aged 18 years. From this diagram it can be seen that bodily movement of the upper incisors to reduce this patient's overjet would not be feasible. Therefore a surgical approach was recommended.

6.8.1 Prognosis tracing

Sometimes it is helpful to be able to determine the type and amount of incisor movement required to correct an increased or reverse overjet. Although the skeletal pattern will give an indication, on occasion compensatory proclination or retroclination (known as dento-alveolar compensation) of the incisors, can confuse the issue. When planning treatment in such a case it may be helpful to carry out a prognosis tracing. This involves 'moving' the incisor(s) to mimic the movements achievable with different treatment approaches to help determine the best course of action for that patient. An example is shown in Fig. 6.12, where it can be seen that bodily retraction of the upper incisors would result in their being retracted out of the palatal bone – obviously not a practical treatment proposition.

Another useful rough guide to assessing tooth movement is to assume that for 2.5° of angular movement (about a point of rotation one-third of the way down the root from the apex) the upper incisor edge will translate approximately 1 mm.

6.8.2 A-Pogonion line

Raleigh Williams noted when he analysed the lateral cephalometric radiographs of individuals with pleasing facial appearances that one feature which they all had in common was that the tip of their lower incisor lay on or just in front of the line connecting point A with Pogonion. He advocated using this position of the lower incisor as a treatment goal to help ensure a good facial profile. While this line may be useful when planning orthodontic treatment, it must be remembered that it is only a guideline to good facial aesthetics, and not an indicator of stability. If the lower incisors are moved from their pretreatment

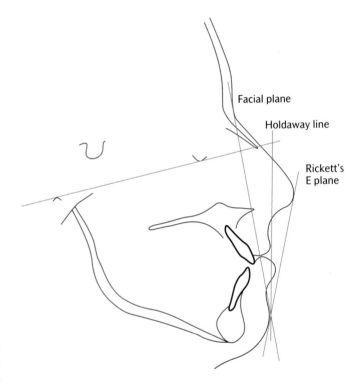

Facial plane

Holdaway line

Rickett's E plane

Fig. 6.13 Soft tissue analysis.

position of labiolingual balance, whatever the rationale, there is a likelihood of appreciable relapse following removal of appliances. This topic is discussed in more detail in Chapters 7 and 10.

6.9 Soft tissue analysis

This is particularly important in diagnosis and planning prior to orthognathic surgery (Chapter 21). As with other elements of cephalometric analysis, there are a large number of different analyses of varying complexity. The following are some of the more commonly used.

6.9.1 The Holdaway line

This is a line from the soft tissue chin to the upper lip. In a well-proportioned face this line, if extended, should bisect the nose (Fig. 6.13).

6.9.2 Rickett's E-plane

This line joins the soft tissue chin and the tip of the nose. In a balanced face the lower lip should lie 2 mm (± 2 mm) anterior to this line with the upper lip positioned a little further posteriorly to the line (Fig. 6.13).

6.9.3 Facial plane

The facial plane is a line between the soft tissue nasion and the soft tissue chin. In a well-balanced face the Frankfort plane should bisect the facial plane at an angle of about 86° and point A should lie on it (Fig. 6.13).

As with other aspects of cephalometrics, but perhaps more pertinently, these analyses should be supplementary to a clinical examination, and it should also be remembered that beauty is in the eye of the beholder.

6.10 Assessing growth and treatment changes

The advantage of standardizing lateral cephalometric radiographs is that it is then possible to compare radiographs either of groups of patients for research purposes or of the same patient over time to evaluate growth and treatment changes. In some cases it may be helpful to monitor growth of a patient over time before deciding upon a treatment plan, particularly if unfavourable growth would result in a malocclusion that could not be treated by orthodontics alone. During treatment it can be helpful to determine the contributions that tooth movements and/or growth have made to the correction and to help ensure that, where possible, a stable result is achieved. For example, in a Class II division 1 malocclusion, correction of an increased overjet can occur by retroclination of the upper incisors and/or proclination of the lower incisors and/or forward growth of the mandible and/or restraint of forward growth of the maxilla. If the major part of the correction is due to proclination of the lower incisors there is an increased likelihood of relapse of the overjet following cessation of appliance therapy owing to soft tissue pressures. If this is determined before appliances are removed, it may be possible to take steps to rectify the situation.

However, in order to be able to compare radiographs accurately it is necessary to have a fixed point or reference line which does not change with time or growth. Unfortunately this poses a dilemma, as there are no natural fixed points or planes within the face and skull. This should be borne in mind when interpreting the differences seen using any of the superimpositions discussed below.

6.10.1 Cranial base

The SN line is taken in cephalometrics as approximating to the cranial base. However, growth does occur at nasion, and therefore superimpositions on this line for the purpose of evaluating changes over time should be based at sella. Unfortunately, growth at nasion does not always conveniently occur along the SN line – if nasion moves upwards or downwards with growth, this will of course introduce a rotational error in comparisons of tracings superimposed on SN. It is more accurate to use the outline of the cranial base (called de Coster's line) as little change occurs in the anterior cranial base after 7 years of age (see Chapter 4). However, a clear radiograph and a good knowledge of anatomy are required to do this reliably.

6.10.2 The maxilla

Growth of the maxilla occurs on all surfaces by periosteal remodelling. For the purpose of interpretation of growth and/or treatment changes the least affected surface is the anterior surface of the palatal vault, although the maxilla is commonly superimposed on the maxillary plane at PNS.

6.10.3 The mandible

It was noted above that there are no natural stable reference points within the face and skull. Bjork overcame this problem by inserting metal markers in the facial skeleton. Whilst this approach is obviously not applicable in the management of patients, it did provide considerable information on patterns of facial growth, indicating that in the mandible the landmarks which change least with growth are as follows (in order of usefulness):

- the innermost surface of the cortical bone of the symphysis;
- the tip of the chin;
- the outline of the inferior dental canal;
- the crypt of the developing third permanent molars from the time of commencement of mineralization until root formation begins.

6.11 Cephalometric errors

As mentioned above cephalometric analysis has its limitations and should only be used as a supplement to the clinical assessment. Cephalometric errors can be sub-divided as follows.

6.11.1 Projection errors

Because a cephalometric radiograph is a slightly enlarged, two-dimensional representation of a three-dimensional patient, angular measurements are generally to be preferred to linear measurements.

6.11.2 Landmark identification

Accurate identification of cephalometric points is often difficult particularly if the radiograph is of poor quality. As described in Section 6.5, some points are more difficult to locate than others, for example Porion is particularly problematic. Where reference planes are constructed between two points, the errors inherent in determining them are compounded.

6.11.3 Measurement errors

All analyses relate cephalometric points and planes to each other so any errors of landmark identification are multiplied. In addition, operator mistakes may contribute to measurement error.

6.12 3D Cephalometric analysis

Spiral and Cone Beam Computerized Tomography is becoming more widely available and as a result 3D cephalometry is now a reality. Although this is still in the early stages of development as this book went to press, without doubt it will become increasingly important, especially for orthognathic planning (see Section 21.10.1) and particularly for those patients with facial asymmetry.

Key point

The wise clinician will always re-evaluate the results of a cephalometric assessment in the light of their clinical assessment. After all, the aim of orthodontic treatment is to improve the patient's appearance, not to move them nearer to a cephalometric norm.

Principal sources and further reading

Ahlqvist, J., Eliasson, S., and Welander, U. (1986). The effect of projection errors on cephalometric length measurements. *European Journal of Orthodontics*, **8**, 141–8.

Ahlqvist, J., Eliasson, S., and Welander, U. (1986). The effect of projection errors on angular measurements on cephalometry. *European Journal of Orthodontics*, **10**, 353–61.

Brown, M. (1981). Eight methods of analysing a cephalogram to establish anteroposterior skeletal discrepancy. *British Journal of Orthodontics*, **8**, 139–46.

This paper admirably illustrates the pitfalls and problems with cephalometric analysis, whilst also briefly presenting some alternative analyses.

Drage, N., Carmichael, F., and Brown, J. (2010). Radiation protection: Protection of patients undergoing cone beam computed tomography examinations. *Dental Update*, **37**, 542–8.

Much of the content on radiation protection is relevant to any radiograph.

Ferguson, J. W., Evans, R. I. W., and Cheng, L. H. H. (1992). Diagnostic accuracy and observer performance in the diagnosis of abnormalities in the anterior maxilla: a comparison of panoramic with intra-oral radiography. *British Dental Journal*, **173**, 265–71.

Houston, W. J. B. (1979). The current status of facial growth prediction. *British Journal of Orthodontics*, **6**, 11–17.

Houston, W. J. B. (1986). Sources of error in measurements from cephalometric radiographs. *European Journal of Orthodontics*, **8**, 149–51.

Isaacson, K. G., Thom, A. R., Horner, K., and Whaites, E. (2008). *Orthodontic Radiographs – Guidelines (third edition)*. British Orthodontic Society, London.

An excellent publication which explains the legislative background to taking radiographs and the need to justify every exposure. It contains several helpful flow charts to assist in deciding whether or not to take a radiograph.

Jacobson, A. (1995). *Radiographic Cephalometry: From Basics to Videoimaging*. Quintessence Publishing, USA.

An authoritative book. Includes a very good section on how to trace a cephalometric radiograph with actual copy films and overlays to aid landmark identification.

Kamoon, A., Dermaut, L., and Verbeek, R. (2001). The clinical significance of error measurement in the interpretation of treatment results. *European Journal of Orthodontics*, **23**, 569–78.

An interesting paper which puts into context cephalometric errors in the interpretation of small reported treatment changes.

Sandham, A. (1988). Repeatability of head posture recordings from lateral cephalometric radiographs. *British Journal of Orthodontics*, **15**, 157–62.

Sedentexct Project (2011) Radiation protection: Cone Beam CT for dental and maxillofacial radiology. www.sedentexct.eu

An important and authoritative document which comprises detailed guidelines prepared by a systematic review of the current available evidence.

References for this chapter can also be found at www.oxfordtextbooks.co.uk/orc/mitchell4e/. Where possible, these are presented as active links which direct you to the electronic version of the work, to help facilitate onward study. If you are a subscriber to that work (either individually or through an institution), and depending on your level of access, you may be able to peruse an abstract or the full article if available.

7 Treatment planning

S. J. Littlewood

Chapter contents

Learning objectives for this chapter

- Understand how to form a logical problem list from the information gathered during the orthodontic assessment
- Recognize the importance of clear treatment aims based on the problem list
- Be familiar with the different approaches to treating a patient with an underlying skeletal pattern
- Appreciate the basic process of formulating an orthodontic treatment plan
- Recognize how space analysis can help provide a disciplined approach to treatment planning, as well as helping to assess the feasibility of treatment aims and aid planning of anchorage and treatment mechanics.
- Understand the importance of informed consent and the orthodontic treatment plan

---

7.1 Introduction

Treatment planning is the most complex area in Orthodontics. In order to formulate an appropriate treatment plan the clinician needs to be competent in history taking, examination of the patient and collection of appropriate records. The clinician also needs to have an understanding of growth and development, facial and dental aesthetics, occlusion, the aetiology of malocclusion, different orthodontic appliances and mechanics, the physiology of tooth movement, the risks and benefits of treatment, retention and relapse. This chapter must therefore be read in conjunction with other relevant chapters. The aim of this chapter is to offer a logical approach to treatment planning.

7.2 General objectives of orthodontic treatment

When planning orthodontic treatment the following areas need to be considered:

- Aesthetics
- Oral health
- Function
- Stability

Ideally, orthodontic treatment should ensure a good aesthetic result, both facially and dentally; it should not compromise dental health; it should promote good function; and it should produce as stable a result as possible. Orthodontic treatment should never compromise dental health or function, but occasionally, it may not be possible to produce a treatment plan that creates ideal aesthetics and the most stable result. In these cases a compromise may need to be reached and this must be discussed with the patient as part of the informed consent process (see Section 7.8).

7.3 Forming an orthodontic problem list

By following a logical process, the clinician can draw up a problem list that will help to provide the information needed to form the treatment plan. This process is shown in Fig. 7.1.

The history, examination and collection of appropriate records are required to identify the problems in any case. This list of problems helps to formulate a diagnosis. Problems can be divided into pathological problems and developmental problems. Pathological problems are problems related to disease, such as caries and periodontal disease, and need to be addressed before any orthodontic treatment is undertaken. Developmental problems are those factors related to the malocclusion and make up the orthodontic problem list. In order to make this problem list more understandable, it can be classified into six sections:

(1) The patient's concerns

(2) Facial and smile aesthetics

(3) Alignment and symmetry within each arch

(4) Skeletal and dental relationships in the transverse plane

(5) Skeletal and dental relationships in the anteroposterior plane

(6) Skeletal and dental relationships in the vertical plane

7.3.1 The patient's concerns

The patient's role in orthodontic treatment success is vital. The following areas need to be considered:

- Patient's concerns
- Patient's expectations
- Patient motivation

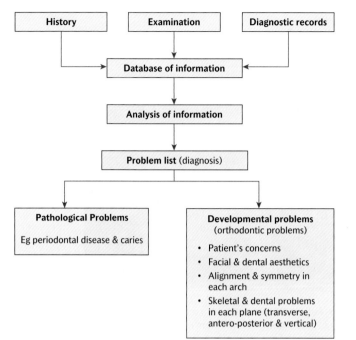

Fig. 7.1 Dividing the problem list into pathological and developmental problems.

A patient will only be satisfied if those aspects of their malocclusion which trouble them are addressed. An appropriate history should reveal which features they are unhappy with and importantly, the result they are hoping for, or expect, at the end of treatment. Where possible the clinician should formulate a plan that addresses the patient's area of complaint. However, occasionally the patient's perception of their problem or expectations may be unrealistic. The role of the orthodontist is then to counsel the patient carefully to explain what can or cannot be achieved. If the patient's expectations are unrealistic, then treatment should not be undertaken.

Undergoing orthodontics requires a great deal of active participation and co-operation from the patient. No matter how skilful the orthodontist, treatment will not succeed unless the patient is sufficiently motivated to co-operate with all aspects of their orthodontic care. If the patient is not sufficiently motivated, then treatment should not be undertaken.

7.3.2 Facial and smile aesthetics

Straight teeth do not necessarily create a good smile and appropriate facial aesthetics. The position of the teeth within the face, and the effects of tooth movements on the overlying soft tissues of the lips, need to be considered. This is a complex area for a number of reasons.

The area of facial aesthetics is affected by personal and cultural factors and also by fashions and trends. There has been a recent trend towards more protrusive profiles, with proclination of both the upper and lower dentitions to produce more lip support. Advocates suggest that this treatment approach leads to increased lip protrusion and can produce a more youthful appearance, but it does not come without potential risks. Firstly, proclination of incisors may move the teeth into areas of increased instability, with a tendency for the lips and cheeks to push the teeth back and cause relapse. In addition, excess expansion and proclination may lead to teeth perforating the buccal plate, causing bony dehiscences and possibly compromising future periodontal health.

The effect of tooth movement on the overlying soft tissues is unpredictable. It is untrue to suggest that extracting teeth and retroclining the upper incisors will automatically compromise the facial aesthetics. However, care must be taken in cases where excessive retroclination of the upper labial segment is being considered, to avoid flattening of the facial profile. This would be particularly contraindicated in patients with an increased nasio-labial angle, large nose and retrognathic mandible (Fig. 7.2).

Smile aesthetics are discussed in Section 5.4.4.

Many aspects of facial or smile aesthetics cannot be influenced by orthodontics alone, and in some cases cannot be influenced at all. This needs to be discussed with the patient, and if appropriate, surgical and restorative options may need to be considered.

7.3.3 Alignment and symmetry in each arch

The amount of crowding or spacing in each arch needs to be assessed, as well as the inclination of the upper and lower incisors and any tooth size discrepancies identified. This will play a major role in assessing the amount of space required to treat the case. The process of determining the amount of space required is called 'space analysis' (see Section 7.8). The shape and symmetry within each arch is also noted.

7.3.4 Skeletal and dental relationships in all three dimensions

Chapter 5 emphasised the importance of assessing the patient in all three dimensions (transverse, anteroposterior and vertical). The aim is to describe the occlusion, distinguishing between the dental and skeletal factors contributing to the malocclusion in each plane. Generally, it is easier to correct malocclusions that are due to dental problems alone – if there are underlying skeletal problems, these are often more difficult to treat. The approaches to treating patients with skeletal problems are discussed in Section 7.5.

7.4 Aims of orthodontic treatment

The orthodontic problem list provides a logical summary of the information collected during the history, examination and taking of diagnostic records. The next stage is to work through the orthodontic problem list deciding which problems will be addressed and which will be accepted. This will result in a list, which contains the aims of treatment. Once the aims have been decided, possible solutions can

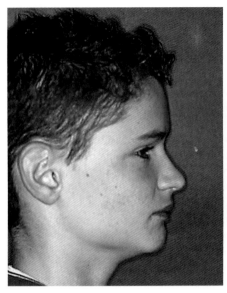
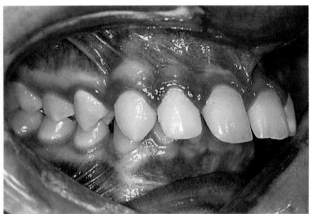

Fig. 7.2 Consideration of facial aesthetics in orthodontic treatment planning. Patient OP presents with a markedly increased overjet of 12 mm. Although the patient complained about the prominent upper teeth, a large proportion of the problem is the retrognathic mandible. Simply retracting the upper labial segment would reduce the overjet, but this would have an unfavourable effect on the facial profile. The soft tissue response to dental movement is unpredictable, but in this case, with such a large dental movement required and the retrognathic mandible, reducing the overjet by reduction of the incisors alone would unfavourably flatten the facial profile. The full treatment of this case is shown in Chapter 19, Fig. 19.1.

be considered, which will lead to the formulation of the final definitive treatment plan (Fig. 7.3).

There is often more than one treatment plan possible for each patient. The clinician must discuss the realistic options available to the patient, explaining the risks and benefits of each approach, including the effects of no treatment at all. This forms the basis of informed consent (Section 7.8).

7.5 Skeletal problems and treatment planning

There are three options for treating malocclusions with underlying skeletal problems:

- Orthodontic camouflage
- Growth modification
- Combined orthodontic and surgical approach

7.5.1 Orthodontic camouflage

Treatment with orthodontic camouflage means that the skeletal discrepancy is accepted, but the teeth are moved into a Class I relationship. The smaller the skeletal contribution to the malocclusion, the more likely that orthodontic camouflage will be possible. It is easier to camouflage anteroposterior skeletal problems than vertical problems, which in turn are easier to camouflage than transverse problems.

7.5.2 Growth modification

This type of treatment is also known as dentofacial orthopaedics and is only possible in growing patients. By use of orthodontic appliances, minor changes can be made to the skeletal pattern. Most growth modification is used to correct anteroposterior discrepancies as it is harder to make changes in the vertical dimension and even more difficult to alter transverse skeletal discrepancies.

There is increasing evidence that any growth modification that does occur is usually minimal. In most cases, growth modification is used for treatment of Class II malocclusions using headgear (Chapters 9 and 15) or functional appliances (Chapter 19). It can also be used for the early treatment of patients with a Class III skeletal pattern with a retrognathic maxilla, using a protraction facemask.

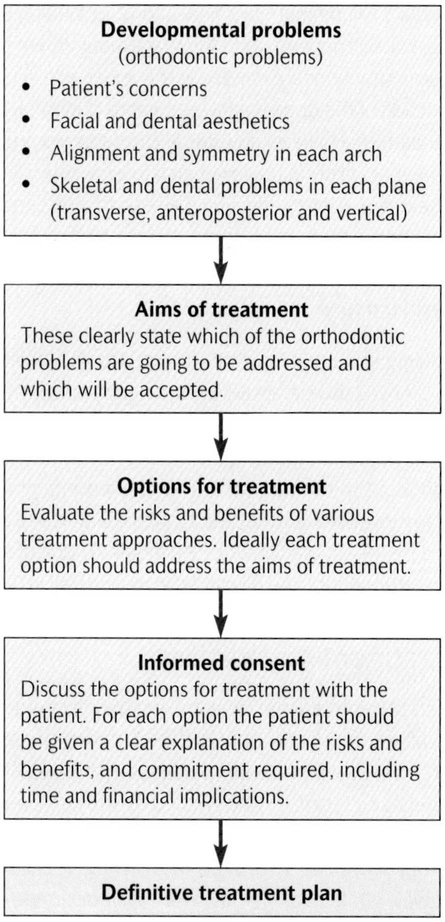

Fig. 7.3 Turning the problem list into a definitive treatment plan.

7.5.3 Combined orthodontic and orthognathic surgical treatment

This involves surgical correction of the jaw discrepancy in combination with orthodontics, to position the dentition to produce optimum dental and facial aesthetics. This is undertaken on patients who are fully grown. This may be indicated for patients with severe skeletal or very severe dento-alveolar problems, who are beyond the scope of orthodontics alone. It is also sometimes indicated if the patient is too old for growth modification, and orthodontic camouflage would produce a compromised facial result. Combined orthodontics and orthognathic surgical treatment is discussed further in Chapter 21.

7.6 Basic principles in orthodontic treatment planning

Once the aims of treatment have been established, treatment planning can begin. Below are some basic principles in orthodontic treatment planning, which can be used in conjunction with space analysis.

7.6.1 Oral health

The first part of any orthodontic treatment plan is to establish and maintain good oral health. While definitive restorations, such as crowns and bridges may be placed after alignment of the teeth, all active disease must be fully treated before beginning any orthodontic treatment.

7.6.2 The lower arch

Traditionally treatment planning has been based around the lower labial segment. Once the position of the lower labial segment is determined, the rest of the occlusion can be planned around this. In most cases it is advisable to maintain the current position of the lower labial segment. This is because the lower labial segment is positioned in an area of relative stability between the tongue lingually, and the lips and cheeks labially and buccally. Any excessive movement of the lower labial segment would increase the risk of relapse. Treatment planning around the lower incisor position is less rigidly adhered to in contemporary orthodontic treatment planning, due to the increasing emphasis on facial and soft-tissue aesthetics, in addition to occlusal goals (see Box 7.1)

Exceptions do exist when the lower labial segment can be either proclined or retroclined, but are best treated by a specialist. Here are some examples of when the lower incisors may be proclined.

- Cases presenting with very mild lower incisor crowding
- Treatment of deep overbites, particularly in Class II division 2 cases (see Chapter 10, Section 10.3)
- Patients who had a digit-sucking habit (where the lower incisors have been held back from their natural position by the habit)
- To prevent unfavourable profile changes in reduction of large overjets when surgery is not indicated or declined

The lower incisors can also be retroclined to camouflage a Class III malocclusion, or in the treatment of bimaxillary dental proclination.

If the anteroposterior position and inclination of lower incisors are moved excessively this may compromise stability. The patient must be aware of this and implications for retention discussed.

Box 7.1 How upper incisor position influences contemporary treatment planning

The objectives of any orthodontic treatment are optimal aesthetics, oral health, function and stability. Traditional orthodontic planning is focused on planning around the lower arch by maintaining its initial position to increase stability. However, with greater awareness of facial and smile aesthetics it has become apparent that this traditional approach may place the upper incisors in a less than ideal aesthetic position in some cases. If the lower arch can be maintained in its current position without compromising aesthetics then this is the best approach. However, in some cases the stability of the lower arch may need to be compromised to allow better positioning of the upper incisors and hence maximizing the aesthetic result. The implications for stability of this approach would then need to be discussed with the patient.

7.6.3 The upper arch

Once the lower arch has been planned, the upper arch position can be planned in order to obtain a Class I incisor relationship. The secret to achieving a Class I incisor relationship is to get the canines into a Class I relationship. It is helpful to anticipate the position of the lower canine once the lower labial segment has been aligned and positioned appropriately. It is then possible to mentally reposition the maxillary canine so that it is in a Class I relationship with the lower canine. This gives the clinician an idea of how much space will be required and how far the upper canine will need to be moved. This will also give an indication of the type of movement and therefore type of appliance required, as well as providing information about anchorage requirements.

7.6.4 Buccal segments

Although the aim is usually to obtain a Class I canine relationship, it is not necessary to always have a Class I molar relationship. If teeth are extracted in the upper arch, but not in the lower, the molars will be in a Class II relationship. Conversely, if teeth are extracted in the lower arch but not in the upper, the molars will be in a Class III relationship. Whether extractions are needed or not will depend upon the space requirement in each arch. Typically, more extractions are needed in the upper arch in Class II cases, to allow retraction of the upper labial segment to camouflage the underlying skeletal pattern. However, in Class III cases treated orthodontically extractions are more likely in the lower arch to allow retroclination of the lower labial segment. Factors affecting the need for and choice of extractions are described in the section on creating space (Section 7.7.1)

7.6.5 Anchorage

Anchorage planning is about resisting unwanted tooth movement. Whenever teeth are moved there is always an equal and opposite reaction. This means that when teeth are moved there is often a side-effect of unwanted tooth movement of other teeth in the arch. When planning a case it is therefore important to decide how to limit the movement of teeth that do not need to move. It is vital that anchorage is understood and planned correctly for a treatment plan to work. Anchorage is one of the most difficult areas in orthodontics and is covered in more detail in Chapter 15.

7.6.6 Treatment mechanics

Once the aims of treatment are clear, the final result could be achieved using many different types of appliances and treatment mechanics. As there is a often a lack of high quality evidence in the area, the choice of treatment mechanics is often determined by the clinician's expertise and experience with different techniques. The clinician should utilise mechanics that produce the desired result in the most efficient and predictable way, while avoiding any risks or undesirable side-effects and minimizing the compliance required from the patient.

It is important to mention that the aims of the treatment should be determined first, and then the appropriate appliances and treatment mechanics chosen to deliver these aims. The appliance system and the treatment mechanics should not be used to determine the treatment aims.

7.6.7 Retention

At the end of orthodontic treatment almost every case needs to be retained to prevent relapse back towards the original malocclusion. It is vital that retention must be considered, planned for and discussed at the beginning of treatment. Wearing retainers requires commitment from the patient and they should be made aware of the need for these retainers before treatment begins (see Chapter 16).

7.7 Space analysis

Space analysis is a process that allows an estimation of the space required in each arch to fulfil the treatment aims. Although not an exact science, it does allow a disciplined approach to diagnosis and treatment planning. It also helps to determine whether the treatment aims are feasible, as well as assisting with the planning of treatment mechanics and anchorage control.

Space planning is carried out in two phases: the first is to determine the space required and the second calculates the amount of space that will be created during treatment. This includes creating space for any planned prostheses.

It must be stressed that space analysis can act only as a guide, albeit a useful one, as many aspects of orthodontics cannot be accurately predicted, such as growth, the individual patient's biological response and patient compliance. Before undertaking a space analysis, the aims of the treatment should be determined as this will affect the amount of space required or created.

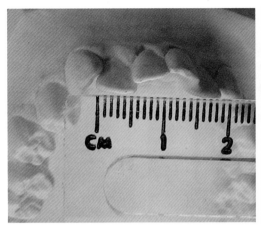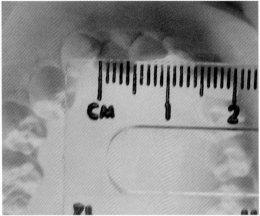

Fig. 7.4 Assessment of crowding. These photographs show the method of assessing the degree of crowding by measuring the width of the misaligned tooth compared with the amount of available space in the arch. In this example, the first photograph shows that the width of the tooth is 6 mm and the second photograph shows that the amount of space available in the arch for this tooth is 4 mm. This suggests crowding of 2 mm for this tooth. This process is repeated for all the misaligned teeth in the arch to give the total extent of crowding. If two adjacent teeth are displaced, then assessment of crowding can be undertaken by measuring the mesiodistal width of each tooth and determining the combined space available.

An example of space analysis used in the treatment planning of a clinical case is shown at the end of the chapter (Fig. 7.10).

7.7.1 Calculating the space requirements

Space is required to correct the following:

- Crowding
- Incisor anteroposterior change (usually obtaining a normal overjet of 2 mm)
- Levelling of occlusal curves
- Arch contraction (expansion will create space)
- Correction of upper incisor angulation (mesiodistal tip)
- Correction of upper incisor inclination (torque)

The space requirements to correct incisor angulation and inclination are usually minimal and will not be discussed further here (see section on Further reading for more details). However, the other aspects are briefly discussed below.

Crowding

The amount of crowding present can be calculated by measuring the mesiodistal widths of any misaligned teeth in relation to the available space in the arch (Fig. 7.4).

The amount of crowding present is often classified as:

- Mild (<4 mm)
- Moderate (4–8 mm)
- Severe (>8 mm)

Incisor anteroposterior change

It is often necessary to alter the anteroposterior position of the upper incisors, particularly when reducing an overjet. If incisors are retracted, this requires space; if incisors are proclined then space is created. The aim is to create an overjet of 2 mm at the end of treatment. Every

millimetre of incisor retraction requires 2 mm of space in the dental arch. Conversely, for every millimetre of incisor proclination 2 mm of space are created in the arch.

For example, if a patient presented with an overjet of 6 mm and the incisors needed to be retracted to create a normal overjet of 2 mm, then this would require space. Every millimetre of retraction requires 2 mm of space. So to reduce the overjet by 4 mm would require 8 mm of space.

As discussed earlier the anteroposterior position of the lower incisors is often accepted for stability reasons. However, situations do occur when the position is altered, and similar space requirements apply in the lower arch.

Levelling occlusal curves

Where there is no occlusal stop the lower incisors may over-erupt. This may result in an occlusal curve which runs from the molars to the incisors and is known as a Curve of Spee as seen in Fig 7.5. The amount of space required to level an increased curve of Spee is controversial, as it is affected by a number of factors, such as the shape of the archform and tooth shape. However, as a guide Table 7.1 gives an estimation of the space required. The depth of curve is assessed from the premolar cusps to a flat plane joining the distal cusps of first permanent molars and incisors (Fig. 7.5).

7.7.2 Creating space

The amount of space that will be created during treatment can also be assessed. The aim is to balance the space required with the space created. Space can be created by one or more of the following:

- Extractions
- Distal movement of molars
- Enamel stripping
- Expansion
- Proclination of incisors
- A combination of any or all of the above

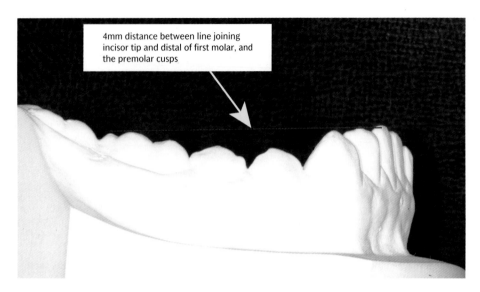

4mm distance between line joining incisor tip and distal of first molar, and the premolar cusps

Fig. 7.5 Assessment of the space requirement for flattening the curve of Spee. It has been decided that the curve of Spee should be flattened in this case, which requires space. The depth of the curve is 4 mm, which requires 1.5 mm of space.

Table 7.1 Approximate space requirement to flatten a curve of Spee

Depth of curve (mm)	Space requirement (mm)
3 or less	1
4	1.5
5 or more	2

7.7.3 Extractions

Before planning extractions of any permanent teeth, it is essential to ensure that all remaining teeth are present and developing appropriately. The following are factors which affect the choice of teeth for extraction:

- Prognosis
- Position
- Amount of space required and where
- Incisor relationship
- Anchorage requirements
- Appliances to be used (if any)
- Patient's profile and aims of treatment

Choosing the appropriate teeth for extraction is a complex decision and requires understanding of all aspects of orthodontic treatment. It is often helpful to obtain a specialist opinion before choosing which teeth to extract.

Incisors

Incisors are rarely the first choice for extraction due to the risk of compromising aesthetics. It can also be difficult to fit four incisors in one arch against three incisors in the opposing arch. However, indications do exist for a lower incisor extraction:

- Incisor has poor prognosis or compromised periodontal support
- Buccal segments are Class I, but there is lower incisor crowding
- Adult patient who has a mild Class III skeletal pattern with well-aligned buccal segments

Fixed appliances are often required to align the teeth following extraction of an incisor and a bonded retainer may be required to maintain the correction.

Management of missing or enforced extraction of upper incisors is discussed in greater detail in Chapter 8.

Canines

Canines form the cornerstone of the arch and are important both aesthetically and functionally (providing canine guidance in lateral movements). However, if severely displaced or ectopic, they may need to be extracted. A reasonable contact between the lateral incisor and first premolar is possible, but rarely occurs without the use of fixed appliances. If a canine is missing, the occlusion must also be checked to ensure that there are no unwanted displacing contacts, caused by a lack of canine guidance.

First premolars

These are often the teeth of choice to extract when the space requirement is moderate to severe. Also, extraction of a first premolar in either arch usually gives the best chance of spontaneous alignment. This is particularly true in the lower arch where, provided the lower canine is mesially inclined, spontaneous alignment of the lower labial segment may occur. This spontaneous improvement is most rapid in the first 6 months after the extraction. In the upper arch the first premolars usually erupt before the upper canines, so the chances of spontaneous improvement in the position of this tooth can be achieved if the first premolar is extracted just before the canine emerges. A space maintainer may be required to keep the space open for the upper canine.

Typically, when using fixed appliances, 40–60 per cent of a first premolar extraction space will be available for the benefit of the labial segment without anchorage reinforcement. The reason why there is some loss of the space available from the extractions is due to mesial movement of the posterior teeth.

Second premolars

Indications for extraction of second premolars include:

- Mild to moderate space requirement (3–8 mm space required)
- Space closure by forward movement of the molars, rather than retraction of the labial segments is indicated
- Severe displacement of the second premolar

Extraction of the second premolars is preferable to first premolars when there is a mild to moderate space requirement. This is because the anchorage balance is altered, favouring space closure by forward movement of the molars. Hence, only about 25–50 per cent of the space created by a second premolar extraction is available to allow labial segment alignment. Fixed appliances are often required to ensure good contact between the first molar and first premolar, particularly in the lower arch.

Early loss of the second deciduous molars often results in crowding of the second premolars palatally in the upper and lingually in the lower. In the upper arch, extraction of the displaced second premolar on eruption is often indicated. Conversely, in the lower arch, extraction of the first premolars is usually easier and in most cases uprighting of the second premolars occurs spontaneously following relief of crowding.

First permanent molars

Extraction of first permanent molars often makes orthodontic treatment more difficult and prolonged. However, their extraction may need to be considered if they have a poor long-term prognosis (Fig. 5.18). Extraction of first permanent molars is discussed in greater detail in Section 3.3.8.

Second permanent molars

Extraction of second permanent molars has been suggested in the following cases:

- To facilitate distal movement of upper buccal segments
- Relief of mild lower premolar crowding
- Provision of additional space for the third permanent molars, thus avoiding the likelihood of their impaction

Extraction of the upper second molar will not provide relief of crowding in the premolar or labial segments, due to mesial drift. Relief of mild crowding in the lower premolar region may be possible, as well as providing additional space for eruption of the third permanent molar. The eruption of the third permanent molars is never guaranteed, but the chances can be improved by the correct timing of extraction of the second molar. The following features should ideally be present (Fig. 7.6):

- Angle between the third permanent molar tooth germ and the long axis of the second molar is 10–30°
- Crypt of developing third molar overlaps the root of the second molar
- The third permanent molar is developed to the bifurcation

Even if these criteria are satisfied, eruption of the lower third molar into occlusion cannot be guaranteed, and it should be made clear to the patient that a course of fixed appliance treatment to upright or align the third molar may be necessary.

Third permanent molars

In the past, early extraction of these teeth has been advocated to prevent lower labial segment crowding. However, it is much more likely that late lower incisor crowding is caused by subtle growth and soft tissue changes that continue to occur throughout life (Chapter 16). It is now not acceptable to extract third molars purely on the grounds of preventing crowding of the lower labial segment (see Chapter 8, Section 8.2.1).

7.7.4 Distal movement of molars

Distal movement of molars in the upper arch is possible. This movement can be achieved with headgear. Extra-oral traction using headgear will usually produce up to 2–3 mm per side (creating 4–6 mm space in total). It therefore tends to be used when there is a mild space requirement where extractions may produce too much space. It can also be used in addition to extractions when there is a very high space requirement.

Examples of clinical situations when it may be used include:

- Class I incisor relationship with mild crowding in the upper arch
- Class II division 1 incisor relationship with minimally increased overjet and molar relationship of less than half a unit Class II
- Where extraction of first premolars does not give sufficient space to complete alignment
- Where unilateral loss of a deciduous molar has resulted in mesial drift of the first permanent molar

Temporary bone anchorage devices (TADS) offer an alternative to headgear in some cases. Appliances attached to these anchorage devices can be used to distalize upper molars. The subject of anchorage, including headgear and TADs, is discussed in more detail in Chapter 15.

Distal movement of the lower first molar is very difficult and in reality the best that can be achieved is uprighting of this tooth.

7.7.5 Enamel stripping

Enamel interproximal reduction or 'stripping' is the removal of a small amount of enamel on the mesial and distal aspect of teeth and is sometimes known as reproximation. In addition to creating space, the process has been advocated for improving the shape and contact points of teeth, and possibly enhancing stability at the end of treatment. On the anterior teeth approximately 0.5 mm can be removed

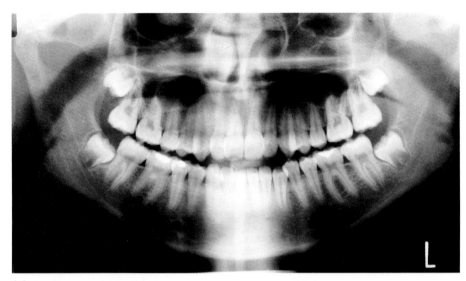

(a)

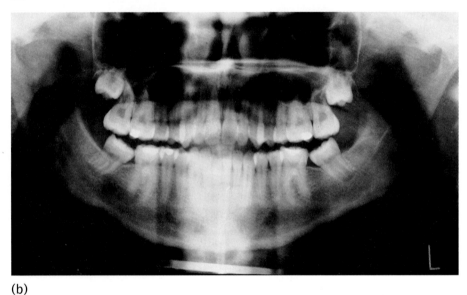

(b)

Fig. 7.6 Example of a case where second permanent molars were extracted. Patient with mild lower arch crowding who had both lower second molars removed in an attempt to treat mild crowding in the lower premolar region. (a) DPT radiograph prior to extraction of both lower second molars (the upper second molars were not extracted because of concerns over the prognosis for the upper first molars); (b) DPT radiograph 2 years after the extractions showing eruption of both lower third molars.

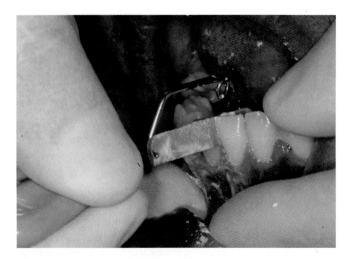

Fig. 7.7 Interproximal stripping using abrasive strips.

on each tooth (0.25 mm mesial and distal) without compromising the health of the teeth. Enamel can be carefully removed with an abrasive strip (Fig. 7.7). The abrasive strip can be used in conjunction with pumice mixed with acid etch, to provide a smoother surface finish. The teeth are treated topically with fluoride following reduction of the enamel.

Air-rotor stripping is a more controversial approach. This is a technique for removing enamel, predominantly from the buccal segments, using a high speed air-turbine handpiece. Advocates of this approach claim to create an additional 3–6 mm of space in each arch. There is potential for damage to both the teeth and the periodontium unless undertaken carefully and therefore should only be considered by a specialist. It is important that teeth are reasonably aligned before starting the procedure, and spaces must be opened up between teeth, either by separators or fixed appliances, before the enamel reduction begins (Fig. 7.8).

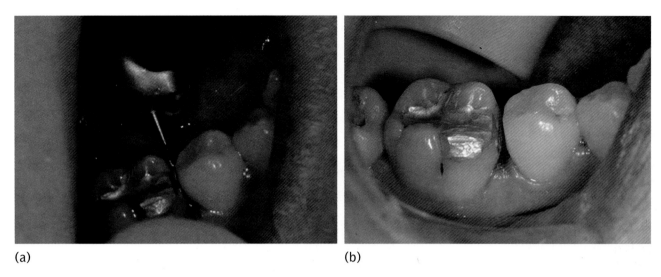

(a)   (b)

Fig. 7.8 Air-rotor stripping (ARS). This technique aims to remove interproximal enamel, predominantly in the buccal segments. (a) A small protective wire lies under the contact point to protect the gingival soft tissues. The teeth are already reasonably well aligned and access space has previously been created by use of a separator. The enamel is carefully removed with an air-rotor from the mesial aspect of the first permanent molar and distal aspect of the second premolar. In this case amalgam is also removed from the mesial side of the first permanent molar. (b) The space has been created and the tooth carefully re-contoured to ensure a good contact point.

7.7.6 Expansion

Space can be created by expanding the upper arch laterally – approximately 0.5 mm is created for every 1 mm of posterior arch expansion. Expansion should ideally only be undertaken when there is a crossbite. Expansion without a crossbite may increase the risk of instability and the risk of perforation of the buccal plate.

Expansion of the lower arch may be indicated if a lingual crossbite of the lower premolars and/or molars exists, but management of this type of malocclusion should be undertaken by the specialist. Any significant expansion in the lower arch, particularly the lower intercanine width, is likely to be unstable.

7.7.7 Proclination of incisors

Space can be created by proclining incisors, but this will be dictated by the aims of the treatment. Each millimetre of incisor advancement creates approximately 2 mm of space within the dental arch.

7.8 Informed consent and the orthodontic treatment plan

Informed consent means the patient is given information to help them to understand the:

- malocclusion
- proposed treatment and alternatives
- commitment required
- duration of treatment
- cost implications

Treatment alternatives, which must always include no treatment as an option, must be clearly explained, with the risks and benefits of each approach carefully discussed.

Patients who are 16 years or older are presumed to have competence to give consent for themselves. Many orthodontic patients are younger than this, but provided that they fully understand the process, they can give consent. If a competent child consents to treatment, a parent cannot override this decision – this is known as 'Gillick competence'.

However, it is preferable to have full parental support for the treatment if possible. If the converse occurs – the parent wants the treatment, but the child does not – then it is best not to proceed. Orthodontic treatment requires a great deal of compliance, and unless the patient is totally committed, it is best to delay until such time as they are.

It is advisable to obtain a written consent for the treatment. A copy should be given to the patient with clear details of the aims of the treatment, risks and benefits, types of appliances to be used, details of any teeth to be extracted, commitment required, likely duration of treatment, any financial implications, as well as long-term retention requirements. When estimating treatment time, it is always better to slightly overestimate the likely treatment duration. If the treatment is completed quicker than first promised, the patient will be pleased. However, if the treatment takes longer, the patient may lose interest, resulting in compliance problems.

As well as providing a written record of the aims of the treatment and the treatment plan, it is useful to give the patient a summary of exactly what is expected from them. This involves not only information about good oral hygiene, appropriate diet and regular attendance, but also any specific requirements relevant to their case, such as headgear wear, turning expansion screws and elastic wear. A fully prepared and committed patient is more likely to result in more successful orthodontic treatment.

7.9 Conclusions

This chapter has discussed how the information collected during the history, examination and record collection can be used to develop a problem list for each patient. Any pathological problems are treated initially and then the developmental or orthodontic problems can be addressed. The orthodontic problems are divided up into patient's concerns, facial and smile aesthetics, the alignment and symmetry of each arch, and occlusal problems transversely, anteroposteriorly and vertically. The skeletal and dental components making up the occlusal problems are identified. Any skeletal problems that are present can be treated by orthodontic camouflage, growth modification or combined orthodontic and orthognathic surgery treatment.

Once the problem list is formed, a list of aims can be drawn up, deciding which of the problems will be addressed and which will be accepted. Throughout the planning process the clinician must consider aesthetics, function, health and stability. Different treatment options should then be considered to address the treatment aims.

Space analysis involves assessment of the space required and methods of creating this space, and although not an exact science, helps to provide a disciplined approach to diagnosis and treatment planning. It also allows the clinician to assess whether the treatment aims are feasible, and also helps in planning the type of mechanics and anchorage control that are required to treat the case.

The final stage, before formulating the definitive treatment plan, is to discuss the options with the patient. This process should lead to informed consent, so the patient is fully aware of their orthodontic problems, how these can be addressed, the risks and benefits of the treatment options, cost implications, the commitment they will need to give and the likely duration of treatment.

The complete treatment planning process is illustrated in the case discussed in Fig. 7.9.

Key points about treatment planning

- The information gathered from the history, examination and collection of records is used to form a problem list or diagnosis
- The problem list is divided into pathological and developmental (orthodontic) problems. Pathological problems are addressed first
- Any skeletal component of the malocclusion can be treated by one of the following: orthodontic camouflage, growth modification or a combination of orthodontics and orthognathic surgery
- By deciding which of the problems will be treated and which accepted, a list of the aims of treatment can be decided upon. Different treatment options can then be considered
- A space analysis can help provide a disciplined approach to diagnosis and treatment planning, as well as assessing the feasibility of treatment aims, and helping to plan anchorage and treatment mechanics
- The options for treatment, including no treatment should be fully discussed with the patient
- Informed consent is obtained by ensuring the patient understands exactly what the treatment will involve, including the risks and benefits, cost implications, the commitment they will need to give and the likely duration of the treatment

7.10 Case study: example case to demonstrate treatment planning

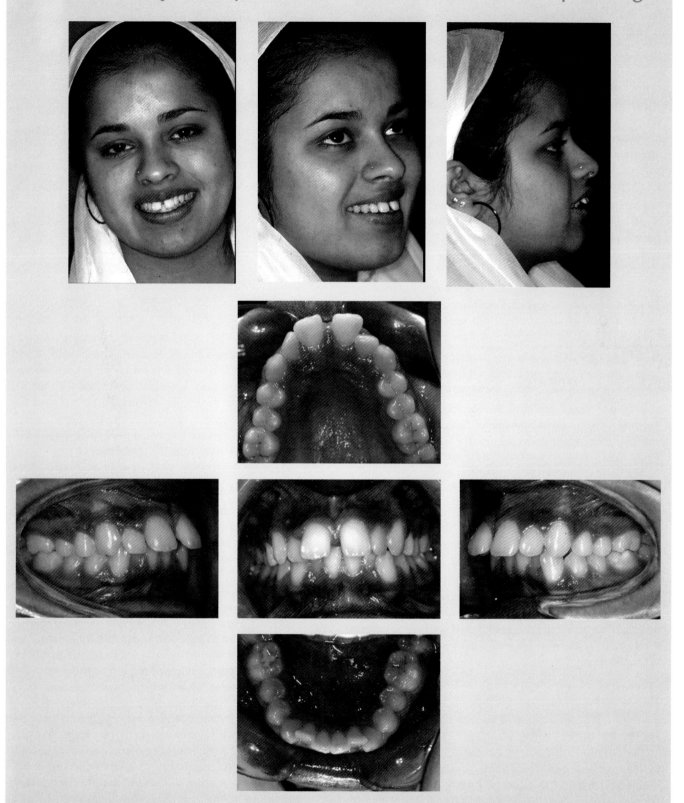

Fig. 7.9 (a) Initial presentation of patient SB Patient SB presented at age 13 years complaining of prominent upper teeth and a gap between her upper incisors. She was happy to wear fixed appliances and her medical history was clear. She was a regular attendee for dental care and her oral health was good. Radiographs confirmed the presence of third permanent molars, but no pathology. A lateral cephalometric radiograph confirmed a mild Class II skeletal pattern (ANB = 5.5°), normal vertical proportions, proclined upper incisors (117°) and normally inclined lower incisors (92°).

Problem list for SB

Pathological problems

None.

Developmental (orthodontic) problems

Patient's concerns: SB was concerned about prominent upper incisors and a space between the upper incisors. She hoped both these problems would be addressed and was happy to wear orthodontic appliances if required. Her expectations were reasonable and her motivation for treatment was good.

Facial and smile aesthetics: She presented with a slightly everted and protruding upper lip. Her vertical show of incisors on full smile was acceptable (nearly total height of upper incisors). Her mandible was very slightly retrognathic, but acceptable.

Alignment and symmetry in each arch: The lower arch was symmetrical and showed 5 mm of crowding. Her lower labial segment was normally inclined. The upper arch was also symmetrical and overall showed 2 mm of spacing (3 mm diastema and 1 mm crowding of the upper left lateral incisor). The upper incisors were proclined at 117°.

Skeletal and dental problems in transverse plane: There was no skeletal asymmetry. The lower centreline was to the left by 1 mm and the upper centreline was correct. There was no posterior crossbites.

Skeletal and dental problems in anteroposterior plane: The mandible was very slightly retrognathic, but clinically acceptable. There was an increased overjet of 8 mm. The buccal segments were $^1/_4$ unit Class II on the left and Class I on the right.

Aims of treatment for SB

The aims of treatment are directly related to the problem list.

Patient's concerns: Address the patient's concerns about the prominent upper teeth and upper midline diastema.

Facial and smile aesthetics: Accept the slightly retrognathic mandible (in other words, use orthodontic camouflage). Orthodontic treatment effects on the soft tissues are unpredictable, but if the upper incisors have to be retracted this will not have an adverse effect on the facial profile. The vertical position of the incisors can be maintained.

Alignment and symmetry in each arch: Relieve the lower crowding, correct the angulation of the upper incisors and close the residual space in the upper arch.

Skeletal and dental problems in transverse plane: Correct the lower centreline.

Skeletal and dental problems in anteroposterior plane: Reduce the overjet by retracting the upper labial segment. The anteroposterior position of the lower incisors will be accepted. This is because

they have normal inclination, maintaining their position will not compromise facial aesthetics and the most stable position is their initial position.

Skeletal and dental problems in the vertical plane: Reduce the overbite by flattening the lower curve of Spee.

Space analysis for SB

The table below shows the amount of space required in each arch to achieve the treatment aims. A negative score shows a space gain, a positive score shows a space requirement.

	Upper	Lower
Crowding or spacing	−2 mm	5 mm
Levelling of curve Spee	0	1 mm
AP movement of incisors	12 mm	0
Total	**10 mm**	**6 mm**

This space analysis shows a larger space requirement in the upper arch, due to the increased overjet. An 8 mm overjet, reduced to a normal overjet of 2 mm, requires 6 mm each side (a total of 12 mm). A curve of Spee of 4 mm in the lower arch requires 1 mm of space for correction.

Now the amount of space required in each arch is known, the methods of creating this space can be considered.

Space creation

The aims of this treatment include achieving an overjet of 2 mm using orthodontic camouflage (i.e. accepting the existing skeletal pattern). Space can be created by extractions, distal movement of molars in the upper arch, enamel stripping, expansion or proclination of incisors.

In the lower arch, 6 mm space is required. Expansion of the arch and proclination of the incisors would be unstable, and enamel stripping would not give sufficient space. Extractions are therefore required. Extraction of lower first premolars would provide too much space, so the lower second premolars will be extracted. Each premolar is 7 mm wide, but after anchorage loss (mesial drift of the teeth distal to the second premolars) extraction will provide the appropriate amount of space.

In the upper arch 10 mm of space requirement is beyond the scope of molar distalization and enamel stripping, and no expansion or incisor proclination is indicated. Therefore extractions are also required in the upper arch. On this occasion more space is required, so the extraction of first premolars is indicated. Although extraction of first premolars creates a total of 14 mm, part of this is lost to mesial drift. To resist forward movements of the upper molars anchorage reinforcement will be required. In this case, a palatal arch will help to partially limit the forward movement of the upper first permanent molars.

Definitive treatment plan for SB

(1) Palatal arch fitted to upper first molars for anchorage

(2) Extraction of upper first premolars and lower second premolars

(3) Upper and lower fixed appliances

(4) Upper and lower vacuum-formed retainers with a bonded retainer on the palatal of the upper incisors

(The bonded retainer is indicated in this case due to the risk of relapse of the upper midline diastema. Retention planning is discussed in more detail in Chapter 16).

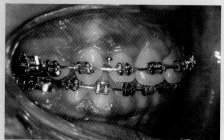 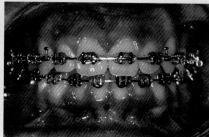 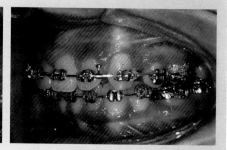

Fig. 7.9 (b) Fixed appliances in place for SB.

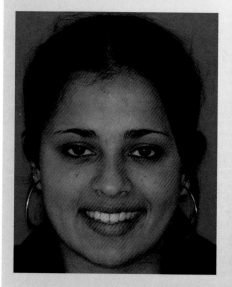 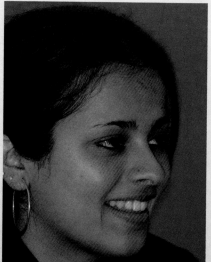 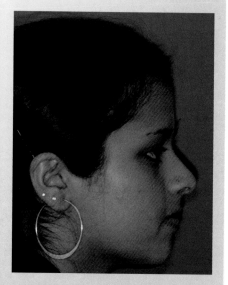

Fig. 7.9 (c) End of treatment extra-oral records for SB.

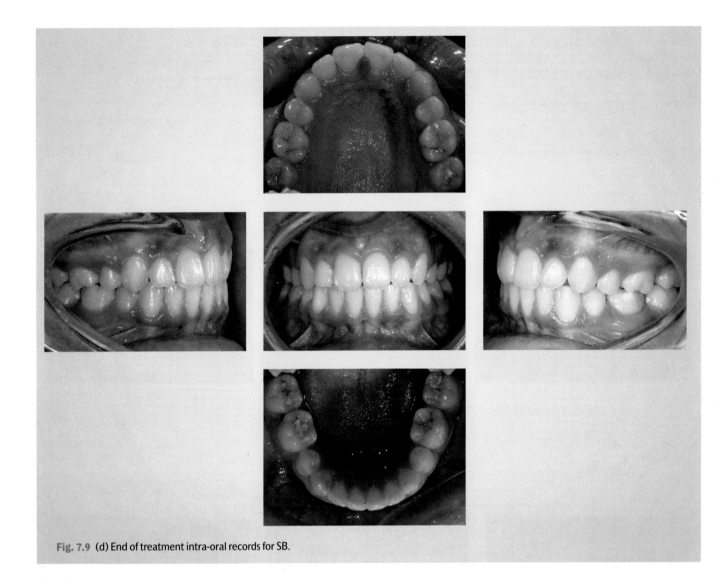

Fig. 7.9 (d) End of treatment intra-oral records for SB.

Principal sources and further reading

Dibiase, A. T. and Sandler, P. J. (2001). Does orthodontics damage faces? *Dental Update*, **28**, 98–102.

The possible unfavourable effects of orthodontics on the face are debated. Of particular relevance to this chapter is the discussion regarding the unpredictability of the effect of extractions on facial profile.

Kirshen, R. H., O'Higgins, E. A., and Lee, R. T. (2000). The Royal London Space Planning: An integration of space analysis and treatment planning. Part 1: Assessing the space required to meet treatment objectives. Part II: The effect of other treatment procedures on space. *American Journal of Orthodontics and Dentofacial Orthopedics*, **118**, 448–55 and 456–61.

These papers describe one possible approach to space analysis.

NHS Centre for Reviews and Dissemination, York (1998). Prophylactic removal of impacted third molars: is it justified? *British Journal of Orthodontics*, **26**, 149–51.

This review makes it clear that extraction of third molars to prevent crowding is no longer indicated.

Proffit, W. R., Fields, H. R., and Sarver, D. M. (2007). *Contemporary Orthodontics*, 4th edn, Mosby, St Louis.

Section III on orthodontic diagnosis and treatment planning provides more detailed information on the development of a problem list as part of the treatment planning process.

Sheridan, J. J. (1987). Air-rotor stripping update. *Journal of Clinical Orthodontics*, **21**, 781–8.

The practical aspects of creating space by air-rotor stripping of the buccal segments are described in this paper.

References for this chapter can also be found at www.oxfordtextbooks.co.uk/orc/mitchell4e/. Where possible, these are presented as active links which direct you to the electronic version of the work, to help facilitate onward study. If you are a subscriber to that work (either individually or through an institution), and depending on your level of access, you may be able to peruse an abstract or the full article if available.

8

Class I

A Class I incisor relationship is defined by the British Standards incisor classification as follows: 'the lower incisor edges occlude with or lie immediately below the cingulum plateau of the upper central incisors'. Therefore Class I malocclusions include those where the anteroposterior occlusal relationship is normal and there is a discrepancy either within the arches and/or in the transverse or vertical relationship between the arches.

8.1 Aetiology

8.1.1 Skeletal

In Class I malocclusions the skeletal pattern is usually Class I, but it can also be Class II or Class III with the inclination of the incisors compensating for the underlying skeletal discrepancy (Fig. 8.1), i.e. dento-alveolar compensation. Marked transverse skeletal discrepancies between the arches are more commonly associated with Class II or Class III occlusions, but milder transverse discrepancies are often seen in Class I cases. Increased vertical skeletal proportions and anterior open bite can also occur where the anteroposterior incisor relationship is Class I.

8.1.2 Soft tissues

In most Class I cases the soft tissue environment is favourable (for example resulting in dento-alveolar compensation) and is not an aetiological factor. The major exception to this is bimaxillary proclination, where the upper and lower incisors are proclined. This may be racial in origin and can also occur because lack of lip tonicity results in the incisors being moulded forwards under tongue pressure.

8.1.3 Dental factors

Dental factors are the main aetiological influences in Class I malocclusions. The most common are tooth/arch size discrepancies, leading to crowding or, less frequently, spacing.

The size of the teeth is genetically determined and so, to a great extent, is the size of the jaws. Environmental factors can also contribute to crowding or spacing. For example, premature loss of a deciduous tooth can lead to a localization of any pre-existing crowding.

Local factors also include displaced or impacted teeth, and anomalies in the size, number, and form of the teeth, all of which can lead to a localized malocclusion. However, it is important to remember that these factors can also be found in association with Class II or Class III malocclusions.

8.2 Crowding

Crowding occurs where there is a discrepancy between the size of the teeth and the size of the arches. Approximately 60 per cent of Caucasian children exhibit crowding to some degree. In a crowded arch loss of a permanent or deciduous tooth will result in the remaining teeth tilting or drifting into the space created. This tendency is greatest when the adjacent teeth are erupting.

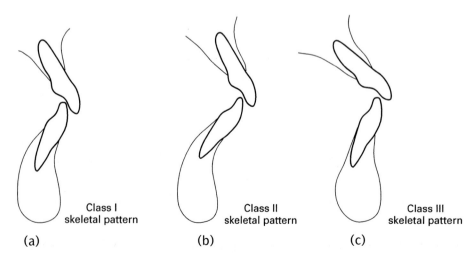

Class I
skeletal pattern

(a)

Class II
skeletal pattern

(b)

Class III
skeletal pattern

(c)

Fig. 8.1 (a) Class I incisor relationship on Class I skeletal pattern; (b) Class I incisor relationship on a Class II skeletal pattern; (c) Class I incisor relationship on a Class III skeletal pattern.

When planning treatment for crowding the following should be considered:

- the position, presence, and prognosis of remaining permanent teeth
- the degree of crowding which is usually calculated in millimetres per arch or quadrant
- the patient's malocclusion and any orthodontic treatment planned, including anchorage requirements
- the patient's age and the likelihood of the crowding increasing or reducing with growth
- the patient's profile

These aspects of treatment planning are considered in more detail in Chapter 7.

After relief of crowding a degree of natural spontaneous movement will take place. In general, this is greater under the following conditions:

- in a growing child
- if the extractions are carried out just prior to eruption of the adjacent teeth
- where the adjacent teeth are favourably positioned to upright if space is made available (for example considerable improvement will often occur in a crowded lower labial segment provided that the mandibular canines are mesially inclined)
- there are no occlusal interferences with the anticipated tooth movement

Most spontaneous improvement occurs in the first 6 months after the extractions. If alignment is not complete after 1 year, then further improvement will require active tooth movement with appliances. Figure 8.2 shows a case which was treated by extraction of all four first premolars without appliances, and Fig. 8.3 shows a patient whose management required extraction of second premolars and the use of fixed appliances. However, for most patients relief of crowding will be an integral of their overall active orthodontic treatment plan (Chapter 7).

8.2.1 Late lower incisor crowding

In most individuals intercanine width increases up to around 12 to 13 years of age, and this is followed by a very gradual diminution throughout adult life. The rate of decrease is most noticeable during the mid to late teens. This reduction in intercanine width results in an increase of any pre-existing lower labial crowding, or the emergence of crowding in arches which were well aligned or even spaced in the early teens. Therefore, to some extent, lower incisor crowding can be considered as an age change. Certainly, patients who have undergone orthodontic treatment (including extractions) are not immune from lower labial segment crowding unless prolonged retention is employed.

The aetiology of late lower incisor crowding is recognized as being multifactorial: the following have all been proposed as influences in the development of this phenomenon.

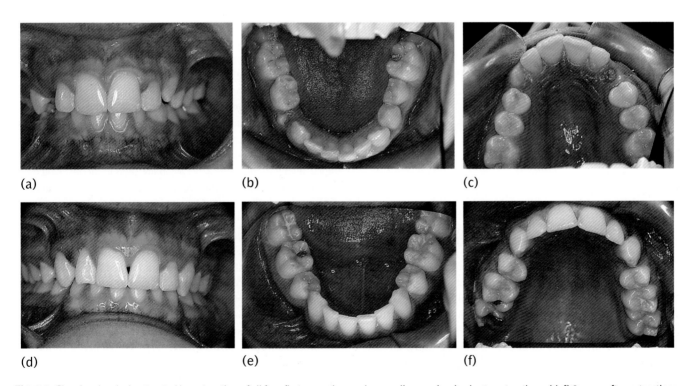

(a)   (b)   (c)

(d)   (e)   (f)

Fig. 8.2 Class I malocclusion treated by extraction of all four first premolars and no appliances: (a–c) prior to extractions; (d–f) 3 years after extractions.

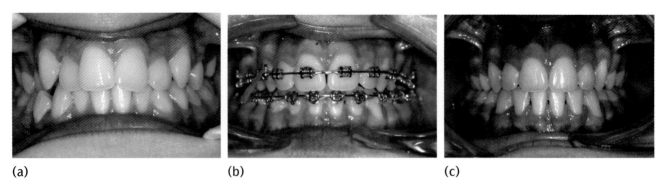

(a)   (b)   (c)

Fig. 8.3 Class I malocclusion with upper arch crowding, treated by extraction of all four second premolars and fixed appliances: (a) pre-treatment; (b) during treatment; (c) at the end of treatment.

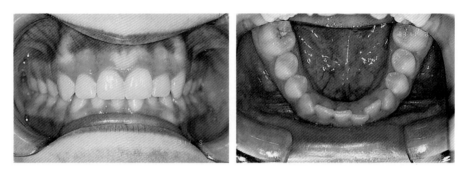

Fig. 8.4 Class I occlusion with acceptable mild lower labial segment crowding.

- Forward growth of the mandible (either horizontally or manifesting as a growth rotation) when maxillary growth has slowed, together with soft tissue pressures, which result in a reduction in lower arch perimeter and labial segment crowding.
- Soft tissue maturation.
- Mesial migration of the posterior teeth owing to forces from the interseptal fibres and/or from the anterior component of the forces of occlusion.
- The presence of an erupting third molar pushes the dentition anteriorly, i.e. the third molar plays an active role.
- The presence of a third molar prevents pressure developed anteriorly (due to either mandibular growth or soft tissue pressures) from being dissipated distally around the arch, i.e. the third molar plays a passive role.

Reviews of the many studies that have been carried out indicate that the third permanent molar has a statistically weak association with late lower incisor crowding. However this crowding can still occur in patients with congenitally absent third molars.

Removal of symptomless lower third molars has been advocated in the past in order to prevent lower labial segment crowding.

Current opinion is that prophylactic removal of lower third molars to prevent lower labial segment crowding cannot be justified – particularly given the associated morbidity with this procedure and this has been enshrined in the recommendations of the National Institute for Heath and Clinical Excellence (NICE). Management of lower labial segment crowding should be considered together with other aspects of the malocclusion (see Chapter 7), bearing in mind the propensity of this problem to worsen with age. However, lower labial segment crowding is occasionally seen in arches, which are otherwise well aligned with a good Class I buccal segment interdigitation and a slightly increased overbite (Fig. 8.4). These cases are best kept under observation until the late teens when the fate of the third permanent molars, if present, has been determined. At that stage mild lower labial segment crowding can be accepted. If the lower labial segment crowding is more marked and upper extractions are contraindicated, one approach may be to consider extraction of the most displaced lower incisor and use of a sectional fixed appliance to align and upright the remaining lower labial segment teeth (Fig. 8.5). However, steps need to be taken to help prevent the labial segments dropping lingually, to the detriment of alignment in the upper arch.

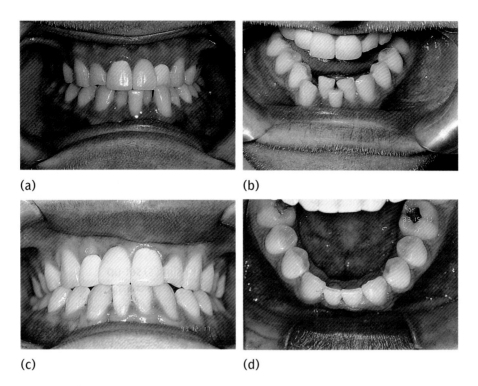

(a)　　　　　　　　　　　(b)

(c)　　　　　　　　　　　(d)

Fig. 8.5 Adult with severe crowding of the lower labial segment despite the previous loss of a lower incisor. Management involved the extraction of the most displaced incisor and a lower sectional fixed appliance: (a, b) pre-treatment; (c, d) post-treatment.

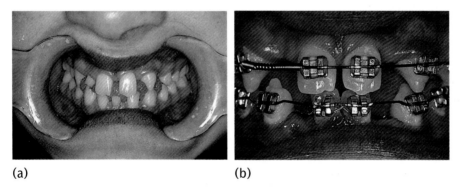

(a)　　　　　　　　　　　(b)

Fig. 8.6 Patient with hypodontia (the upper right second premolar and all four lateral incisors were absent) and generalized spacing. Treated with fixed appliances to localize space for prosthetic replacements: (a) pre-treatment; (b) showing fixed appliances.

8.3 Spacing

Generalized spacing is rare and is due to either hypodontia or small teeth in well-developed arches. Orthodontic management of generalized spacing is frequently difficult as there is usually a tendency for the spaces to re-open unless permanently retained. In milder cases it may be wiser to encourage the patient to accept the spacing, or if the teeth are narrower than average, acid-etch composite additions or porcelain veneers can be used to widen them and thus improve aesthetics. In severe cases of hypodontia a combined orthodontic–restorative approach to localize space for the provision of prostheses, or implants, may be required (Fig. 8.6).

Localized spacing may be due to hypodontia; or loss of a tooth as a result of trauma; or because extraction was indicated because of displacement, morphology, or pathology. This problem is most noticeable if an upper incisor is missing as the symmetry of the smile is affected, a feature which is usually noticed more by the lay public than other aspects of a malocclusion.

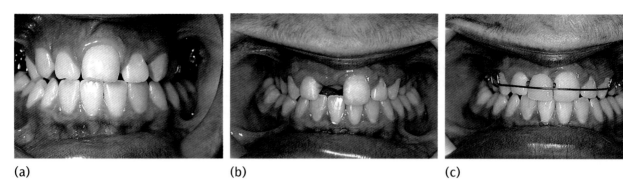

(a)   (b)   (c)

Fig. 8.10 (a) Patient with early traumatic loss of 1/ and partial space closure. Space for prosthetic replacement of 1/ was gained using a fixed appliance. (b) Result on completion of active treatment. (c) Partial denture cum retainer (NB. Stops were placed mesial to both 2/ and /1 to help prevent relapse).

> **Box 8.3 Requirements for the placement of implant to replace missing upper incisor**
>
> - Growth rate slowed to adult levels
> - Adequate bone height
> - Adequate bone width
> - Adequate space between roots of adjacent teeth
> - Adequate space for crown between adjacent crowns and occlusally

which showed that in growing patients 11 per cent of orthodontically re-positioned roots relapsed (see also Box 8.3).

Autotransplantation

This is the surgical repositioning of a tooth into a surgically created socket within the same patient. In recent years the success rate of this procedure has improved in tandem with the understanding of the underlying biology – this is good as autotransplantation has a number of advantages over other methods of tooth replacement:

- Biological replacement – avoids the need for a prosthesis
- Creates alveolar bone
- Has a natural periodontal membrane and better gingival contour
- Can erupt in synchrony with adjacent teeth
- Can be moved orthodontically once healing complete
- Suitable for growing patient

  However, there are also disadvantages:

- Only feasible if there is a suitable tooth which is planned for extraction
- Increased burden of care + general anaesthetic required for procedure
- Requires skilled surgical technique
- Transplanted tooth may undergo resorption and/or ankylosis

It is now appreciated that the timing of the transplant in terms of the root development of the tooth to be transplanted and a careful surgical technique are important (Box 8.4). When these are satisfied

success rates of the order of 85 to 90 per cent have been reported by a number of studies. If a patient has premolar crowding then the teeth of choice for transplanting are the lower premolars or upper second premolars, because of their single root (Fig. 8.11). Third molars are useful teeth for transplantation, but are too bulky for use in the labial segments.

Some centres use trauma titanium splints. A tooth with a closed apex can be used, but root canal treatment should be instituted 7–10 days after transplantation.

8.3.3 Median diastema

A median diastema is a space between the central incisors, which is more common in the upper arch (Fig. 8.12). A diastema is a normal physiological stage in the early mixed dentition when the fraenal attachment passes between the upper central incisors to attach to the incisive papilla. In normal development, as the lateral incisors and canines erupt this gap closes and the fraenal attachment migrates labially to the attached mucosa. If the upper arch is spaced or the lateral incisors are diminutive or absent, there is less pressure forcing the upper central incisors together and the diastema will tend to persist. Rarely, the fraenal attachment appears to prevent the central incisors from moving together. In these cases, blanching of the incisive papilla can be observed if tension is applied to the fraenum, and on radiographic examination a V-shaped notch of the interdental bone can be seen between the incisors indicating the attachment of the fraenum (see Chapter 3, Fig. 3.26). The aetiology of median diastema is considered in Section 3.3.9.

Management
See also Chapter 3, Section 3.3.9

It is important to take a periapical radiograph to exclude the presence of a supernumerary tooth which, if present, should be removed before closure of the diastema is undertaken. As median diastemas tend to reduce or close with the eruption of the canines, management can be subdivided as follows.

- Before eruption of the permanent canines intervention is only necessary if the diastema is greater than 3 mm and there is a lack of space for the lateral incisors to erupt. Care is required not to cause resorption of the incisor roots against the unerupted canines.

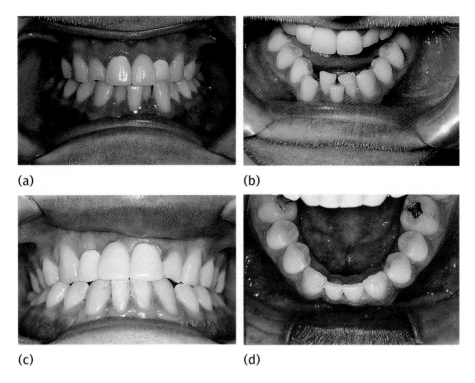

(a) (b)

(c) (d)

Fig. 8.5 Adult with severe crowding of the lower labial segment despite the previous loss of a lower incisor. Management involved the extraction of the most displaced incisor and a lower sectional fixed appliance: (a, b) pre-treatment; (c, d) post-treatment.

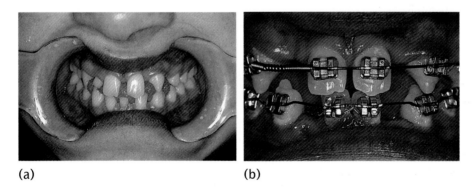

(a) (b)

Fig. 8.6 Patient with hypodontia (the upper right second premolar and all four lateral incisors were absent) and generalized spacing. Treated with fixed appliances to localize space for prosthetic replacements: (a) pre-treatment; (b) showing fixed appliances.

8.3 Spacing

Generalized spacing is rare and is due to either hypodontia or small teeth in well-developed arches. Orthodontic management of generalized spacing is frequently difficult as there is usually a tendency for the spaces to re-open unless permanently retained. In milder cases it may be wiser to encourage the patient to accept the spacing, or if the teeth are narrower than average, acid-etch composite additions or porcelain veneers can be used to widen them and thus improve aesthetics. In severe cases of hypodontia a combined orthodontic–restorative approach to localize space for the provision of prostheses, or implants, may be required (Fig. 8.6).

Localized spacing may be due to hypodontia; or loss of a tooth as a result of trauma; or because extraction was indicated because of displacement, morphology, or pathology. This problem is most noticeable if an upper incisor is missing as the symmetry of the smile is affected, a feature which is usually noticed more by the lay public than other aspects of a malocclusion.

8.3.1 Hypodontia

Hypodontia is defined as the congenital absence of one or more teeth (Box 8.1). The prevalence in a Caucasian population (excluding the third molars) has been reported as being between 3.5 to 6.5 per cent. The third molars are missing in approximately 25–35 per cent of the population. The next most commonly missing teeth are the second premolars (3 per cent) followed by the upper lateral incisors (2 per cent). Recent work has demonstrated a polygenic aetiology (Box 8.2). Missing teeth are also found more commonly in patients with a cleft lip and/or palate.

8.3.2 Management of missing upper incisors

Upper central incisors are rarely congenitally absent. They can be lost as a result of trauma, or occasionally their extraction may be indicated because of dilaceration. Upper lateral incisors are congenitally absent in approximately 2 per cent of a Caucasian population, but can also be lost following trauma. Both can occur unilaterally, bilaterally, or together. Whatever the reason for their absence, there are two treatment options:

- closure of the space (and camouflage the adjacent teeth)
- opening of the space and placement of a fixed or removable prosthesis

The choice for a particular patient will depend upon a number of factors, which are listed below. However, this is a difficult area of treatment planning and specialist advice should be sought.

- Skeletal relationship: if the skeletal pattern is Class III, space closure in the upper labial segment may compromise the incisor relationship; conversely, for a Class II division 1 pattern space closure may be preferable as it will aid overjet reduction.
- Smile line.
- Number and site of missing teeth. Are incisors missing unilateral or bilaterally?
- Presence of crowding or spacing.
- Colour and form of adjacent teeth: if the permanent canines are much darker than the incisors and/or particularly caniniform in shape, modification to make them resemble lateral incisors will be difficult; also, if a

lateral incisor is to be brought forward to replace a missing single upper central incisor, an aesthetically pleasing result will only be possible if the lateral is fairly large and has a broad gingival circumference.

- The inclination of adjacent teeth, as this will influence whether it is easier to open or close the space.
- The desired buccal segment occlusion at the end of treatment; for example if the lower arch is well aligned and the buccal segment relationship is Class I, space opening is preferable.
- The patient's wishes and ability to co-operate with complex treatment: some patients have definite ideas about whether they are willing to proceed with appliance treatment, and whether they wish to have the space closed or opened for a prosthetic replacement.
- Long-term maintenance/ replacement of a prosthesis.

Trial (Kesling's) set-up

To investigate the feasibility of different options a trial set-up can be carried out using duplicate models. The teeth to be moved are cut off the model and repositioned in the desired place using wax (Fig. 8.7). This allows any number of options to be tested and also gives an opportunity to evaluate in more detail the amount and nature of any orthodontic and restorative treatment required by a particular option. This exercise is often helpful in describing the outcome of different options to the patient.

After assessment of the above factors a provisional plan can be discussed with the patient. It is often possible to draw up more than one plan and these should all be thoroughly discussed, including the advantages and disadvantages, and the long-term maintenance of any prosthetic replacements.

Space closure

This can be facilitated by early extraction of any deciduous teeth to allow forward movement of the first permanent molars in that quadrant(s). Fixed appliances are required to complete alignment and correct the axial inclinations. If any masking procedures (for example contouring a canine incisally, palatally, and interproximally to resemble a lateral incisor) or acid-etch composite additions are required, these should be

---

Box 8.1 Hypodontia

Mild: one to two teeth missing

Moderate: three to five teeth missing

Severe: more than six teeth missing

Box 8.2 Features associated with hypodontia

- Familial tendency
- Association with syndromes (e.g. ectodermal dysplasia)
- Reduced lower facial height and increased overbite
- Small teeth
- Delayed dental development
- Retained deciduous teeth

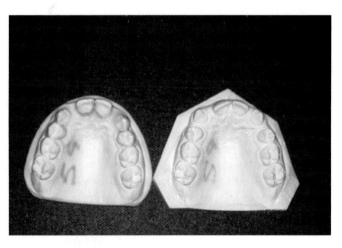

Fig. 8.7 Trial (Kesling's) set-up.

carried out prior to the placement of appliances to facilitate final tooth alignment (although definitive restorations e.g. crowns or veneers, are best deferred until treatment is completed). Temporary anchorage screws may be helpful where large spaces need to be closed. Placement of a bonded retainer post-treatment is advisable in the majority of cases (Fig. 8.8).

Space maintenance or opening

In cases with congenitally absent upper lateral incisors early extraction of the deciduous predecessor may be indicated. The rationale for this is that the permanent canine is encouraged to erupt mesially then when it is subsequently retracted during active space opening a greater volume of alveolar bone is achieved.

If an incisor is extracted electively or a patient seen soon after loss has occurred, ideally a space maintainer should be fitted forthwith.

Definitive treatment when the permanent dentition is established will require fixed appliances to open the space (Fig. 8.9). Whenever space is opened prior to bridgework, it is important to retain with a partial denture for at least 3 to 6 months (Fig. 8.10), particularly if an adhesive acid-etch retained bridge is to be used. Research has shown that acid-etch bridges placed immediately after the completion of tooth movement, have a greater incidence of failure than those placed following a period of retention with a removable retainer.

Implants are becoming more widely available but for most patients are still relatively expensive. When planning space opening for placement of an implant it is wise to bear in mind the results of a recent study

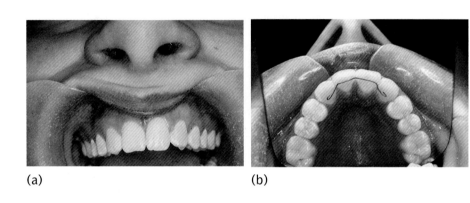

(a) (b)

Fig. 8.8 (a) Patient with missing lateral incisors treated by space closure and modification of the upper canines. (b) Occlusal view of same patient to show bonded retainer.

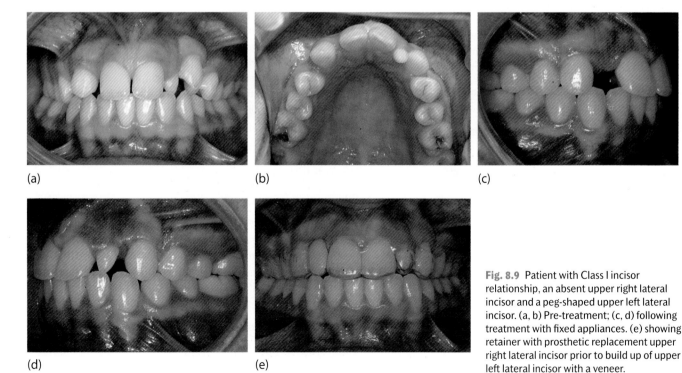

(a) (b) (c)

(d) (e)

Fig. 8.9 Patient with Class I incisor relationship, an absent upper right lateral incisor and a peg-shaped upper left lateral incisor. (a, b) Pre-treatment; (c, d) following treatment with fixed appliances. (e) showing retainer with prosthetic replacement upper right lateral incisor prior to build up of upper left lateral incisor with a veneer.

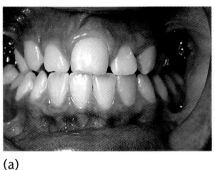 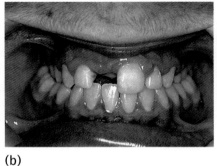 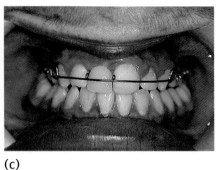

(a)   (b)   (c)

Fig. 8.10 (a) Patient with early traumatic loss of 1/ and partial space closure. Space for prosthetic replacement of 1/ was gained using a fixed appliance. (b) Result on completion of active treatment. (c) Partial denture cum retainer (NB. Stops were placed mesial to both 2/ and /1 to help prevent relapse).

> **Box 8.3 Requirements for the placement of implant to replace missing upper incisor**
>
> - Growth rate slowed to adult levels
> - Adequate bone height
> - Adequate bone width
> - Adequate space between roots of adjacent teeth
> - Adequate space for crown between adjacent crowns and occlusally

which showed that in growing patients 11 per cent of orthodontically re-positioned roots relapsed (see also Box 8.3).

Autotransplantation

This is the surgical repositioning of a tooth into a surgically created socket within the same patient. In recent years the success rate of this procedure has improved in tandem with the understanding of the underlying biology – this is good as autotransplantation has a number of advantages over other methods of tooth replacement:

- Biological replacement – avoids the need for a prosthesis
- Creates alveolar bone
- Has a natural periodontal membrane and better gingival contour
- Can erupt in synchrony with adjacent teeth
- Can be moved orthodontically once healing complete
- Suitable for growing patient

However, there are also disadvantages:

- Only feasible if there is a suitable tooth which is planned for extraction
- Increased burden of care + general anaesthetic required for procedure
- Requires skilled surgical technique
- Transplanted tooth may undergo resorption and/or ankylosis

It is now appreciated that the timing of the transplant in terms of the root development of the tooth to be transplanted and a careful surgical technique are important (Box 8.4). When these are satisfied

success rates of the order of 85 to 90 per cent have been reported by a number of studies. If a patient has premolar crowding then the teeth of choice for transplanting are the lower premolars or upper second premolars, because of their single root (Fig. 8.11). Third molars are useful teeth for transplantation, but are too bulky for use in the labial segments.

Some centres use trauma titanium splints. A tooth with a closed apex can be used, but root canal treatment should be instituted 7–10 days after transplantation.

8.3.3 Median diastema

A median diastema is a space between the central incisors, which is more common in the upper arch (Fig. 8.12). A diastema is a normal physiological stage in the early mixed dentition when the fraenal attachment passes between the upper central incisors to attach to the incisive papilla. In normal development, as the lateral incisors and canines erupt this gap closes and the fraenal attachment migrates labially to the attached mucosa. If the upper arch is spaced or the lateral incisors are diminutive or absent, there is less pressure forcing the upper central incisors together and the diastema will tend to persist. Rarely, the fraenal attachment appears to prevent the central incisors from moving together. In these cases, blanching of the incisive papilla can be observed if tension is applied to the fraenum, and on radiographic examination a V-shaped notch of the interdental bone can be seen between the incisors indicating the attachment of the fraenum (see Chapter 3, Fig. 3.26). The aetiology of median diastema is considered in Section 3.3.9.

Management
See also Chapter 3, Section 3.3.9

It is important to take a periapical radiograph to exclude the presence of a supernumerary tooth which, if present, should be removed before closure of the diastema is undertaken. As median diastemas tend to reduce or close with the eruption of the canines, management can be subdivided as follows.

- Before eruption of the permanent canines intervention is only necessary if the diastema is greater than 3 mm and there is a lack of space for the lateral incisors to erupt. Care is required not to cause resorption of the incisor roots against the unerupted canines.

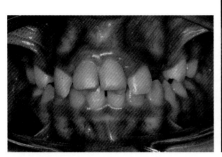
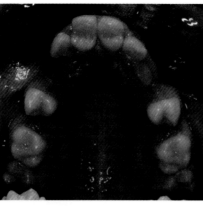
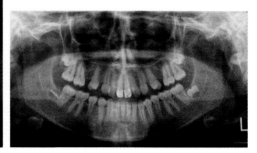

Fig. 8.11 This patient lost both upper central incisors due to trauma. Both upper second premolars were transplanted to replace the missing incisors. The facial surfaces have been modified with composite to improve the appearance. Permanent aesthetic modifications were deferred until orthodontic treatment had been completed and growth had slowed to adult levels. Pictures printed with the kind permission of Nadine Houghton.

Box 8.4 Criteria for successful autotransplantation

- Root development of tooth to be transplanted – $^2/_3$ to $^3/_4$ complete
- Sufficient space in arch and occlusally to accommodate transplanted tooth
- Careful preparation of donor site to ensure good root to bone adaptation
- Careful surgical technique to avoid damage to root surface of transplanted tooth
- Transplanted teeth positioned at same level as donor site and splinted for 7–10 days

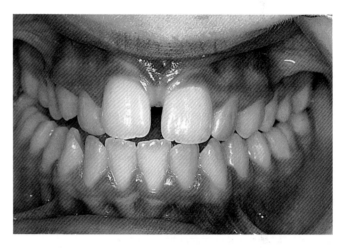

Fig. 8.12 Upper midline diastema with low frenal attachment.

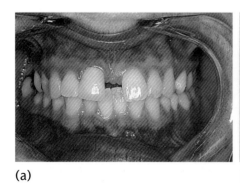
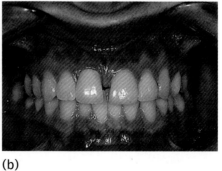

      (a)   (b)

Fig. 8.13 Adult with narrow proclined upper central incisors with a midline diastema. An upper removable appliance was used to reduce the overbite, and then to retract and move 1/1 a little closer together: (a) pre-treatment; (b) at the completion of active appliance therapy, following veneering of 21/1.

- After eruption of the permanent canines space closure is usually straightforward. Fixed appliances are required to achieve uprighting of the incisors after space closure. Prolonged retention is usually necessary as diastemas exhibit a great tendency to re-open, particularly if there is a familial tendency, the upper arch is spaced or the initial diastema was greater than 2 mm. In view of this it may be better to accept a minimal diastema, particularly if no other orthodontic treatment is required. Alternatively, if the central incisors are narrow a restorative solution, for example veneers, can be considered (Fig. 8.13).

If it is thought that the fraenum is a contributory factor, then fraenectomy should be considered. Opinions differ as to whether this should be done before treatment; during space closure; or following completion of closure of the diastema. There is currently no strong evidence upon which to base the timing of this procedure.

8.4 Displaced teeth

Teeth can be displaced for a variety of reasons including the following.

- Abnormal position of the tooth germ: canines (Chapter 14) and second premolars are the most commonly affected teeth. Management depends upon the degree of displacement. If this is mild, extraction of the associated primary tooth plus space maintenance, if indicated, may result in an improvement in position in some cases. Alternatively, exposure and the application of orthodontic traction may be used to bring the mildly displaced tooth into the arch. If the displacement is severe, extraction is usually necessary.

- Crowding: lack of space for a permanent tooth to erupt within the arch can lead to or contribute to displacement. Those teeth that erupt last in a segment, for example upper lateral incisors, upper canines (Fig. 8.14), second premolars, and third molars, are most commonly affected. Management involves relief of crowding, followed by active tooth movement where necessary. However, if the displacement is severe it may be prudent to extract the displaced tooth (Fig. 8.15).

- Retention of a deciduous predecessor: extraction of the retained primary tooth should be carried out as soon as possible provided that the permanent successor is not displaced.

- Secondary to the presence of a supernumerary tooth or teeth (see Chapter 3): management involves extraction of the supernumerary followed by tooth alignment, usually with fixed appliances. Displacements due to supernumeraries have a tendency to relapse and prolonged retention is required.

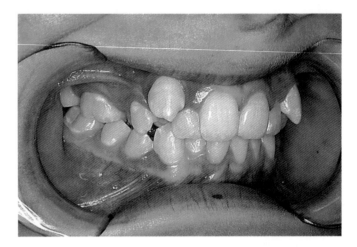

Fig. 8.14 Class I malocclusion with mild lower and marked upper arch crowding. In crowded arches the last teeth in a segment to erupt, in this case the upper canines, are the most likely to be short of space. The maxillary second premolars are also crowded, probably owing to early loss of the upper second deciduous molars.

- Caused by a habit (see Chapter 9).

- Secondary to pathology, for example a dentigerous cyst. This is the rarest cause.

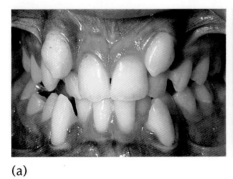 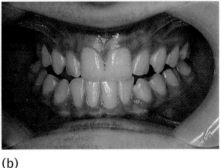

(a)   (b)

Fig. 8.15 Occasionally it may be prudent to extract the most displaced tooth. In this case all four canines were extracted: (a) prior to extractions; (b) after extractions (NB. Patient is posturing forwards to show lower arch alignment).

8.5 Vertical discrepancies

Variations in the vertical dimension can occur in association with any anteroposterior skeletal relationship. Increased vertical skeletal proportions are discussed in Chapter 9 in relation to Class II division 1, in Chapter 11 in relation to Class III, and in Chapter 12 on anterior open bite.

8.6 Transverse discrepancies

A transverse discrepancy between the arches results in a cross-bite and can occur in association with Class I, Class II, and Class III malocclusions. Classification and management of crossbite is discussed in Chapter 13.

8.7 Bimaxillary proclination

As the name suggests, bimaxillary proclination is the term used to describe occlusions where both the upper and lower incisors are proclined. Bimaxillary proclination is seen more commonly in some racial groups (for example Afro-Caribbean), and this needs to be borne in mind during assessment (including cephalometric analysis) and treatment planning.

When bimaxillary proclination occurs in a Class I malocclusion the overjet is increased because of the angulation of the incisors (Fig. 8.16). Management is difficult because both upper and lower incisors need to be retroclined to reduce the overjet. Retroclination of the lower labial segment will encroach on tongue space and therefore has a high likelihood of relapse following removal of appliances. For these reasons, treatment of bimaxillary proclination should be approached with caution and consideration should be given to accepting the incisor relationship. If the lips are incompetent, but have a good muscle tone and are likely to achieve a lip-to-lip seal if the incisors are retracted, the chances of a stable result are increased. However, the patient should still be warned that the prognosis for stability is guarded. Where bimaxillary proclination is associated with competent lips, or with grossly incompetent lips which are unlikely to retain the corrected incisor position, permanent retention is advisable.

Bimaxillary proclination can also occur in association with Class II division 1 and Class III malocclusions.

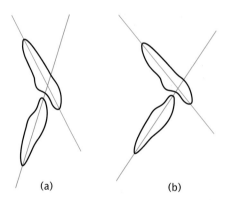

(a)   (b)

Fig. 8.16 (a) Class I incisor relationship with normal axial inclination (inter-incisal angle is 137°); (b) Class I incisor relationship with bimaxillary inclination showing increased overjet (inter-incisal angle is 107°).

Key points

- Class I incisor relationships can occur in association with any skeletal pattern (AP, vertical, transverse)
- With the exception of bimaxillary proclination, in Class I incisor relationships are usually associated with a favourable soft tissue environment

Principal sources and further reading

Bishara, S. E. (1999). Third molars: a dilemma: Or is it? *American Journal of Orthodontics and Dentofacial Orthopedics*, **115**, 628–33.

Harradine, N. W. T., Pearson, M. H., and Toth, B. (1998). The effect of extraction of third molars on late lower incisor crowding: A randomised controlled trial. *British Journal of Orthodontics*, **25**, 117–22.

This excellent study is essential reading.

Hobkirk, J.A., Gill, D.S., Jones, S.P., Hemmings, G., Bassi, S., O'Donnell, A.L., and Goodman, J.R. (2011). *Hypodontia: A Team Approach to Management*. Wiley-Blackwell.

Lewis, B. R.K., Gahan, M.J., Hodge, T. M., and Moore, D. (2010). The orthodontic-restorative interface: 2 Compensating for variations in tooth number and shape. *Dental Update*, **37**, 138–52.

Little, R. M., Reidel, R. A., and Artun, J. (1981). An evaluation of changes in mandibular anterior alignment from 10–20 years postretention. *American Journal of Orthodontics and Dentofacial Orthopedics*, **93**, 423–8.

Classic paper. The authors found that lower labial segment crowding tends to increase even following extractions and appliance therapy.

Kokich, K. (2001). Managing orthodontic-restorative treatment for the adolescent patient. *Orthodontics and Dentofacial Orthopedics* (Chapter 25). Needham Press, Michigan.

Mittal, M., Murray, A.M., and Sandler, J. (2011). Maxillary labial frenectomy: indications and technique. *Dental Update*, **38**, 159–62.

Polder, B. J., Van't Hof, M. A., Van der Linden, F. P. G. M., and Kuijpers-Jagtman, A. M. (2004). A meta-analysis of the prevalence of dental agenesis of permanent teeth. *Community Dentistry, Oral Epidemiology*, **32**, 217–26.

Robertsson, S. and Mohlin, B. (2000). The congenitally missing upper lateral incisor. A retrospective study of orthodontic space closure versus restorative treatment. *European Journal of Orthodontics*, **22**, 697–710.

This interesting study concluded that space closure produced outcomes that were well accepted by patients, not detrimental to TMJ function and better for the periodontium compared with prosthetic replacement.

Shashua, D. and Artun, J. (1999). Relapse after orthodontic correction of maxillary median diastema: a follow-up evaluation of consecutive cases. *The Angle Orthodontist*, **69**, 257–63.

Thilander, B. (2008). Orthodontic space closure versus implant placement in subjects with missing teeth. *Journal of Oral Rehabilitation*, **35**, 64–71.

The author would also recommend an excellent pair of point/counterpoint articles which neatly summarize the opposing views in relation to the decision whether to open or close space when the upper lateral incisors are absent:

Kokich, K. O. Jr., Kinzer, G.A., and Janakievski, J. (2011). Congenitally missing maxillary lateral incisors: canine substitution. *American Journal of Orthodontics and Dento-facial Orthopedics*, **139**, 435–45.

Zachrisson, B.U., Rosa, M., and Toreskog, S. (2011). Congenitally missing maxillary lateral incisors: canine substitution. *American Journal of Orthodontics and Dento-facial Orthopedics*, **139**, 434.

 References for this chapter can also be found at www.oxfordtextbooks.co.uk/orc/mitchell4e/. Where possible, these are presented as active links which direct you to the electronic version of the work, to help facilitate onward study. If you are a subscriber to that work (either individually or through an institution), and depending on your level of access, you may be able to peruse an abstract or the full article if available.

9

Class II division 1

Chapter contents

Learning objectives for this chapter

- Gain an understanding of the aetiological factors which contribute to the development of a Class II division 1 incisor relationship
- Gain an appreciation of the management of increased overjet based on an understanding of the probable aetiology

The British Standards classification defines a Class II division 1 incisor relationship as follows: 'the lower incisor edges lie posterior to the cingulum plateau of the upper incisors, there is an increase in overjet and the upper central incisors are usually proclined'. In a Caucasian population the incidence of Class II division 1 incisor relationship is approximately 15–20 per cent.

Prominent upper incisors, particularly when the lips are incompetent, are at increased risk of being traumatized. It has been shown that children with an overjet greater than 3 mm have twice the risk of injury to their anterior teeth than those with overjets less than 3 mm and that the risk increases as the overjet increases.

9.1 Aetiology

9.1.1 Skeletal pattern

A Class II division 1 incisor relationship is usually associated with a Class II skeletal pattern, commonly due to a retrognathic mandible (Fig. 9.1). However, proclination of the upper incisors and/or retroclination of the lower incisors by a habit or the soft tissues can result in an increased overjet on a Class I (Fig. 9.2), or even a Class III skeletal pattern.

A Class II division 1 incisor relationship is found in association with a range of vertical skeletal patterns. Management of those patients with significantly increased or significantly reduced vertical proportions is usually difficult and is the province of the specialist.

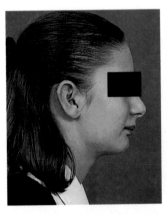
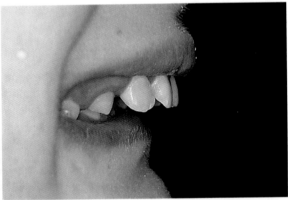

Fig. 9.1 A Class II division 1 incisor relationship on a Class II skeletal pattern with a retrognathic mandible.

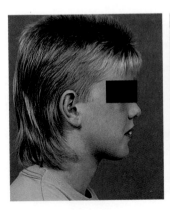
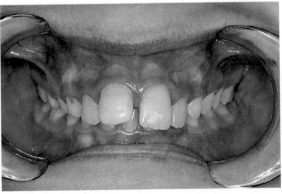

Fig. 9.2 A Class II division 1 incisor relationship on a Class I skeletal pattern.

9.1.2 Soft tissues

The influence of the soft tissues on a Class II division 1 malocclusion is mainly mediated by the skeletal pattern, both anteroposteriorly and vertically. Nevertheless, the resting position of the patient's soft tissues and their functional activity are important.

In a Class II division 1 malocclusion the lips are typically incompetent owing to the prominence of the upper incisors and/or the underlying skeletal pattern. If the lips are incompetent, the patient will try to achieve an anterior oral seal in one of the following ways:

- circumoral muscular activity to achieve a lip-to-lip seal (Fig. 9.3);
- the mandible is postured forwards to allow the lips to meet at rest;
- the lower lip is drawn up behind the upper incisors (Fig. 9.4);
- the tongue is placed forwards between the incisors to contact the lower lip, often contributing to the development of an incomplete overbite;
- a combination of these.

Where the patient can achieve lip-to-lip contact by circumoral muscle activity or the mandible is postured forwards, the influence of the soft tissues is often to moderate the effect of the underlying skeletal pattern by dento-alveolar compensation. More commonly the lower lip functions by being drawn up behind the upper incisors, which leads to retroclination of the lower labial segment and/or proclination of the upper incisors with the result that the incisor relationship is more severe than the underlying skeletal pattern.

However, if the tongue habitually comes forward to contact the lower lip, proclination of the lower incisors may occur, helping to compensate for the underlying skeletal pattern. This type of soft tissue behaviour is often associated with increased vertical skeletal proportions and/or grossly incompetent lips, or a habit which has resulted in an increase in overjet and an anterior open bite. In practice, it is often difficult to determine the degree to which this is adaptive tongue behaviour, or whether a rarer endogenous tongue thrust exists (see Chapter 12).

Infrequently, a Class II division 1 incisor relationship occurs owing to retroclination of the lower incisors by a very active lower lip (Fig. 9.5).

9.1.3 Dental factors

A Class II division 1 incisor relationship may occur in the presence of crowding or spacing. Where the arches are crowded, lack of space may result in the upper incisors being crowded out of the arch labially and thus to exacerbation of the overjet. Conversely, crowding of the lower labial segment may help to compensate for an increased overjet in the same manner.

9.1.4 Habits

See also Section 12.2.3

A persistent digit-sucking habit will act like an orthodontic force upon the teeth if indulged in for more than a few hours per day. The severity of the effects produced will depend upon the duration and the intensity, but the following are commonly associated with a determined habit (Fig. 9.6):

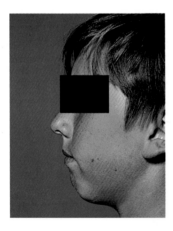

Fig. 9.3 Marked circumoral muscular activity is visible as this patient attempts to achieve an anterior oral seal by a lip-to-lip seal.

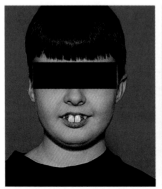
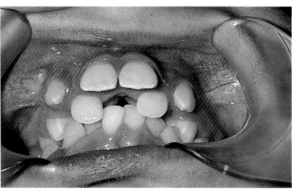

Fig. 9.4 In this patient with a Class II division 1 malocclusion the lower lip lies behind the upper central incisors which have been proclined, and in front of the lateral incisors which have been retroclined as a result.

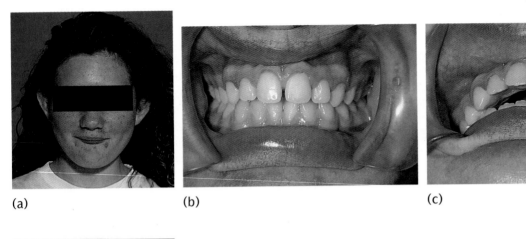

(a) (b) (c)

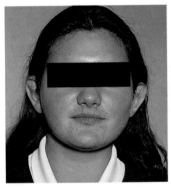

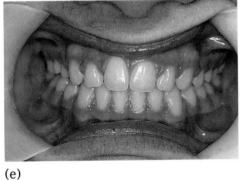

(d) (e)

Fig. 9.5 A Class II division 1 malocclusion due mainly to retroclination of the lower labial segment by an active lower lip. This patient achieved an anterior oral seal by contact between the tongue and the lower lip. (a–c) Pre-treatment; (d, e) post-treatment.

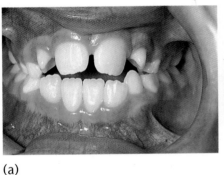

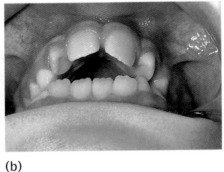

(a) (b)

Fig. 9.6 The effects of a persistent digit-sucking habit on the occlusion: the upper incisors have been proclined and the lower incisors retroclined.

- proclination of the upper incisors;
- retroclination of the lower labial segment;
- an incomplete overbite or a localized anterior open bite;
- narrowing of the upper arch thought to be mediated by the tongue taking up a lower position in the mouth and the negative pressure generated during sucking of the digit.

The first two effects will contribute to an increase in overjet.

The effects of a habit will be superimposed upon the child's existing skeletal pattern and incisor relationship, and thus can lead to an increased overjet in a child with a Class I or Class III skeletal pattern, or can exacerbate a pre-existing Class II malocclusion. The effects may be asymmetric if a single finger or thumb is sucked (Fig. 9.7).

9.2 Occlusal features

The overjet is increased, and the upper incisors may be proclined, perhaps as the result of the influence of the soft tissues or a habit; or upright, with the increased overjet reflecting the skeletal pattern. The overbite is often increased, but may be incomplete as a result of a forward adaptive tongue position, a habit, or increased vertical skeletal proportions. If the latter two factors are marked, an anterior open bite may result. If the lips are grossly incompetent and are habitually apart at rest, drying of the gingivae may lead to an exacerbation of any pre-existing gingivitis.

The molar relationship usually reflects the skeletal pattern unless early deciduous tooth loss has resulted in mesial drift of the first permanent molars.

9.3 Assessment of and treatment planning in Class II division 1 malocclusions

9.3.1 Factors influencing a definitive treatment plan

Before deciding upon a definitive treatment plan the following factors should be considered.

The patient's age

This is of importance in relation to facial growth: first whether further facial growth is to be expected, and second, if further growth is anticipated, whether this is likely to be favourable or unfavourable. In the 'average' growing child, forward growth of the mandible occurs during the pubertal growth spurt and the early teens. This is advantageous in the management of Class II malocclusions. However, correction of the incisor relationship in a child with increased vertical skeletal proportions and a backward-opening rotational pattern of growth has a poorer prognosis for stability. This is because the anteroposterior discrepancy will worsen with growth, and in addition an increase in the lower face height may reduce the likelihood of lip competence at the end of treatment.

In the adult patient, a lack of growth will reduce the range of skeletal Class II malocclusions that can be treated by orthodontic means alone and will also make overbite reduction more difficult.

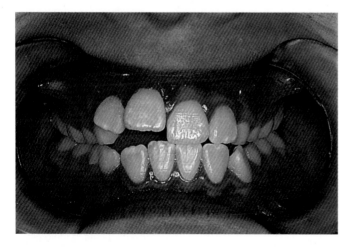

Fig. 9.7 An asymmetrical increase in overjet in a patient with a habit of sucking one finger.

The difficulty of treatment

The skeletal pattern is the major determinant of the difficulty of treatment. Those cases with a marked anteroposterior discrepancy and/or significantly increased or reduced vertical skeletal proportions will require careful evaluation, an experienced orthodontist, and possibly surgery for a successful result.

The results of a recent retrospective study of over 1200 consecutively treated Class II division 1 malocclusions found that patients with large overjets and more upright incisors were less likely to achieve an excellent outcome.

The likely stability of overjet reduction

Before planning treatment it is often helpful to try to determine those factors that have contributed to the development of that particular Class II division 1 malocclusion and the degree to which they can be modified or corrected by treatment. The soft tissues are the major determinant of stability following overjet reduction. For example, the patient shown in Fig. 9.8 has an increased overjet on a Class I skeletal pattern with a lower lip trap. In the absence of a habit, it is probable that the upper incisors were deflected labially as they erupted, and it is likely that retraction of the upper incisors within the control of the lower lip would be stable as the lips would then be competent. In contrast, the patient shown in Fig. 9.9 has a Class II skeletal pattern with increased vertical skeletal proportions and markedly incompetent lips. In this case overjet reduction is unlikely to be stable as, following retraction the upper labial segment would not be controlled by the lower lip.

Ideally, at the end of overjet reduction the lower lip should act on the incisal one-third of the upper incisors and be able to achieve a competent lip seal. If this is not possible, consideration should be given as to whether treatment is necessary (if alignment is acceptable and the overjet is not significantly increased) and, if indicated, whether prolonged retention or even surgery is required.

The patient's facial appearance

In some cases a consideration of the profile may help to make the decision between two alternative modes of treatment. For example, in a case with a Class II skeletal pattern due to a retrusive mandible, a functional appliance may be preferable to distal movement of the upper buccal

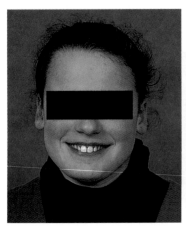 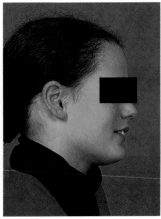 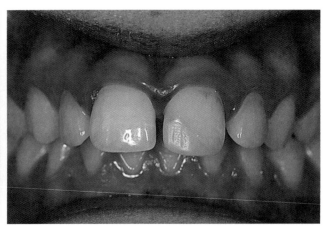

Fig. 9.8 Following overjet reduction, this patient's lips will probably be competent. Therefore the prognosis for stability of the corrected incisor relationship is good.

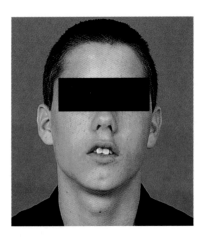

Fig. 9.9 Class II division 1 malocclusion with a poor prognosis for the stability of overjet reduction owing to the markedly incompetent lips and increased vertical proportions. Prolonged retention would be advisable.

Box 9.1 Treatment in the following situations is challenging and best managed by an experienced operator (Fig. 9.10):

- Significant skeletal discrepancy

- The lips are grossly incompetent

- The molar relationship is Class II and the lower arch is crowded as the extraction of one unit in each quadrant in the upper arch will not give sufficient space for relief of crowding and overjet reduction

- The molar relationship is greater than one unit Class II

---

segments with headgear (see Fig. 19.1). The profile may also influence the decision whether or not to relieve mild crowding by extractions.

Occasionally, although management by orthodontics alone is feasible, this will be to the detriment of the facial appearance and acceptance of the increased overjet or a surgical approach may be preferred. Features which may lead to this scenario include an obtuse nasolabial angle or excessive upper incisor show (Box 9.1).

9.3.2 Practical treatment planning

Treatment planning in general is discussed in Chapter 7. In particular the reader is directed to Sections 7.3.1 and 7.3.2.

The decision as to whether extractions are required will depend upon the presence of crowding, the tooth movements planned, and their anchorage requirements. Class II division 1 malocclusions are commonly associated with increased overbite, which must be reduced before the overjet can be reduced. Overbite reduction requires space (see Table 7.1) and allowance for this must be made when planning space requirements in the lower arch (see Section 7.7.1). Significantly increased overbites will require more space and fixed appliances, or even surgery. Overbite reduction is also considered in more detail in Chapter 10 (Section 10.3.1).

Where the lower arch is well aligned and the molar relationship is Class II, space for overjet reduction can be gained by distal movement of the upper buccal segments or by extractions. Where possible, a Class I buccal segment relationship is preferable. If extractions are carried out in the upper arch only, the molar relationship at the end of treatment will be Class II. This is functionally satisfactory, but as half a molar width is narrower than a premolar, there will be a slight space discrepancy between the arches with a little excess space to close in the upper arch. However with fixed appliances, the upper first molar can be rotated mesiopalatally to take up this space by virtue of its rhomboid shape.

Distal movement by means of headgear is discussed in more detail in Chapter 7 (Section 7.7.4), and is usually considered if the molar relationship is half a unit Class II or less, although a full unit of space can be

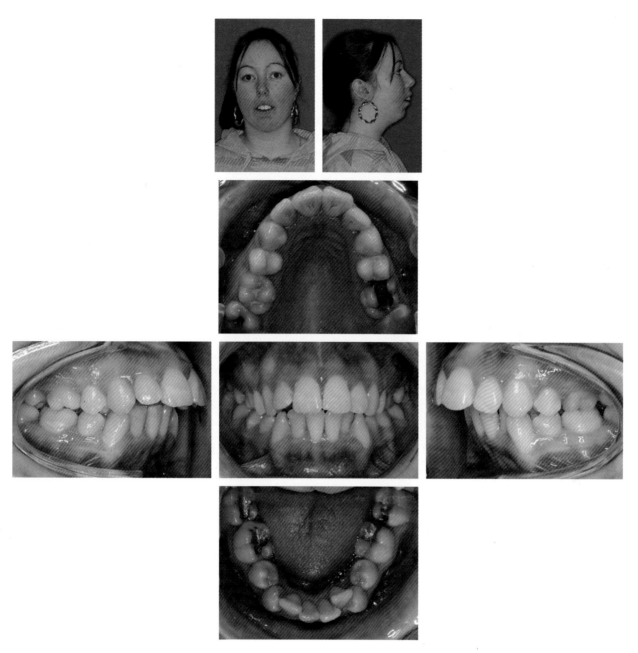

Fig. 9.10 Patient with a marked Class II skeletal pattern, increased vertical skeletal proportions, obtuse nasolabial angle and grossly incompetent lips. This patient also showed an excessive amount of upper incisor show at rest and when smiling. The buccal segment relationship was Class II and the lower arch was crowded. Not a straightforward case.

gained in a co-operative, growing patient. If the prognosis for overjet reduction is guarded, it may be advisable to gain space in the upper arch by distal movement of the upper buccal segments rather than by extractions. Then, should relapse occur this will not result in a re-opening of the extraction space.

It is fair to say that headgear is associated with compliance problems; to try and eliminate this a number of 'non-compliance' appliances have been developed which aim to produce distal movement of the molars. These can be classified as follows:

- Intramaxillary: anchorage derived from within the arch – anterior teeth, premolars, coverage of palatal vault.

- Intermaxillary: anchorage derived from opposing arch. In Class II cases this is the lower arch.

- Absolute anchorage: anchorage derived from implants (TADs). Examples include temporary anchorage screws and plates (see Section 15.4).

The latter category is the only one which does not result in movement of the anchorage unit, which in most cases is undesirable. For example, if movement of the upper molars is pitted against the upper anterior teeth, then some increase in overjet is likely, which in a Class II division malocclusion is undesirable. The main drawback to the use of TADs for anchorage is the need for the procedures to place and then remove the screw or plate. However, modern designs of the screw type can be placed and removed relatively easily. Use of TADs has increased the envelope of cases that can be treated by orthodontics alone.

9.4 Early treatment

Given the susceptibility of prominent incisors to trauma and for children to tease, early treatment is a tempting proposition. In the UK and America a number of large, randomized, controlled clinical trials have been carried out to look at the timing of treatment for Class II malocclusions. Pre-adolescent children were randomized to either early treatment with a functional appliance (or in some studies headgear) or a period of observation followed by functional appliance treatment in the early permanent dentition. Patients in both groups then underwent comprehensive treatment with fixed appliances in the permanent dentition. Following completion of all treatment, little difference, if any, was detectable between the early and the later treatment groups in the quality of the final result. However, the overall treatment time was considerably longer for those children who underwent early treatment, plus a period of "retention" was required between completion of the functional appliance phase and the commencement of fixed appliances which was problematic to manage.

As a result many clinicians feel that treatment for Class II division 1 malocclusions is best deferred until the late mixed/early permanent dentition where the transition from the functional to the fixed appliance can be made straightaway without having to wait for teeth to erupt; space can be gained for relief of crowding and reduction of the overjet by the extraction of permanent teeth (if indicated), and soft tissue maturity increases the likelihood of lip competence. In the interim a custom-made mouthguard can be worn for sports. However, if the upper incisors are thought to be at particular risk of trauma during the mixed dentition, treatment with a functional appliance can be considered (Fig. 9.11).

9.5 Management of an increased overjet associated with a Class I or mild Class II skeletal pattern

Fixed appliances, with extractions if indicated, will give good results in skilled hands in this group (Fig. 9.12). In patients with moderately crowded arches, lower second premolars and upper first premolars are a common extraction pattern as this favours forward movement of the lower molar to aid correction of the molar relationship and retraction of the upper labial segment.

A functional appliance can be used to reduce an overjet in a co-operative child with well-aligned arches and a mild to moderate Class II skeletal pattern, provided that there is still some growth remaining. If the arches are crowded, anteroposterior correction can be achieved with a functional appliance followed by extractions, and then fixed appliances can be used to achieve alignment and to detail the occlusion.

In a very limited number of cases with good arch alignment, no crowding and proclined upper incisors a removable appliance can be considered (Fig. 9.13), but most patients benefit from comprehensive treatment with fixed appliances.

9.6 Management of an increased overjet associated with a moderate to severe Class II skeletal pattern

Management of the more severe case is the province of the experienced operator. There are three possible approaches to treatment.

(1) **Growth modification** by attempting restraint of maxillary growth, by encouraging mandibular growth, or by a combination of the two (Fig. 9.14). Headgear can be used to try and restrain growth of the maxilla horizontally and/or vertically, depending upon the direction of force relative to the maxilla. Functional appliances appear to produce limited restraint of maxillary growth whilst encouraging mandibular growth. However, a number of recent studies have shown that the actual amount of growth modification achieved is limited; and success is dependent upon favourable growth and an enthusiastic patient. Recent work has suggested that predictors of a successful outcome are

- Mandibular retrusion (Pogonion to Nasion perpendicular >7 mm)
- The angle between the ramus and the lower border of the mandible (Condylion-Gonion-Menton) is <123°

For a more detailed discussion please see Chapter 19. There is some evidence to show that discluding the arches with appliances results

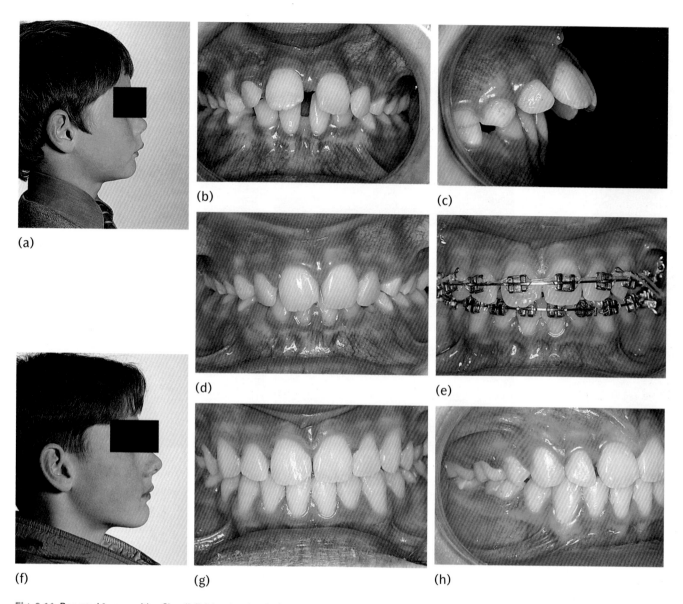

Fig. 9.11 Boy aged 9 years with a Class II division 1 malocclusion on a Class II skeletal pattern. As the upper incisors were at risk of trauma, treatment was started early with a functional appliance. Following eruption of the permanent dentition, definitive treatment involving the extraction of all four second premolars and the use of fixed appliances was carried out to correct the inter-incisal angle and alleviate the crowding: (a–c) pre-treatment (age 9 years); (d) at end of treatment with functional appliance (note the retroclination of the upper incisors as most of the reduction of the overjet has been achieved by dento-alveolar change); (e) following extraction of second premolars fixed appliances were placed; (f–h) following removal of fixed appliances (age 15 years).

in favourable mandibular growth being expressed as anteroposterior change of the mandible to the maxilla (in effect a degree of 'growth modification'), but further work is required to evaluate this effect.

(2) **Orthodontic camouflage** using fixed appliances to achieve bodily retraction of the upper incisors (Fig. 9.15). The severity of the case that can be approached in this way is limited by the availability of cortical bone palatal to the upper incisors and by the patient's facial profile.

(3) **Surgical correction** (see Chapter 21).

As mandibular growth predominates over maxillary growth during the pubertal growth spurt, more Class II malocclusions than Class III

malocclusions can be managed with orthodontics alone. Research indicates that the amount of growth modification that can be achieved is limited, but even a small amount of skeletal change can be helpful. In practice, the child with a moderately severe Class II skeletal pattern can often be managed by a combination of approaches 1 and 2, provided that growth is not unfavourable. This usually involves initially functional appliance therapy carried out during the pubertal growth spurt, after which fixed appliances are used, plus extractions if indicated.

Orthodontic camouflage can also be achieved by proclination of the lower labial segment. In the main this movement is inherently unstable, but it can be stable in a small number of cases where the lower incisors have been trapped lingually by an increased overbite or pushed

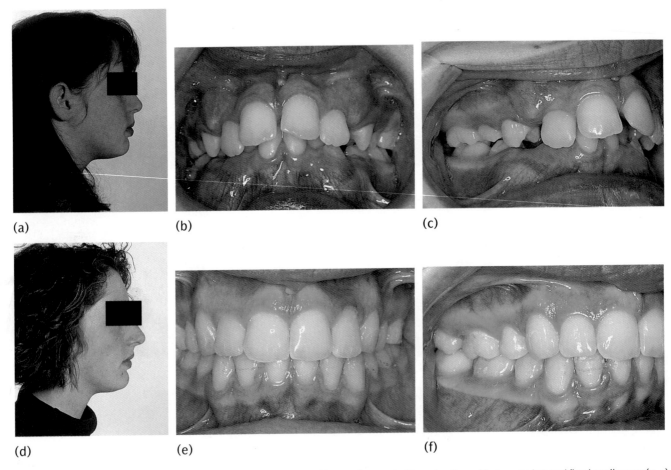

(a) (b) (c)

(d) (e) (f)

Fig. 9.12 Class II division 1 malocclusion on a Class I skeletal pattern with crowding treated by extraction of first premolars and fixed appliances: (a–c) pre-treatment; (d–f) post-treatment.

lingually by a habit or by a lower lip trap. Diagnosis of these cases is difficult and the inexperienced operator should avoid proclination of the lower labial segment. Experienced operators may plan to move the lower labial segment to improve facial and smile aesthetics and/or avoid a surgical option (see Section 7.6.2).

Unfortunately, 'gummy' smiles associated with increased vertical skeletal proportions and/or a short upper lip will often worsen as the incisors are retracted. Therefore active steps should be taken to manage this problem. Milder cases are best managed by either the use of high-pull headgear to either a functional type of appliance or a removable appliance, for example, a Maxillary Intrusion Splint (see Section 12.3.1) to try and restrain maxillary vertical development while the rest of the face grows. In severe cases of vertical maxillary excess or where there is an excessive amount of upper incisor show in an adult patient, surgery to impact the maxilla is advisable.

In cases with a severe Class II skeletal pattern, particularly where the lower facial height is significantly increased or reduced, a combination of orthodontics and surgery may be required to produce an aesthetic and stable correction of the malocclusion (see Chapter 21). The threshold for surgery is lower in adults because of a lack of growth.

9.7 Retention

Relapse encompasses the return following treatment of the original features of the malocclusion as well as long-term growth and soft tissue changes. Unfortunately it is not possible to accurately predict those patients who will relapse and so retention must be discussed with, and planned, for every patient. To aid stability, full reduction of the overjet and the achievement of lip competence are advisable. If the overjet is not fully reduced there is the risk that the lower lip will continue to function behind the upper incisors, with a subsequent relapse in incisor position. Retention is discussed more fully in Chapter 16.

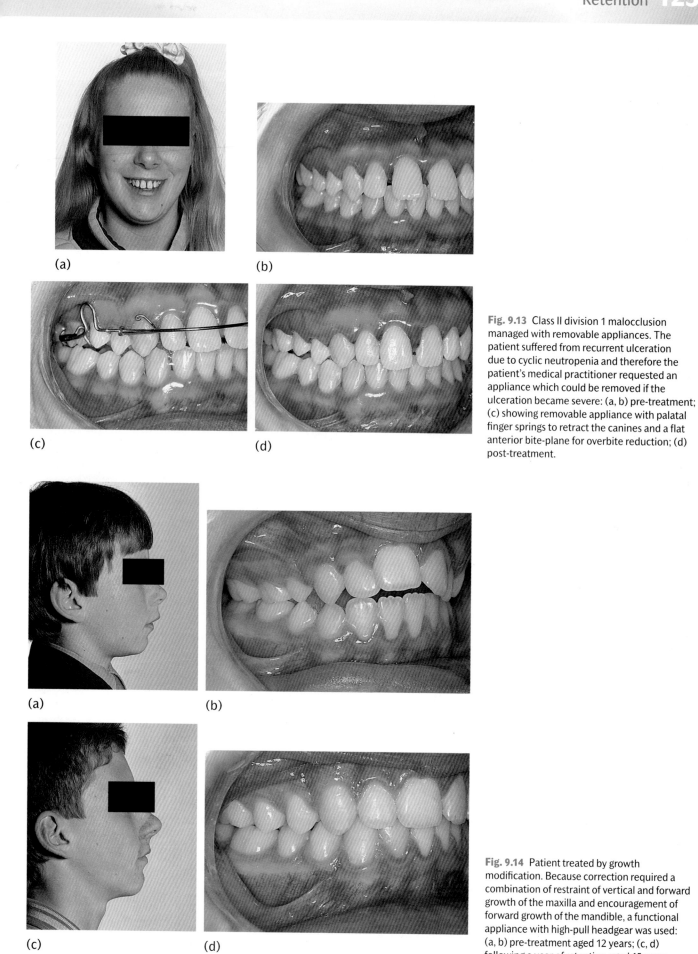

(a)

(b)

(c)

(d)

Fig. 9.13 Class II division 1 malocclusion managed with removable appliances. The patient suffered from recurrent ulceration due to cyclic neutropenia and therefore the patient's medical practitioner requested an appliance which could be removed if the ulceration became severe: (a, b) pre-treatment; (c) showing removable appliance with palatal finger springs to retract the canines and a flat anterior bite-plane for overbite reduction; (d) post-treatment.

(a)

(b)

(c)

(d)

Fig. 9.14 Patient treated by growth modification. Because correction required a combination of restraint of vertical and forward growth of the maxilla and encouragement of forward growth of the mandible, a functional appliance with high-pull headgear was used: (a, b) pre-treatment aged 12 years; (c, d) following a year of retention aged 15 years.

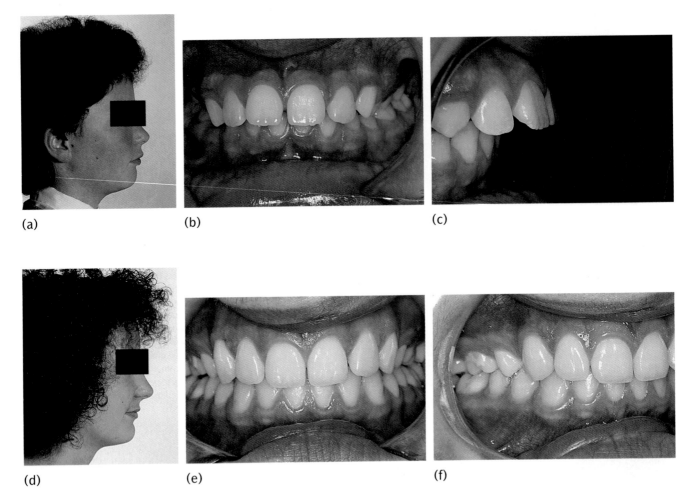

(a) (b) (c)

(d) (e) (f)

Fig. 9.15 Patient with Class II division 1 malocclusion on a moderately severe Class II skeletal pattern treated by orthodontic camouflage in which both upper first premolars were extracted to gain space for overjet reduction and fixed appliances were used for bodily retraction of the upper incisors: (a–c) pre-treatment (note the upright upper incisors); (d–f) post-retention.

Key points

- Class II/1 malocclusions are commonly associated with an underlying Class II skeletal pattern with a retrusive mandible
- For cases with an underlying Class II skeletal pattern the options are growth modification, camouflage or surgery
- Research evidence would suggest that growth modification produces limited skeletal effects over and above normal growth
- Research indicates that early (two-phase) treatment does not have any benefits over conventional treatment

---

Relevant Cochrane reviews:

Orthodontic treatment for prominent upper front teeth in children

Harrison, J.E. *et al.* (2008)

http://onlinelibrary.wiley.com/doi/10.1002/14651858.CD003452.pub2/abstract;jsessionid=8E74BEB3B88B94E94FB3DEF174A11EC4.d03t01

The evidence suggests that providing early orthodontic treatment for children with prominent upper front teeth is no more effective than providing one course of orthodontic treatment when the child is in early adolescence.

Principal sources and further reading

Banks, P. A. (1986). An analysis of complete and incomplete overbite in Class II division 1 malocclusions (an analysis of overbite incompleteness). *British Journal of Orthodontics*, **13**, 23–32.

Cozza, P., Baccetti, T., Franchi, L., De Toffo, L., and McNamara Jnr., J. A. (2006). Mandibular changes produced by functional appliances in Class II malocclusion: a systematic review. *American Journal of Orthodontics and Dentofacial Othopedics*, **129**, 559.el–12 (online article).

Marsico, E., Gatto, E., Burrascano, M., Matarese, G., and Cordasco, G. (2011). Effectiveness of orthodontic treatment with functional appliances on mandibular growth in the short term. *American Journal of Orthodontics and Dentofacial Orthopedics*, **139**, 24–36.

McGuinness, N.J.P., Burden D. J., Hunt, O.T., Johnstone, C.D., and Stevenson, M. (2011). Long-term occlusal and soft-tissue profile outcomes after treatment of Class II division 1 malocclusion treated with fixed appliances. *American Journal of Orthodontics and Dentofacial Orthopedics*, **139**, 362–8.

Nguyen, Q.V., Bezemer, P.D., Habets, L., and Prahl-Andersen, B. (1999). A systematic review of the relationship between overjet size and traumatic dental injuries. *Eurpoena Journal of Orthodontics*, **21**, 503–15.

O'Brien, K., Wright, J., Conboy, F. *et al.* (2009). Early treatment for Class II Division 1 malocclusion with the Twin-block appliance: A multicenter, randomized, controlled trial. *American Journal of Orthodontics and Dentofacial Orthopedics*, **135**, 573–9.

Tulloch, C. J. F., Proffit, W. R., and Phillips, C. (2004). Outcomes in a 2-phase randomized clinical trial of early Class II treatment. *American Journal of Orthodontics and Dentofacial Orthopedics*, **125**, 657–67.

The results of this important trial are essential reading for any clinician involved in treating patients with Class II malocclusions.

You, Z-H., Fishman, L. S., Rosenblum, R. E., and Subtelny, J. D. (2001). Dento-alveolar changes related to mandibular forward growth in untreated Class II persons. *American Journal of Orthodontics and Dentofacial Orthopedics*, **120**, 598–607.

An interesting paper which suggests that disarticulating the occlusion (for example with a functional appliance) allows normal favourable mandibular growth to be harnessed to help in the treatment of Class II malocclusions. In the absence of this freeing of the occlusion, the effects of favourable mandibular growth are masked by dento-alveolar compensation.

The British Orthodontic Society also produce two excellent Advice Sheets entitled: *Mouthguards* and *Dummy and digit sucking* which unfortunately are only available to members (so you may need to track down a BOS member and ask nicely!)

 References for this chapter can also be found at www.oxfordtextbooks.co.uk/orc/mitchell4e/. Where possible, these are presented as active links which direct you to the electronic version of the work, to help facilitate onward study. If you are a subscriber to that work (either individually or through an institution), and depending on your level of access, you may be able to peruse an abstract or the full article if available.

10

Class II division 2

Learning objectives for this chapter

- Gain an understanding of the aetiological factors which contribute to the development of a Class II division 2 incisor relationship
- Gain an appreciation of the management of Class II division 2 malocclusions based on an understanding of the probable aetiology

A Class II incisor relationship is defined by the British Standards classification as being present when the lower incisor edges occlude posterior to the cingulum plateau of the upper incisors. Class II division 2 includes those malocclusions where the upper central incisors are retroclined. The overjet is usually minimal, but may be increased. The prevalence of this malocclusion in a Caucasian population is approximately 10 per cent.

10.1 Aetiology

The majority of Class II division 2 malocclusions arise as a result of a number of interrelated skeletal and soft tissue factors.

10.1.1 Skeletal pattern

Class II division 2 malocclusion is commonly associated with a mild Class II skeletal pattern, but may also occur in association with a Class I or even a Class III dental base relationship. Where the skeletal pattern is more markedly Class II the upper incisors usually lie outside the control of the lower lip, resulting in a Class II division 1 relationship, but where the lower lip line is high relative to the upper incisors a Class II division 2 malocclusion can result.

The vertical dimension is also important in the aetiology of Class II division 2 malocclusions, and typically is reduced. A reduced lower face height occurring in conjunction with a Class II jaw relationship often results in the absence of an occlusal stop to the lower incisors, which then continue to erupt leading to an increased overbite (Fig. 10.1).

A reduced lower facial height is associated with a forward rotational pattern of growth (Chapter 4). This usually means that the mandible becomes more prognathic with growth. While this pattern of growth is helpful in reducing the severity of a Class II skeletal pattern, it also has the effect of increasing overbite (Fig. 10.2) unless an occlusal stop is created by treatment to limit further eruption of the lower incisors and to shift the axis of growth rotation to the lower incisal edges.

10.1.2 Soft tissues

The influence of the soft tissues in Class II division 2 malocclusions is usually mediated by the skeletal pattern. If the lower facial height is reduced, the lower lip line will effectively be higher relative to the crown of the upper incisors (more than the normal one-third coverage). A high lower lip line will tend to retrocline the upper incisors (Fig. 10.3). In some cases the upper lateral incisors, which have a shorter crown length, will escape the action of the lower lip and therefore lie at an average inclination, whereas the central incisors are retroclined (Fig. 10.4).

Class II division 2 incisor relationships may also result from bimaxillary retroclination caused by active muscular lips (Fig. 10.5), irrespective of the skeletal pattern.

10.1.3 Dental factors

As with other malocclusions, crowding is commonly seen in conjunction with a Class II division 2 incisor relationship. In addition, any pre-existing

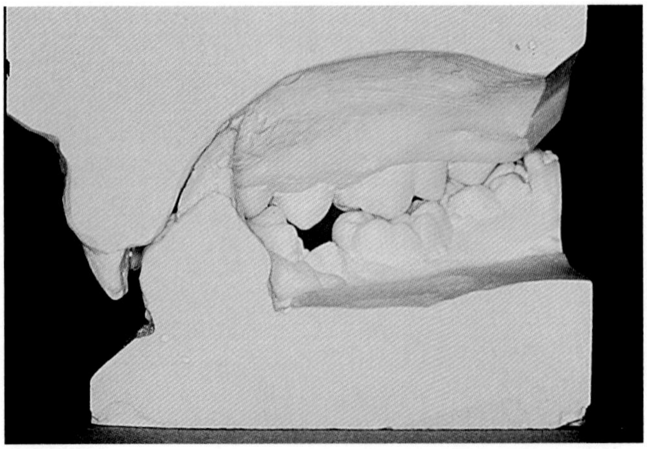

Fig. 10.1 A cross-sectional view through the study models of a patient with a very severe Class II division 2 incisor relationship. Lack of an occlusal stop allowed the incisors to continue erupting, leading to a significantly increased overbite.

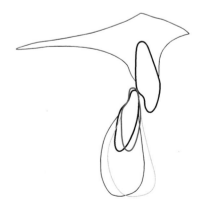

Fig. 10.2 Diagram showing how, despite a forward pattern of facial growth, the overbite can become worse in an untreated Class II division 2 incisor relationship.

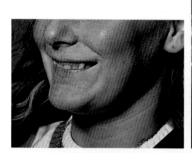

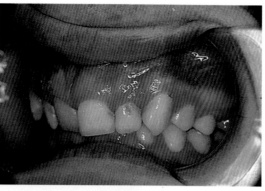

Fig. 10.3 Class II division 2 malocclusion with retroclination of all the upper incisors owing to a high lower lip line which is evident in the view of the patient smiling.

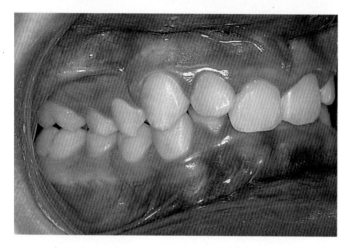

Fig. 10.4 Typical Class II division 2 malocclusion with retroclination of the upper central incisors. The lateral incisors, which are shorter, escape the effect of the lower lip and lie at an average inclination, albeit slightly mesiolabially rotated and crowded.

crowding is exacerbated because retroclination of the upper central incisors results in them being positioned in an arc of smaller circumference. In the upper labial segment this usually manifests in a lack of space for the upper lateral incisors which are crowded and are typically rotated mesiolabially out of the arch. In the same manner lower arch crowding is often exacerbated by retroclination of the lower labial segment. This can occur because the lower labial segment becomes 'trapped' lingually to the upper labial segment by an increased overbite (Fig. 10.6).

Lack of an effective occlusal stop to eruption of the lower incisors may result in their continued development, giving rise to an increased overbite. This may be due to a Class II skeletal pattern or retroclination of the incisors as a result of the action of the lips, leading to an increased inter-incisal angle. In addition, it has been found that in some Class II division 2 cases the upper central incisors exhibit a more acute crown and root angulation. However, rather than being the cause, this crown–root angulation could itself be due to the action of a high lower lip line causing deflection of the crown of the tooth relative to the root after eruption.

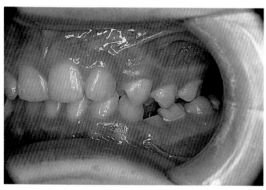

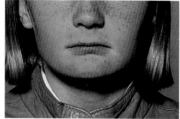

Fig. 10.5 Patient with bimaxillary retroclination due to the action of the lips.

10.2 Occlusal features

Classically, the upper central incisors are retroclined and the lateral incisors are at an average angulation or are proclined, depending upon their position relative to the lower lip (see Fig. 10.4). Where the lower lip line is very high the lateral incisors may be retroclined (see Fig. 10.3). The more severe malocclusions occur either where the underlying skeletal pattern is more Class II or where the lip musculature is active, causing bimaxillary retroclination.

In mild cases the lower incisors occlude with the upper incisors, but in patients with a more severe Class II skeletal pattern the overbite may be complete onto the palatal mucosa. In a small proportion of cases the

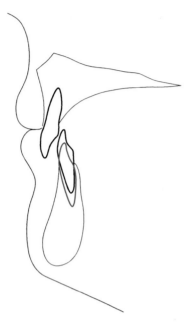

Fig. 10.6 'Trapping' of the lower incisor teeth behind the cingulum of the upper incisors in a Class II division 2 malocclusion. Note the space created labial to the lower incisor crown by reduction of the overbite (the blue line) within the soft tissue environment.

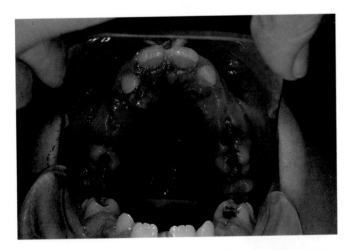

Fig. 10.7 Ulceration of the palatal mucosa of 1/1 caused by the occlusion of the lower incisor edges – an example of a traumatic overbite.

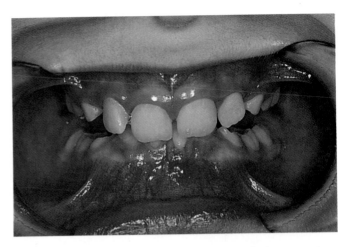

Fig. 10.8 Stripping of the labial gingivae of the lower incisors caused by the severely retroclined upper incisors – an example of a traumatic overbite.

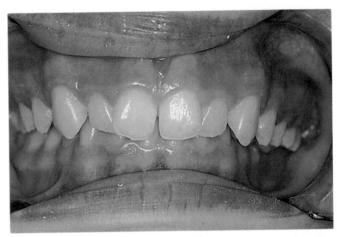

Fig. 10.9 Particularly severe lingual crossbite of the entire left buccal segment owing to a Class II skeletal pattern resulting in wider portion of upper arch occluding with narrower section of lower arch.

lower incisors may cause ulceration of the palatal tissues (Fig. 10.7), and in some patients retroclination of the upper incisors leads to stripping of the labial gingivae of the lower incisors (Fig. 10.8). In these cases the overbite is described as traumatic, but fortunately both are comparatively rare.

Another feature associated with a more severe underlying Class II skeletal pattern is lingual crossbite of the first and occasionally the second premolars (Fig. 10.9) owing to the relative positions and widths of the arches, and possibly to trapping of the lower labial segment within a retroclined upper labial segment.

10.3 Management

Stable correction of a Class II division 2 incisor relationship is difficult as it requires not only reduction of the increased overbite (discussed in Section 10.3.1), but also reduction of the inter-incisal angle which classically is increased (Fig. 10.10). If re-eruption of the incisors and therefore an increase in overbite is to be resisted, the inter-incisal angle needs to be reduced, preferably close to 135°, so that an effective occlusal stop is created (Fig. 10.11). In addition, it has been shown that stability is increased if at the end of treatment the lower incisor edge lies 0–2 mm anterior to the mid-point of the root axis of the upper incisors (this is known as the centroid; see also Section 16.3.2).

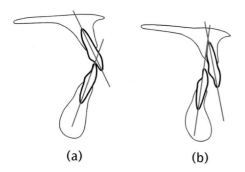

Fig. 10.10 (a) A Class I incisor relationship with an average inter-incisal angle of around 135°; (b) a Class II division 2 relationship where the inter-incisal angle is increased.

The inter-incisal angle in a Class II division 2 malocclusion can be reduced in a number of ways:

- Torquing the incisor roots palatally/lingually with a fixed appliance (Fig. 10.12).
- Proclination of the lower labial segment (Fig. 10.13). This approach should only be employed by the experienced practitioner as, although it provides additional space for alignment of the lower incisor teeth, any excessive movement of the lower arch would increase the risk of relapse.
- Proclination of the upper labial segment followed by use of a functional appliance to reduce the resultant overjet and achieve intermaxillary correction (Fig. 10.14).
- A combination of the above approaches.
- Orthognathic surgery. This approach may be the only alternative for patients with a marked Class II skeletal pattern and/or reduced vertical skeletal proportions.

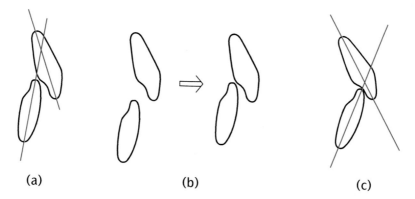

Fig. 10.11 If a Class II division 2 incisor relationship is to be corrected not only the overbite but also the inter-incisal angle must be reduced to prevent re-eruption of the incisors post-treatment: (a) Class II division 2 incisor relationship; (b) reduction of the overbite alone will not be stable as the incisors will re-erupt following removal of appliances; (c) reduction of the inter-incisal angle in conjunction with reduction of the overbite has a greater chance of stability.

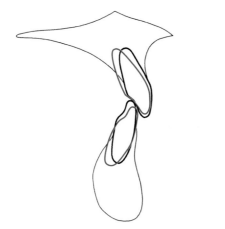

Fig. 10.12 Correction of a Class II division 2 incisor relationship by reducing the overbite and torquing the incisors lingually/palatally. Fixed appliances are necessary.

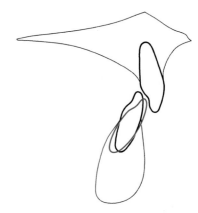

Fig. 10.13 Correction of a Class II division 2 incisor relationship by proclination of the lower labial segment.

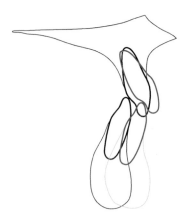

Fig. 10.14 Correction of a Class II division 2 incisor relationship by an initial phase involving proclination of the upper incisors, followed by reduction of the resultant overjet with a functional appliance.

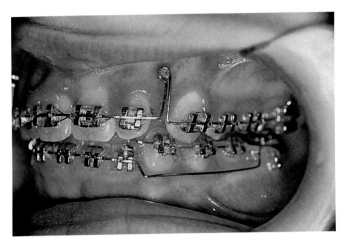

Fig. 10.15 Lower utility arch for overbite reduction. Note the difference in level between the lower incisor brackets and the buccal segment teeth.

The treatment approach chosen for a particular patient will depend upon the aetiology of the malocclusion, the presence and degree of crowding, the patient's profile, their age and their wishes.

Consideration of the approach to be used for correcting the incisor relationship will influence decisions regarding anchorage requirements and whether extractions are required to relieve crowding and to provide space for incisor alignment. Some practitioners have argued that closure of excess extraction space in a Class II division 2 malocclusion will result in further retroclination of the labial segments and a 'dished-in profile'. This claim is usually made in association with the presentation of isolated case reports. However, research using groups of carefully matched patients has shown that there is little difference in the amount of retraction of the lips between extraction and non-extraction treatment approaches. Nevertheless, it would seem advisable in the management of Class II division 2 malocclusions to minimize lingual movement of the lower incisors in order to avoid any possibility of worsening the patient's overbite; indeed, it may be preferable to accept some proclination of the lower incisors and permanent retention rather than run this risk. Certainly, extraction of permanent teeth in the lower arch in Class II division 2 malocclusions should be approached with caution, and if any doubt exists specialist advice should be sought. In addition, clinical experience suggests that space closure occurs less readily in patients with reduced vertical skeletal proportions, which are commonly associated with Class II division 2 malocclusions, than in those with increased lower face heights. In view of this, it is not surprising that Class II division 2 malocclusions are managed more frequently on a non-extraction basis, particularly in the lower arch, than are other types of malocclusion.

Proclination of the lower incisors is helpful in reducing both overbite and the inter-incisal angle. In general, proclination of the lower labial segment should be considered unstable, but it has been argued that in some Class II division 2 malocclusions due to the increased overbite, the lower labial segment is trapped behind the upper labial segment, resulting in retroclination of the lower incisors and constriction of the lower intercanine width with growth. This means that a limited increase in intercanine width and a degree of proclination of the lower labial segment can be stable in such cases. However, in the majority of patients

movement of the lower labial segment labially increases the likelihood of relapse therefore patients need to be advised of and accept the need for prolonged retention (Chapter 16). It is also advisable to assess the lower labial supporting tissues to avoid iatrogenic gingival recession.

This discussion will have highlighted some of the difficulties in managing Class II division 2 malocclusions. It is also worth noting that a recent Cochrane review could not advocate any treatment approach over another.

10.3.1 Approaches to the reduction of overbite

Intrusion of the incisors

Actual intrusion of the incisors is difficult to achieve. Fixed appliances are necessary and the mechanics employed pit intrusion of the incisors against extrusion of the buccal segment teeth; as it is easier to move the molars occlusally than to intrude the incisors into bone, the former tends to predominate. In practice, the effects achieved are relative intrusion, where the incisors are held still while vertical growth of the face occurs around them, plus extrusion of the molars.

Increasing anchorage by using temporary anchorage screws or by reinforcing the anchorage unit posteriorly by including second permanent molars (or even third molars in adults) will aid intrusion of the incisors and help to limit extrusion of the molars. Arches which bypass the canines and premolars to pit the incisors against the molars, for example the utility arch (Fig. 10.15), are employed with some success to reduce overbite by intrusion of the incisors, although some molar extrusion does occur.

Eruption of the molars

Use of a flat anterior bite-plane on an upper removable appliance to free the occlusion of the buccal segment teeth will, if worn conscientiously, limit further occlusal movement of the incisors and allow the lower molars to erupt, thus reducing the overbite. This method requires a growing patient to accommodate the increase in vertical dimension that results, otherwise the molars will re-intrude under the forces of occlusion once the appliance is withdrawn. However, this tendency can be resisted to a degree if the treatment creates an effective occlusal stop and reduction of the inter-incisal angle.

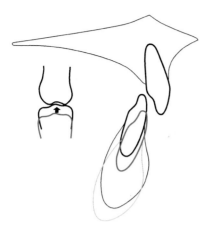

Fig. 10.16 Diagram to show spontaneous proclination of the lower labial segment following placement of a flat anterior bite-plane which has reduced the overbite by eruption of the lower molars.

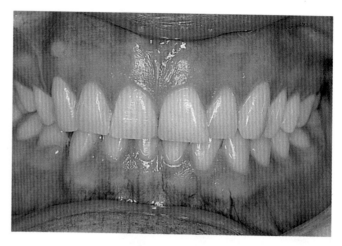

Fig. 10.17 An acceptable mild Class II division 2 incisor relationship.

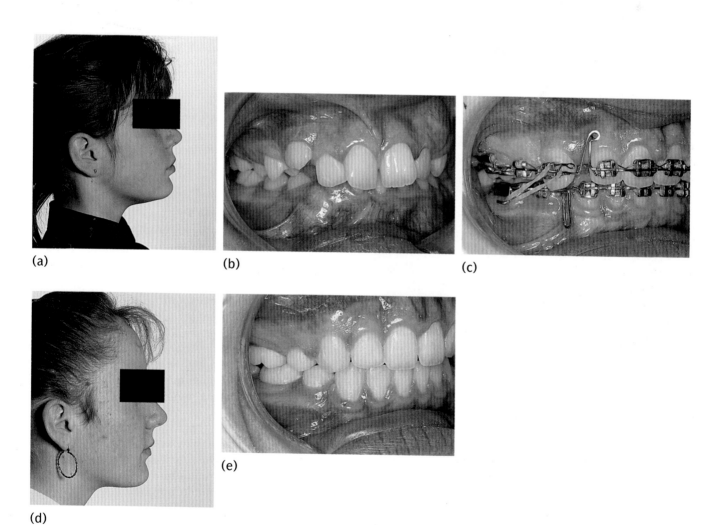

(a)   (b)   (c)

(d)   (e)

Fig. 10.18 Patient aged 12 years with a Class II division 2 incisor relationship on a Class I skeletal pattern with crowded and rotated incisors. The second premolars were extracted and fixed appliances were used to achieve alignment and correction of the incisor relationship: (a, b) pre-treatment; (c) during treatment; (d, e) at end of treatment (note favourable mandibular growth).

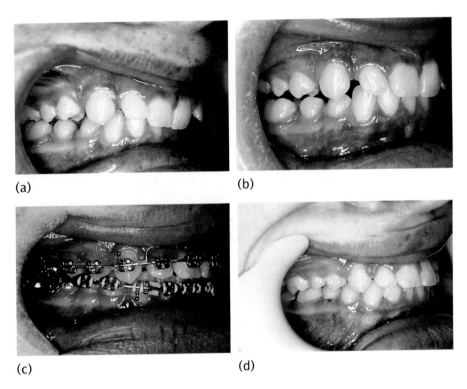

(a)

(b)

(c)

(d)

Fig. 10.19 Class II division 2 malocclusion treated initially with a twin-block appliance, which incorporated a double cantilever spring to procline the retroclined upper central incisors. Then fixed appliances were used to detail the occlusion: (a) pre-treatment; (b) at end of the functional phase; (c) fixed appliance phase; (d) end of active treatment.

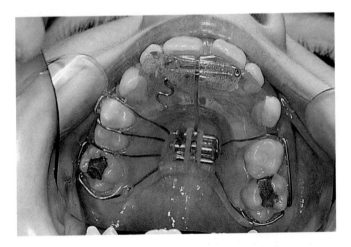

Fig. 10.20 An upper removable appliance used to expand the upper arch and procline retroclined upper incisors prior to functional appliance therapy.

Extrusion of the molars

As mentioned above, the major effect of attempting intrusion of the incisors is often extrusion of the molars. This may be advantageous in Class II division 2 cases as this type of malocclusion is usually associated with reduced vertical proportions. Again, vertical growth is required if the overbite reduction achieved in this way is to be stable.

Proclination of the lower incisors

Advancement of the lower labial segment anteriorly will result in a reduction of overbite as the incisors tip labially. This approach should only be carried out by the experienced orthodontist (see Section

10.3.2). However, in a few cases where the lower incisors have been trapped behind the upper labial segment by an increased overbite, fitting of an upper bite-plane appliance may allow the lower labial segment to procline spontaneously (Fig. 10.16).

Surgery

In adults with a markedly increased overbite and those patients where the underlying skeletal pattern is more markedly Class II, a combination of orthodontics and surgery is required.

10.3.2 Practical management

In milder cases, where the overbite is slightly increased, the arches are not significantly crowded and the aesthetics acceptable, it may be prudent to accept the malocclusion (Fig. 10.17).

Where treatment is indicated there are three possible treatment modalities as described below. The use of temporary skeletal anchorage devices has allowed clinicians to successfully treat more severe Class II/2 maloccusions with orthodontics alone.

Fixed appliances

When fixed appliances are used the inter-incisal angle can be reduced by palatal/lingual root torque or by proclination of the lower incisors. The relative role of these two approaches in the management of a particular malocclusion is a matter of fine judgement.

Torquing of incisor apices is dependent upon the presence of sufficient cortical bone palatally/lingually and places a considerable strain on anchorage. This type of movement is also more likely to result in resorption of the root apices than other types of tooth movement.

Mild crowding in the lower arch may be eliminated by forward movement of the lower labial segment and/or interdental stripping.

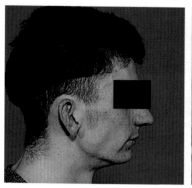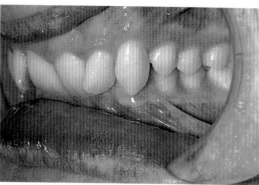

Fig. 10.21 Adult patient with severe Class II division 2 malocclusion on a marked Class II skeletal pattern with reduced vertical proportions. It was decided that a combined orthodontic and orthognathic surgery approach was required to correct this malocclusion.

Key points

- Careful assessment of the aetiological factors contributing to the incisor relationship and the degree to which they can be reduced or eliminated is essential if treatment is to be successful
- The threshold for extractions in the lower arch is raised compared with other malocclusions
- To increase the chances of a stable reduction in overbite, the inter-incisal angle needs to be reduced and an adequate occlusal stop for the lower incisors created

---

If crowding is more marked, extractions will be required and a lower fixed appliance used to ensure that space closure occurs without movement of the lower incisor edges lingually (Fig. 10.18). For this reason lower second premolars are often extracted rather than first premolars.

Space for correction of the incisor relationship and for relief of crowding, if indicated, can be gained by upper arch extractions or by distal movement of the upper buccal segments. If headgear is used for anchorage or distal movement, a direction of pull below the occlusal plane (cervical pull) is usually indicated in Class II division 2 malocclusions as the vertical facial proportions are reduced. A lingual crossbite, if present, usually affects the first premolars only. If extraction of the upper first premolars is not indicated, or if the second premolars are involved, elimination of the crossbite will involve a combination of contraction across the affected upper teeth and expansion of the lower premolar width. Following treatment, the prognosis for the corrected position is good as cuspal interlock will help to prevent relapse.

The retention phase is particularly important in Class II division 2 malocclusions, with regard to the following:

- to prevent an increase in overbite
- to retain any de-rotated teeth, for example, the upper lateral incisors
- to maintain alignment of the lower labial segment, particularly if it has been proclined during treatment

For further details see Chapter 16.

Functional appliances

See also Section 19.6.2

Functional appliances can be utilized in the correction of Class II division 2 malocclusions in growing patients with a mild to moderate Class II skeletal pattern (Fig. 10.19). Reduction of the inter-incisal angle is achieved mainly by proclination of the upper incisors, although some proclination of the lower labial segment may occur as a result of the functional appliance. If the upper incisors are retroclined it may be helpful to have a pre-functional phase to procline them and, if indicated to ensure the correct buccolingual

arch relationship at the end of treatment, to expand the upper arch. This can be achieved using a removable appliance (Fig. 10.20) which is known as an ELSAA (Expansion and Labial Segment Alignment Appliance). If a twin-block functional appliance is used, then a spring to procline the incisors can be incorporated into the upper appliance (see Fig. 19.2). Alternatively a sectional-fixed appliance can be placed on the upper labial segment teeth to achieve their alignment during the functional phase.

After anteroposterior correction with the functional appliance, fixed appliances are required to detail the occlusion. If the lower incisors have been proclined, the stability of their position should be assessed and, if doubtful, permanent retention should be instituted.

Surgery

See Chapter 20

A stable aesthetic orthodontic correction may not be possible in patients with an unfavourable skeletal pattern anteroposteriorly and/or vertically, particularly if growth is complete (Fig. 10.21). In these cases surgery may be necessary (see Chapter 21). A phase of presurgical orthodontics is required to align the teeth. However, arch levelling is usually not completed as extrusion of the molars is much more easily accomplished after surgery (see Section 21.8.2).

Relevant Cochrane reviews:

Orthodontic treatment for deep bite and retroclined upper front teeth in children.
Millett, D. T. *et al.* (2009).
http://onlinelibrary.wiley.com/doi/10.1002/14651858.CD005972.pub2/full
Authors concluded it was not possible to provide any evidence-based guidance to clinicians and patients with respect to the management of this malocclusion in children.

Principal sources and further reading

Baccetti, T., Franchi, L., and McNamara, J. (2011). Longitudinal growth changes in subjects with deepbite. *American Journal of Orthodontics and Dentofacial Orthopedics*, **140**, 202–9.

Burstone, C. R. (1977). Deep overbite correction by intrusion. *American Journal of Orthodontics*, **72**, 1–22.

A useful paper for the more experienced orthodontist using fixed appliances.

Dyer, F. M., McKeown, H. F., and Sandler, P. J. (2001). The modified twin block appliance in the treatment of Class II division 2 malocclusions. *Journal of Orthodontics*, **28**, 271–80.

Describes with beautiful illustrations the management of two Class II division 2 cases treated with functional and fixed appliances.

Lee, R. T. (1999). Arch width and form: a review. *American Journal of Orthodontics and Dentofacial Orthopedics*, **115**, 305–13.

A classic article.

Leighton, B. C. and Adams, C. P. (1986). Incisor inclination in Class II division 2 malocclusions. *European Journal of Orthodontics*, **8**, 98–105.

Kim, T. W. and Little, R. M. (1999). Post retention assessment of deep overbite correction in Class II division 2 malocclusion. *Angle Orthodontist*, **69**, 175–86.

Melsen, B. and Allais, D. (2005). Factors of importance for the development of dehiscences during labial movement of mandibular incisors: a retrospective study of adult orthodontic patients. *American Journal of Orthodontics and Dentofacial Orthopedics*, **127**, 552–61.

Although this is a retrospective study, it does have a sample size of 150 adults. The authors concluded that thin gingivae pre-treatment, presence of plaque and inflammation were useful predictors of gingival recession.

Millett, D.T., Cunningham, S., O'Brien, D., Benson, P., and de Oliveira, C.M. (2012). Treatment and stability of Class II Division 2 malocclusion in children and adolescents: A systematic review. *American Journal of Orthodontics and Dentofacial Orthopedics*, **142**, 159–69. e9

http://www.ajodo.org/article/S0889-5406(12)00404-0/abstract

Ng, J., Major, P. W., Heo, G., and Flores-Mir, C. (2005). True incisor intrusion attained during orthodontic treatment: A systematic review and meta-analysis. *American Journal of Orthodontics and Dentofacial Orthopedics*, **128**, 212–19.

Authors found limited true incisor intrusion in non-growing patients.

Selwyn-Barnett, B. J. (1991). Rationale of treatment for Class II division 2 malocclusion. *British Journal of Orthodontics*, **18**, 173–81.

This paper contains a carefully constructed argument for management of Class II division 2 malocclusion by proclination of the lower labial segment rather than extractions, in order to avoid detrimental effects upon the profile.

References for this chapter can also be found at www.oxfordtextbooks.co.uk/orc/mitchell4e/. Where possible, these are presented as active links which direct you to the electronic version of the work, to help facilitate onward study. If you are a subscriber to that work (either individually or through an institution), and depending on your level of access, you may be able to peruse an abstract or the full article if available.

11

Class III

Chapter contents

The British Standards definition of Class III incisor relationship includes those malocclusions where the lower incisor edge occludes anterior to the cingulum plateau of the upper incisors. Class III malocclusions affect around 3 per cent of Caucasians.

11.1 Aetiology

11.1.1 Skeletal pattern

The skeletal relationship is the most important factor in the aetiology of most Class III malocclusions, and the majority of Class III incisor relationships are associated with an underlying Class III skeletal relationship. Cephalometric studies have shown that, compared with Class I occlusions, Class III malocclusions exhibit the following:

• increased mandibular length;

• a more anteriorly placed glenoid fossa so that the condylar head is positioned more anteriorly leading to mandibular prognathism;

• reduced maxillary length;

• a more retruded position of the maxilla leading to maxillary retrusion.

The first two of these factors are the most influential. Figure 11.1 shows a patient with a Class III malocclusion with mandibular prognathism and Fig. 11.2 illustrates maxillary retrognathia (maxillary retrusion).

Class III malocclusions occur in association with a range of vertical skeletal proportions, ranging from increased to reduced. A backward opening rotation pattern of facial growth will tend to result in a reduction of overbite; however, a forward rotating pattern of facial growth will lead to an increase in the prominence of the chin.

There is evidence to indicate that Class III skeletal patterns exhibit less maxillary growth and more mandibular growth than Class I skeletal patterns.

11.1.2 Soft tissues

In the majority of Class III malocclusions the soft tissues do not play a major aetiological role. In fact the reverse is often the case, with the soft tissues tending to tilt the upper and lower incisors towards each other so that the incisor relationship is often less severe than the underlying skeletal pattern. This dento-alveolar compensation occurs in Class III malocclusions because an anterior oral seal can frequently be achieved by upper to lower lip contact. This has the effect of moulding the upper and lower labial segments towards each other. The main exception occurs in patients with increased vertical skeletal proportions where the lips are more likely to be incompetent and an anterior oral seal is often accomplished by tongue to lower lip contact.

11.1.3 Dental factors

Class III malocclusions are often associated with a narrow upper arch and a broad lower arch, with the result that crowding is seen more commonly, and to a greater degree, in the upper arch than in the lower. Frequently, the lower arch is well aligned or even spaced.

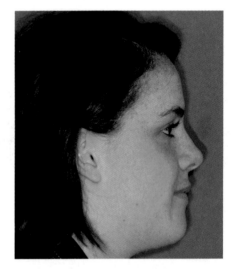

Fig. 11.1 Patient with mandibular prognathism.

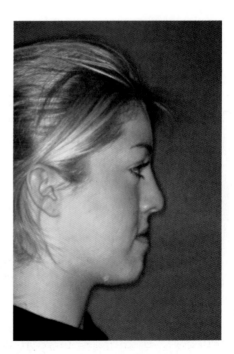

Fig. 11.2 Patient with maxillary retrognathia.

11.2 Occlusal features

By definition Class III malocclusions occur when the lower incisors are positioned more labially relative to the upper incisors. Therefore an anterior crossbite of one or more of the incisors is a common feature of Class III malocclusions. As with any crossbite, it is essential to check for a displacement of the mandible on closure from a premature contact into maximal interdigitation. In Class III malocclusions this can be ascertained by asking the patient to try to achieve an edge-to-edge incisor position. If such a displacement is present, the prognosis for correction of the incisor relationship is more favourable. In the past it was thought that such a displacement led to overclosure and greater prominence of the mandible, with the condylar head displaced forward. In fact cephalometric studies suggest that in most cases, although there is a forward displacement of the mandible to disengage the premature contact of the incisors as closure into occlusion occurs, the mandible moves backwards until the condyles regain their normal position within the glenoid fossa (Fig. 11.3).

Another common feature of Class III malocclusions is buccal crossbite, which is usually due to a discrepancy in the relative width of the arches. This occurs because the lower arch is positioned relatively more anteriorly in Class III malocclusions and is often well developed, while the upper arch is narrow. This is also reflected in the relative crowding within the arches with the upper arch commonly more crowded (Fig. 11.4).

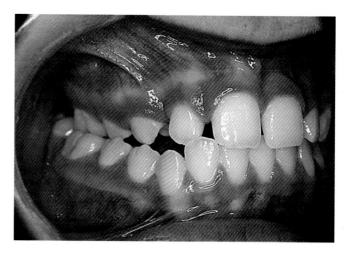

Fig. 11.4 A Class III malocclusion with a narrow crowded upper arch and a broader less crowded lower arch with associated buccal crossbite.

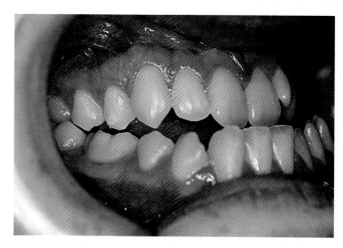

Fig. 11.5 Dento-alveolar compensation.

As mentioned above, Class III malocclusions often exhibit dento-alveolar compensation with the upper incisors proclined and the lower incisors retroclined, which reduces the severity of the incisor relationship (Fig. 11.5).

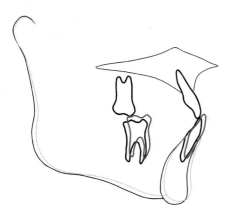

Fig. 11.3 Diagram illustrating the path of closure in a Class III malocclusion from an edge-to-edge incisor relationship into maximal occlusion. Although the mandible is displaced forwards from the initial contact of the incisors to achieve maximal interdigitation, the condylar head is not displaced out of the glenoid fossa.

11.3 Treatment planning in Class III malocclusions

A number of factors should be considered before planning treatment.

The patient's opinion regarding their occlusion and facial appearance must be taken into account. This subject needs to be approached with some tact.

The severity of the skeletal pattern, both anteroposteriorly and vertically, should be assessed. This is the major determinant of the difficulty and prognosis of orthodontic treatment.

The amount and expected pattern of future growth, both anteroposteriorly and vertically, should be considered. It is important to remember that average growth will tend to result in a worsening of the relationship between the arches, and a significant deterioration can be anticipated if growth is unfavourable. When evaluating the likely direction and extent of facial growth, the patient's age, sex, facial pattern and family history of Class III malocclusions should be taken into consideration (see Chapter 4). Children with increased vertical skeletal proportions often continue to exhibit a vertical pattern of growth, which will have the effect of reducing incisor overbite. For patients on the borderline between different management regimes it is wise to err on the side of pessimism (as growth will often prove this to be correct).

In Class III malocclusions a normal or increased overbite is an advantage, as sufficient vertical overlap of the upper incisors with the lower incisors post-treatment is vital for stability.

If the patient can achieve an edge-to-edge incisor contact and then displaces forwards into a reverse overjet, this increases the prognosis for correction of the incisor relationship.

In general, orthodontic management of Class III malocclusion will aim to increase dento-alveolar compensation. Therefore, if considerable dento-alveolar compensation is already present, trying to increase it further may not be an aesthetic or stable treatment option. Cephalometrically it has been suggested that an upper incisor angle of 120° to the maxillary plane and a lower incisor angle of 80° to the mandibular plane, are the limits of acceptable compromise.

The degree of crowding in each arch should be considered. In Class III malocclusions crowding occurs more frequently, and to a greater degree, in the upper arch than in the lower. Extractions in the upper arch only should be resisted as this will often lead to a worsening of the incisor relationship. Where upper arch extractions are necessary, it is advisable to extract at least as far forwards in the lower arch.

Using headgear for distal movement of the upper buccal segments to gain space for alignment is inadvisable in Class III malocclusions as this will have the effect of restraining growth of the maxilla.

Functional appliances are less widely used in Class III malocclusions because it is difficult for patients to posture posteriorly to achieve an active working bite. However, they can be useful in mild cases in the mixed dentition where a combination of proclination of the upper incisors together with retroclination of the lower incisors is required.

In patients with a severe Class III skeletal pattern and/or reduced overbite, the possibility that a surgical approach may ultimately be required must be considered, particularly before any permanent extractions are undertaken (see Section 11.4.4).

Box 11.1 summarizes those features which need to be considered when planning treatment in Class III patients.

11.4 Treatment options

11.4.1 Accepting the incisor relationship

In mild Class III malocclusions, particularly those cases where the overbite is minimal, it may be preferable to accept the incisor relationship and direct treatment towards achieving arch alignment (Fig. 11.6).

Also some patients with more severe Class III incisor relationships are unwilling to undergo comprehensive treatment involving orthognathic surgery which would be required to correct their incisor relationship and opt instead for upper arch alignment only.

11.4.2 Early orthopaedic treatment

This is an area of orthodontics that is attracting considerable attention. Orthopaedic correction of Class III malocclusions aims to enhance or encourage maxillary growth and/or restrain or re-direct mandibular growth. Although a number of different treatment modalities have been shown to be successful in the short to mid-term, given the propensity for unfavourable growth in skeletal Class III, the results of long-term follow-up are awaited with interest. There is an increasing body of evidence that orthopaedic correction treatment is more likely to be successful if it is carried out prior to the pubertal growth spurt.

- Protraction face-mask used to advance the maxilla. The forces applied in this technique are in the region of 400 g per side and a

co-operative patient is necessary to achieve the 14 hours per day wear required (Fig. 11.7). A recent multi-centre randomized controlled trial in patients under the age of 10 years showed a success rate of 70 per cent in terms of achieving a positive overjet over a follow-up period of 15 months. A number of workers advocate the use of

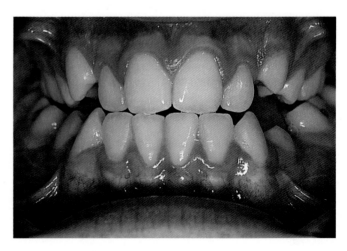

Fig. 11.6 Mild Class III case where it was decided to accept the incisor relationship and direct treatment towards alignment of the arches only.

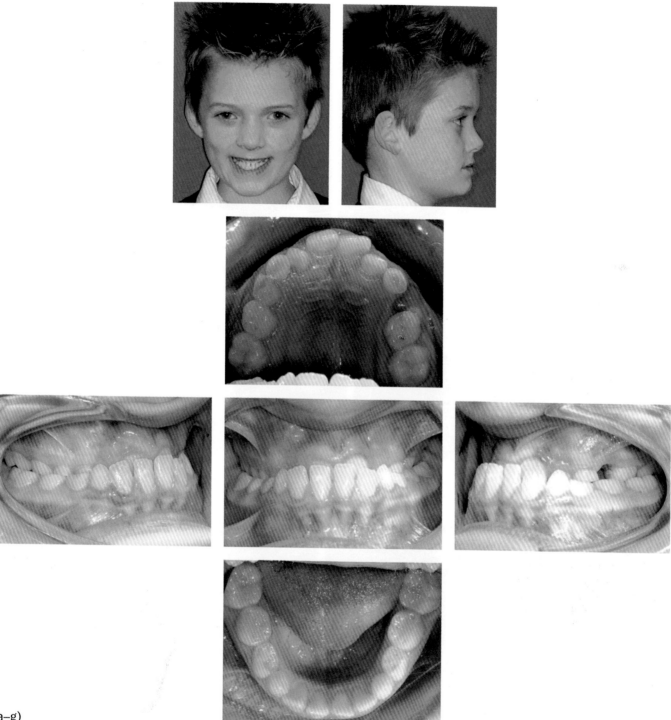

(a–g)

Fig. 11.7 Patient treated by reverse head-gear and rapid maxillary expansion. (a–g) pre-treatment; (h–k) showing face mask and rapid maxillary expansion appliance which was cemented in position. Elastic traction was applied from the hooks on the intra-oral appliance adjacent to the first deciduous molars to hooks on the face frame; (l–n) after 10 months of treatment; (o–s) 2 years after completion of treatment showing good stability. Case treated by and reproduced with the kind permission of Simon Littlewood.

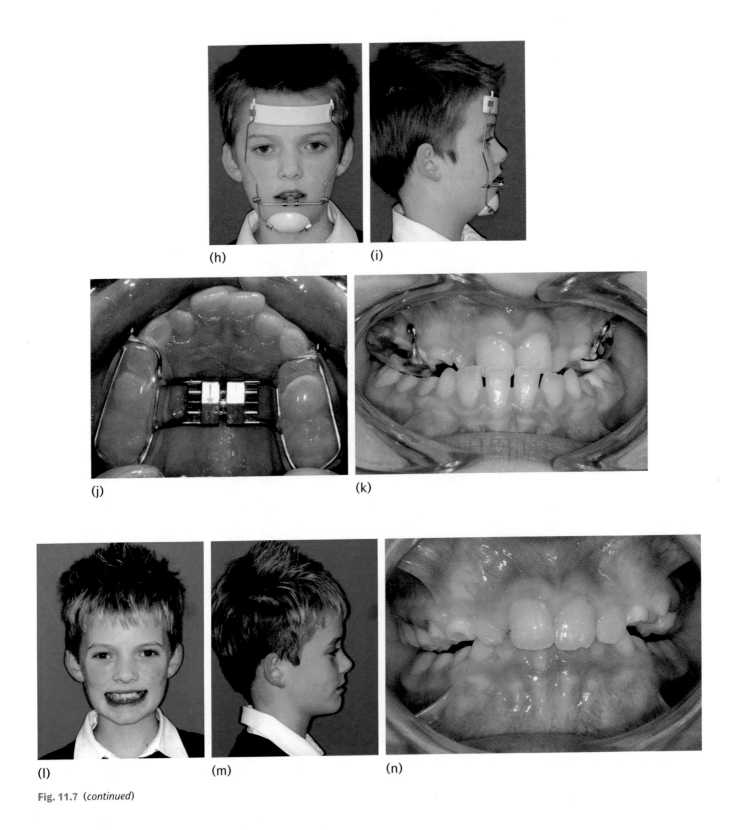

(h)

(i)

(j)

(k)

(l)

(m)

(n)

Fig. 11.7 (*continued*)

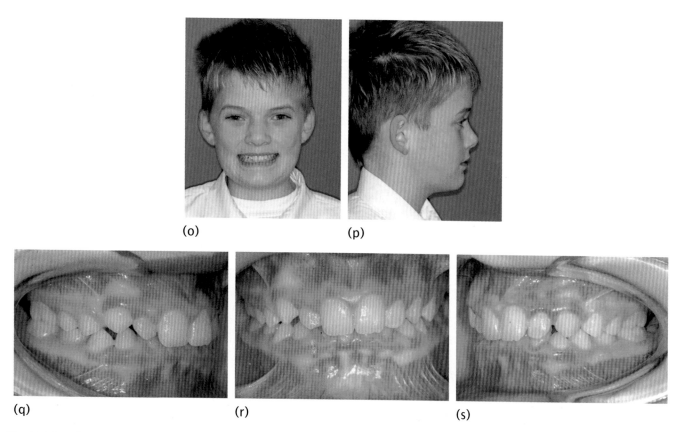

(o)   (p)

(q)   (r)   (s)

Fig. 11.7 (*continued*)

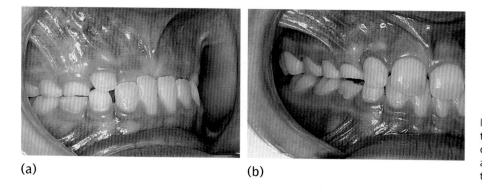

(a)   (b)

Fig. 11.8 Mild Class III malocclusion that was treated in the mixed dentition by proclination of the upper labial segment with a removable appliance: (a) pre-treatment; (b) post-treatment.

rapid maxillary expansion (see Section 13.4.5) in conjunction with protraction face-mask therapy, however, more recent work has suggested that this additional appliance is not essential to success.

- Bone anchored maxillary protraction (known as BAMP). Screws or mini-plates are used in the posterior maxilla and anterior mandible for Class III elastics. There is some evidence to show that a greater degree of maxillary advancement is achieved than with face-mask therapy alone.

- A combination of these two techniques – elastics are run between skeletal anchorage in the maxilla and a face mask.

- Chin-cup – this has the effect of rotating the mandible downwards and backwards with a reduction of overbite so is largely historic.

11.4.3 Orthodontic camouflage

Correction of an anterior crossbite in a Class I or mild Class III skeletal pattern can be undertaken in the mixed dentition when the unerupted permanent canines are high above the roots of the upper lateral incisors (Fig. 11.8). Extraction of the lower deciduous canines at the same time may allow the lower labial segment to move lingually slightly. Early correction of a Class III incisor relationship has the advantage that further forward mandibular growth may be counter-balanced by dento-alveolar compensation (Fig. 11.9). Later in the mixed dentition when the developing canines drop down into a buccal position relative to the lateral incisor root there may be a risk of resorption if the incisors are moved labially. In this situation correction is then best deferred until the permanent canines have erupted.

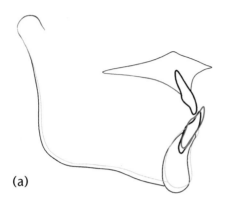

(a)

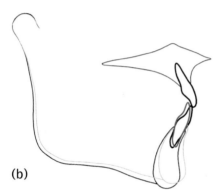

(b)

Fig. 11.9 (a) Forward growth rotation is the most common pattern of mandibular growth. In a Class III malocclusion this will lead to a worsening of the skeletal pattern and the incisor relationship. (b) If a Class III incisor relationship is corrected in the mixed dentition, dento-alveolar compensation may help to mask the effects of further growth provided that this is not marked.

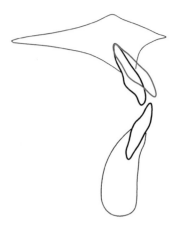

Fig. 11.10 Diagram to show how proclination of the upper incisors results in a reduction of overbite.

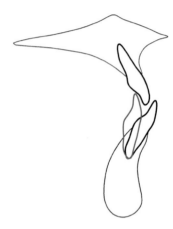

Fig. 11.11 Diagram to show how retroclination of the lower incisors results in an increase of overbite.

Orthodontic correction of a Class III incisor relationship can be achieved by proclination of the upper incisors, retroclination of the lower incisors or a combination of both. Proclination of the upper incisors reduces the overbite (Fig. 11.10) whereas retroclination of the lower incisors helps to increase overbite (Fig. 11.11). Although the pitfalls of significant movement of the lower labial segment have been emphasized in earlier chapters, in the correction of Class III malocclusions the positions of the upper and lower incisors are changed around within the zone of soft tissue balance and, provided that there is an adequate overbite and further growth is not unfavourable, the corrected incisor relationship has a good chance of stability. Although functional appliances can be used to advance the upper incisors and retrocline the lower incisors, in practice these tooth movements are accomplished more efficiently with fixed appliances.

Space for relief of crowding in the upper arch can often be gained by expansion of the arch anteriorly to correct the incisor relationship and/or buccolingually to correct buccal segment crossbites. Therefore, it may be prudent to delay permanent extractions until after the crossbite is corrected and the degree of crowding is reassessed. Expansion of the upper arch to correct a crossbite will have the effect of reducing overbite, which is a disadvantage in Class III cases. This reduction in overbite occurs because expansion of the upper arch is achieved primarily by tilting the upper premolars and molars buccally, which results in the palatal cusps of these teeth swinging down and 'propping open' the occlusion (see Fig. 13.9). Therefore, if upper arch expansion is indicated and the overbite is reduced, expansion should be achieved using rectangular archwires with buccal root torque added to try and minimize this sequelae.

Space is required in the lower arch for retroclination of the lower labial segment, and therefore extractions may be required unless the arch is naturally spaced. Use of a round archwire in the lower arch and a rectangular arch in the upper arch along with judicious space closure can be used to help correct the incisor relationship (Fig. 11.12).

Intermaxillary Class III elastic traction (see Chapter 15, Section 15.4.6) from the lower labial segment to the upper molars (Fig. 11.13) can also be used to help move the upper arch forwards and the lower arch backwards, but care is required to avoid extrusion of the molars which will reduce overbite.

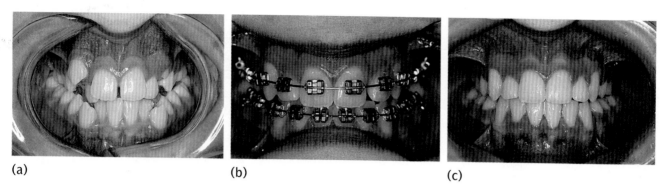

(a)   (b)   (c)

Fig. 11.12 Correction of a Class III malocclusion by retroclination of the lower incisors and proclination of the upper incisors using fixed appliances with relief of crowding by the extraction of all four first premolars: (a) pre-treatment; (b) fixed appliances *in situ* (note the use of rectangular archwire in the upper arch and a round wire in the lower arch during space closure to help achieve the desired movements); (c) post-treatment result.

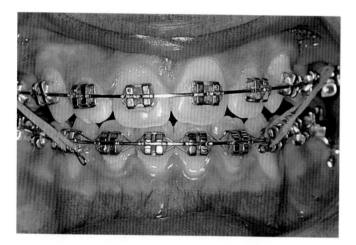

Fig. 11.13 Class III intermaxillary traction.

Recent work has shown good outcomes if headgear to the mandibular dentition is used in conjunction with conventional fixed appliance treatment.

A patient treated using orthodontic camouflage is shown in Fig. 11.14.

11.4.4 Surgery

In a proportion of cases the severity of the skeletal pattern and/or the presence of a reduced overbite or an anterior open bite preclude orthodontics alone, and surgery is necessary to correct the underlying skeletal discrepancy. It is impossible to produce hard and fast guidelines as to when to choose surgery rather than orthodontic camouflage, but it

has been suggested that surgery is almost always required if the value for the ANB angle is below –4° and the inclination of the lower incisors to the mandibular plane is less than 80°. However, the cephalometric findings, in all three planes of space, should be considered in conjunction with the patient's concerns and facial appearance.

For those patients where orthodontic treatment will be challenging owing to the severity of the skeletal pattern and/or a lack of overbite, a surgical approach should be considered before any permanent extractions are carried out, and preferably before any appliance treatment. The reason for this is that management of Class III malocclusions by orthodontics alone involves dento-alveolar compensation for the underlying skeletal pattern. However, in order to achieve a satisfactory occlusal and facial result with a surgical approach, any dento-alveolar compensation must first be removed or reduced (Fig. 11.15). For example, if lower premolars are extracted in an attempt to retract the lower labial segment but this fails and a surgical approach is subsequently necessary, the pre-surgical orthodontic phase will probably involve proclination of the incisors to a more average inclination with re-opening of the extraction spaces. This is a frustrating experience for both patient and operator.

Because the actual surgery needs to be delayed until the growth rate has diminished to adult levels, planning and commencement of a combined orthodontic and orthognathic approach is best delayed until age 15 years in girls and age 16 years in boys. This has the advantage that the patient is of an age when they can make up their own mind as to whether they wish to proceed with a combined approach. An example of a patient treated by a combination of orthodontics and surgery is shown in Fig. 11.16. Surgical approaches to the correction of Class III malocclusions are considered in Chapter 21.

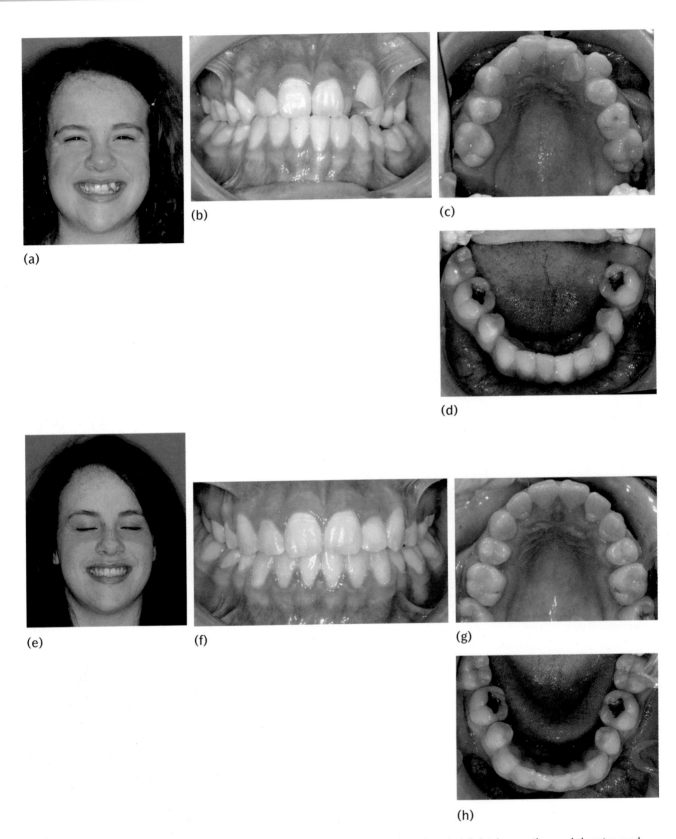

Fig. 11.14 Patient with Class III malocclusion on a mild Class III skeletal pattern with increased vertical skeletal proportions and absent second premolars. Orthodontic camouflage was the approach used and involved the extraction of the retained upper left second deciduous molar and fixed appliances (a–d) pre-treatment; (e–h) post-treatment.

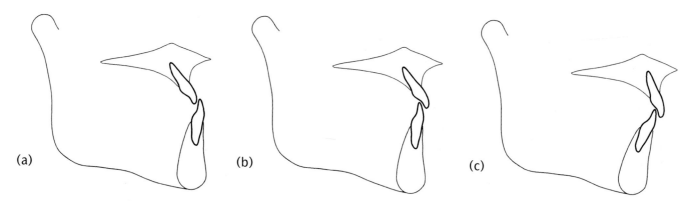

Fig. 11.15 (a) Severe Class III malocclusion with dento-alveolar compensation. (b) Without reduction of the dento-alveolar compensation, surgery to produce a Class I incisor relationship will only achieve a limited correction of the underlying skeletal pattern, thus constraining the overall aesthetic result. (c) Decompensation of the incisors to bring them nearer to their correct axial inclination allows a complete correction of the underlying skeletal pattern.

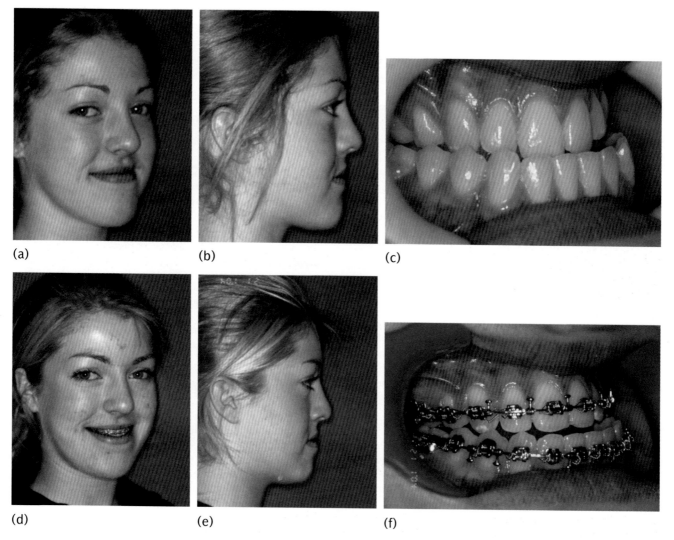

Fig. 11.16 Patient treated with a combination of orthodontics and bimaxillary orthognathic surgery: (a–c) pre-treatment; (d–f) at end of pre-surgical orthodontic alignment; (g–i) post-treatment.

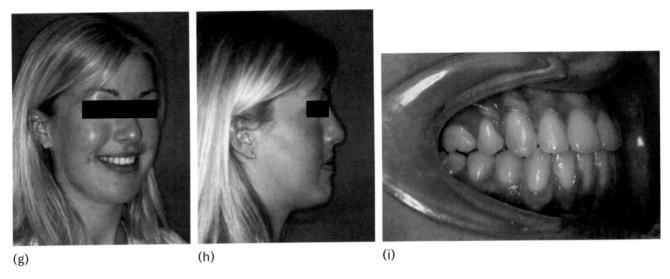

(g)　　　　　　　　　　(h)　　　　　　　　　　(i)

Fig. 11.16 (*continued*)

Key points

- Growth is often unfavourable in Class III malocclusions

- If orthopaedic treatment might be an option then it is important to refer the patient to a specialist before 10 years of age

---

Principal sources and further reading

Baccetti T., Rey, D., Oberti, G., Stahl, F., and McNamara, J.A. (2009). Long-term outcomes of Class III treatment with mandibular cervical headgear followed by fixed appliances. *Angle Orthodontist*, **79**, 828–34.

The patients in the treatment group were followed up over 5 years. The favourable dento-skeletal changes seen were maintained.

Battagel, J. M. (1993). The aetiological factors in Class III malocclusion. *European Journal of Orthodontics*, **15**, 347–70.

Bryant, P. M. F. (1981). Mandibular rotation and Class III malocclusion. *British Journal of Orthodontics*, **8**, 61–75.

This paper is worth reading for the introduction alone, which contains a very good discussion of growth rotations. The study itself looks at the effect of growth rotations and treatment upon Class III malocclusions.

Cevidanes, L., Baccetti, T., Franchi, L., McNamara, J.A., and De Clerk, H. (2010). Comparison of two protocols for maxillary expansion: bone anchors versus face mask with rapid maxillary expansion. *Angle Orthodontist*, **80**, 799–806.

An interesting paper.

De Toffol, L., Pavoni, C. Baccetti, T., Franchi, L., and Cozza, P. (2008). Orthopedic treatment outcomes in Class III malocclusion. *Angle Orthodontist*, **78**, 561–73.

Unfortunately like many systematic reviews the available evidence on this topic at the time of this review was not strong.

Gravely, J. F. (1984). A study of the mandibular closure path in Angle Class III relationship. *British Journal of Orthodontics*, **11**, 85–91.

A very readable and clever article which examines the displacement element of Class III malocclusions.

Kerr, W. J. S., Miller, S., and Dawber, J. E. (1992). Class III malocclusion: surgery or orthodontics? *British Journal of Orthodontics*, **19**, 21–4.

An interesting study which compares the pre-treatment lateral cephalometric radiographs of two groups of Class III cases treated by either surgery or orthodontics alone. The authors report the thresholds for three cephalometric values which would indicate when surgery is required.

Kim, J. H. *et al.* (1999). The effectiveness of protraction face mask therapy: a meta-analysis. *American Journal of Orthodontics and Dentofacial Orthopedics*, **115**, 675–85.

Mandall, N. *et al.* (2010). Is early Class III protraction facemask treatment effective? A randomized, controlled trial: 15-month follow-up. *Journal of Orthodontics*, **37**, 149–61.

A well-designed multi-centre RCT. One of the few studies in this area to look at patient-related outcomes, but interestingly found that early treatment did not result in a clinically significant psychosocial benefit.

Vaughan, G.A., Mason, B., Moon, H.B., and Turley, P. K. (2005). The effects of maxillary protraction therapy with or without rapid palatal expansion: a prospective randomized clinical trial. *American Journal of Orthodontic and Dentofacial Orthopedics*, **132**, 467–74.

 References for this chapter can also be found at www.oxfordtextbooks.co.uk/orc/mitchell4e/. Where possible, these are presented as active links which direct you to the electronic version of the work, to help facilitate onward study. If you are a subscriber to that work (either individually or through an institution), and depending on your level of access, you may be able to peruse an abstract or the full article if available.

12

Anterior open bite and posterior open bite

12.1 Definitions

• **Anterior open bite (AOB):** there is no vertical overlap of the incisors when the buccal segment teeth are in occlusion (Fig. 12.1).

• **Posterior open bite (POB):** when the teeth are in occlusion there is a space between the posterior teeth (Fig. 12.2).

• **Incomplete overbite:** the lower incisors do not occlude with the opposing upper incisors or the palatal mucosa when the buccal segment teeth are in occlusion (Fig. 12.3). The overbite may be decreased or increased.

12.2 Aetiology of anterior open bite

In common with other types of malocclusion, both inherited and environmental factors are implicated in the aetiology of anterior open bite. These factors include skeletal pattern, soft tissues, habits, and localized failure of development. In many cases the aetiology is multifactorial, and in practice it can be difficult to determine the relative roles of these influences as the presenting malocclusion is similar. However, a thorough history and examination, perhaps with a period of observation, may be helpful (Box 12.1).

Box 12.1 Prevalence differs between racial groups:

Caucasians: 2–4%
Afro-Caribbean: 5–10%

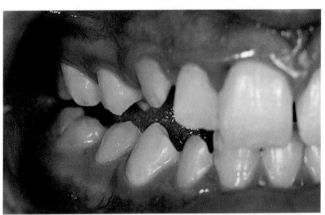

Fig. 12.2 Posterior open bite.

12.2.1 Skeletal pattern

Individuals with a tendency to vertical rather than horizontal facial growth exhibit increased vertical skeletal proportions (see Chapter 4). Where the lower face height is increased there will be an increased inter-occlusal distance between the maxilla and mandible. Although the labial segment teeth appear to be able to compensate for this to a limited extent by further eruption, where the inter-occlusal distance exceeds this compensatory ability an anterior open bite will result. If the

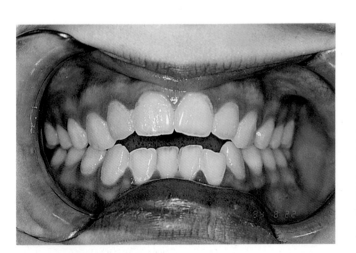

Fig. 12.1 Anterior open bite.

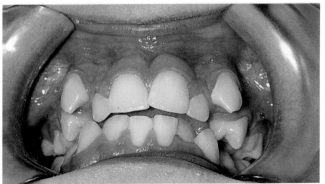

Fig. 12.3 Incomplete overbite.

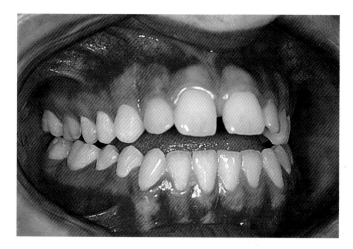

Fig. 12.4 Patient with increased vertical skeletal proportions and an anterior open bite.

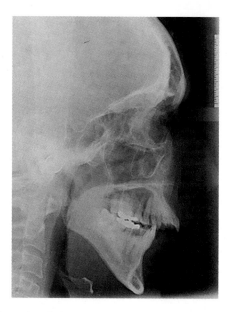

Fig. 12.5 Lateral cephalometric radiograph of a patient with a marked Class II division 1 malocclusion on a Class II skeletal pattern with increased vertical skeletal proportions. Note the thin dento-alveolar processes.

vertical, downwards, and backwards pattern of growth continues, the anterior open bite will become more marked.

In this group of patients the anterior open bite is usually symmetrical and in the more severe cases may extend distally around the arch so that only the posterior molars are in contact when the patient is in maximal interdigitation (Fig. 12.4). The vertical development of the labial segments results in typically extended alveolar processes when viewed on a lateral cephalometric radiograph (Fig. 12.5).

12.2.2 Soft tissue pattern

In order to be able to swallow it is necessary to create an anterior oral seal. In younger children the lips are often incompetent and a proportion will achieve an anterior seal by positioning their tongue forward between the anterior teeth during swallowing. Individuals with increased vertical skeletal proportions have an increased likelihood of incompetent lips and may continue to achieve an anterior oral seal in this manner even when the soft tissues have matured. This type of swallowing pattern is also seen in patients with an anterior open bite due to a digit-sucking habit (see Section 12.2.3). In these situations the behaviour of the tongue is adaptive. An endogenous or primary tongue thrust is rare, but it is difficult to distinguish it from an adaptive tongue thrust as the occlusal features are similar (Fig. 12.6). However, it has been suggested that an endogenous tongue thrust is associated with sigmatism (lisping), and in some cases both the upper and lower incisors are proclined by the action of the tongue.

12.2.3 Habits

See also Section 9.1.4

The effects of a habit depend upon its duration and intensity. If a persistent digit-sucking habit continues into the mixed and permanent dentitions, this can result in an anterior open bite due to restriction of development of the incisors by the finger or thumb (Fig. 12.7). Characteristically, the anterior open bite produced is asymmetrical (unless the patient sucks two fingers) and it is often associated with a posterior crossbite. Constriction of the upper arch is believed to be caused by cheek pressure and a low tongue position.

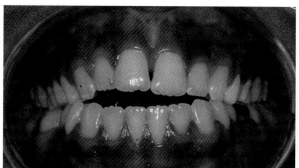

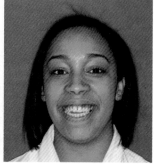

Fig. 12.6 Patient with an anterior open bite which was believed to be due to an endogenous tongue thrust. Both upper and lower incisors were proclined. The patient did not have a digit-sucking habit.

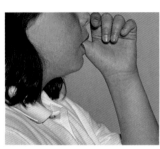
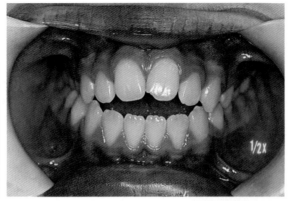

Fig. 12.7 The occlusal effects of a persistent digit-sucking habit. Note the anterior open bite and the unilateral posterior crossbite.

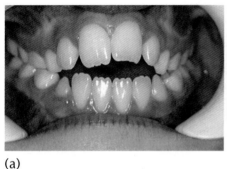
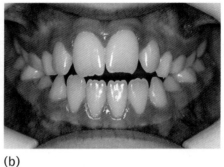

(a)   (b)

Fig. 12.8 A patient aged 10 years with a dummy-sucking habit: (a) at presentation; (b) 4 months after habit stopped.

After a sucking habit stops the open bite tends to resolve (Fig. 12.8), although this may take several months. During this period the tongue may come forward during swallowing to achieve an anterior seal. In a small proportion of cases where the habit has continued until growth is complete the open bite may persist.

12.2.4 Localized failure of development

This is seen in patients with a cleft of the lip and alveolus (see also Fig 22.3), although rarely it may occur for no apparent reason.

12.2.5 Mouth breathing

It has been suggested that the open-mouth posture adopted by individuals who habitually mouth breathe, either due to nasal obstruction or habit, results in overdevelopment of the buccal segment teeth. This leads to an increase in the height of the lower third of the face and consequently a greater incidence of anterior open bite. In support of this it has been shown that patients referred for tonsillectomy and adenoidectomy had significantly increased lower facial heights compared with controls, and that post-operatively the disparity between the two groups diminished. However, the differences demonstrated were small. Other workers have shown that children referred to ear, nose, and throat clinics exhibit the same range of malocclusions as the normal population, and no relationship has been demonstrated between nasal airway resistance and skeletal pattern in normal individuals.

On balance, it would appear that mouth breathing *per se* does not play a significant role in the development of anterior open bite in most patients.

12.3 Management of anterior open bite

Notwithstanding the difficulties faced in determining aetiology, treatment of anterior open bite is one of the more challenging aspects of orthodontics. Management of an anterior open bite due purely to a digit-sucking habit can be straightforward, but where the skeletal pattern, growth, and/or soft tissue environment are unfavourable, correction without resort to orthognathic surgery may not be possible.

In the mixed dentition, a digit-sucking habit that has resulted in an anterior open bite should be gently discouraged. If a child is keen to stop, a removable appliance can be fitted to act as a reminder. However, if the child derives support from his habit, forcing him to wear an appliance to discourage it is unlikely to be successful. Although a number of barbaric designs have been described (for example, involving wire projections), a simple removable plate with a long labial bow for anterior retention will usually suffice if a habit-breaker is indicated. After fitting, the acrylic behind the upper incisors should be trimmed to allow any spontaneous alignment. Once the permanent dentition is established, more active steps can be taken, usually in combination with treatment for other aspects of the malocclusion.

A period of observation may be helpful in the management of children with an anterior open bite which is not associated with a digit-sucking habit. In some cases an anterior open bite may reduce spontaneously, possibly because of maturation of the soft tissues and improved lip competence, or favourable growth. Skeletal open bites with increased vertical proportions are often associated with a downward and backward rotation of the mandible with growth. Obviously, if growth is unfavourable, it is better to know this before planning treatment rather than experiencing difficulties once treatment is under way.

There is no evidence to show that correction of anterior open bite improves lisping/speech problems.

The best predictor of stability following correction is the extent of the anterior open bite at the outset. Some advocate active retention for example, continuing with high-pull headgear if this has been used during treatment. Certainly there is some evidence to suggest that this is advisable when molar intrusion has been achieved using temporary anchorage devices (see Section 12.3.1).

12.3.1 Approaches to the management of anterior open bite

There are three possible approaches to management.

Acceptance of the anterior open bite

In this case treatment is aimed at relief of any crowding and alignment of the arches. This approach can be considered in the following situations (particularly if the AOB does not present a problem to the patient):

- mild cases
- where the soft tissue environment is not favourable, for example where the lips are markedly incompetent and/or an endogenous tongue thrust is suspected

- more marked malocclusions where the patient is not motivated towards surgery

Orthodontic correction of the anterior open bite

If growth and the soft tissue environment are favourable, an orthodontic solution to the anterior open bite can be considered. A careful assessment should be carried out, including the anteroposterior and vertical skeletal pattern, the feasibility of the tooth movements required, and post-treatment stability.

Extrusion of the incisors to close an anterior open bite is inadvisable, as the condition will relapse once the appliances are removed. Rather, treatment should aim to try and intrude the molars, or at least control their vertical development (Box 12.2).

In the milder malocclusions the use of high-pull headgear during conventional treatment may suffice. In cases with a more marked anterior open bite associated with a Class II skeletal pattern, a removable appliance or a functional appliance incorporating buccal blocks and high-pull headgear can be used to try to restrain vertical maxillary growth. In order to achieve true growth modification it is necessary to apply an intrusive force to the maxilla for at least 14–16 hours per day during the pubertal growth spurt, and preferably continuing until the growth rate has slowed. This is only achievable with excellent patient co-operation and favourable growth. The maxillary intrusion splint and the buccal intrusion splint are removable appliances which were developed by Orton. The former incorporates acrylic coverage of all the teeth in the upper arch and high-pull headgear (Fig. 12.9). The buccal intrusion splint is similar, except that only the buccal segment teeth are capped.

Box 12.2 Methods of intruding the molars

- High-pull headgear
- Fixed appliance mechanics
- Buccal capping on a removable/functional appliance
- Repelling magnets
- Temporary anchorage devices (TADs)

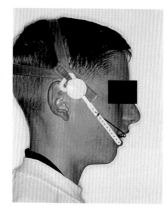
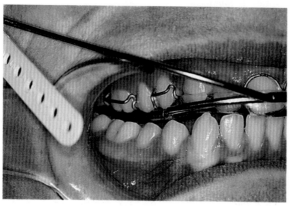

Fig. 12.9 A patient wearing a maxillary intrusion splint and high-pull headgear. The face-bow of the headgear slots into tubes embedded in the acrylic of the occlusal capping, which extends to cover all the maxillary teeth.

Functional appliances are also used for Class II malocclusions with increased vertical proportions. A number of designs have been described, but usually they incorporate high-pull headgear and buccal capping. The van Beek appliance is shown in Fig. 12.10. The Twin-Block appliance (see Chapter 18) with the addition of high-pull headgear is also used. After the functional phase, fixed appliances are then used to complete arch alignment, together with extractions if indicated.

Successful reduction of AOB has been achieved using fixed appliance mechanics that tip the molars teeth distally. This can be achieved using multi-loop archwires or continuous 'rocking-horse' archwires in conjunction with anterior vertical elastics. The rationale is that as the molars tip distally the posterior vertical dimensions reduce and the vertical elastics bring the incisors together as this happens.

The introduction of skeletal anchorage devices has also expanded the envelope in terms of the severity of AOB that can be treated non-surgically (Fig. 12.11). A greater degree of molar intrusion can be achieved utilizing bone anchorage either with screws or plates. There is a risk of tipping the molars buccally with the traction force so some advocate using both palatal and buccal implants. Not surprisingly the evidence suggests that relapse following this mode of treatment is greatest in the first year, so active retention is advocated. This involves continuing with an intrusive force from the skeletal anchorage to the retention appliances. Further work is required to determine if this just offsets the timing of, rather than the extent of, relapse.

In cases with bimaxillary crowding and proclination, relief of crowding and retraction and alignment of the incisors can result in reduction of an open bite. Stability of this correction is more likely if the lips were incompetent prior to treatment but become competent following retroclination of the incisors.

If it is difficult to ascertain the exact aetiology of an anterior open bite but a primary tongue thrust is suspected, even though these are uncommon, it is wise to err on the side of caution regarding treatment objectives (and extractions) and to warn patients of the possibility of relapse.

Surgery

This option can be considered once growth has slowed to adult levels for severe problems with a skeletal aetiology and/or where dental compensation will not give an aesthetic or stable result. In some patients an anterior open bite is associated with a 'gummy' smile which can be difficult to reduce by orthodontics alone necessitating a surgical approach. The assessment and management of such cases is discussed in Chapter 21.

12.3.2 Management of patients with increased vertical skeletal proportions and reduced overbite

The specifics of treatment of patients with increased vertical skeletal proportions will obviously be influenced by the other aspects of their malocclusion (see appropriate chapters), but management requires careful planning to try and prevent an iatrogenic deterioration of the vertical excess. The following points should be borne in mind:

- Space closure appears to occur more readily in patients with increased vertical skeletal proportions.

- Avoid extruding the molars as this will result in an increase of the lower facial height. If headgear is required, a direction of pull above the occlusal plane is necessary, i.e. high-pull headgear. Cervical-pull headgear is contraindicated.

- If overbite reduction is required, this should be achieved by intrusion of the incisors rather than extrusion of the molars. For this reason anterior bite-planes should be avoided.

- Avoid upper arch expansion. When the upper arch is expanded the upper molars are tilted buccally which results in the palatal cusps being tipped downwards (see Fig. 13.9). If arch expansion is required, this is best achieved using a fixed appliance so that buccal root torque can be used to limit downward tipping of the palatal cusps.

- Avoid Class II or Class III intermaxillary traction as this may extrude the molars.

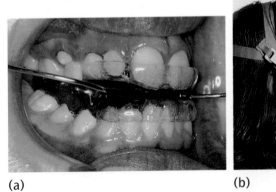
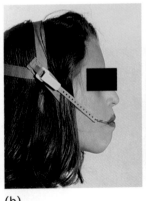
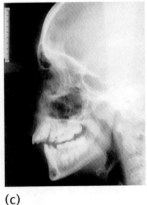
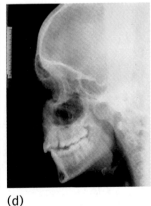

(a)   (b)   (c)   (d)

Fig. 12.10 (a) Intra-oral view of a van Beek appliance; (b) extra-oral view showing the high-pull headgear; (c) lateral cephalometric radiograph of the patient prior to treatment; (d) lateral cephalometric radiograph of the same patient 1 year later.

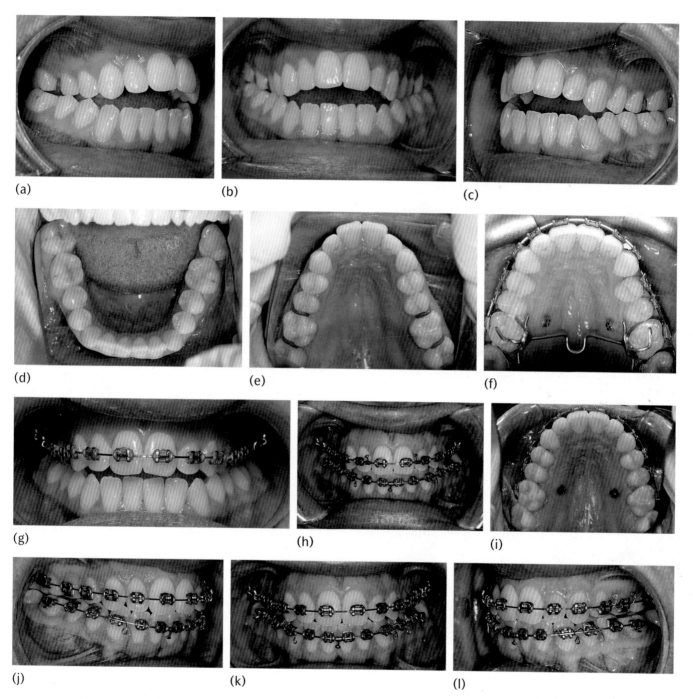

Fig. 12.11 Patient with an anterior open bite treated using temporary screw anchorage (TADs) in the upper arch and fixed appliances: (a–e) pretreatment; (f) posterior intrusion using elastic chain between the TADs and the transpalatal arch (NB. TPA is stepped 5 mm away from the palate and incorporates stops on the upper first permanent molars). The upper rectangular stainless steel archwire is segmented distal to the canines to prevent incisor extrusion during leveling: (g) mid-treatment; (h) a continuous archwire is placed after sufficient posterior intrusion has been achieved; (i) the TADs are retained for the duration of active treatment in case additional posterior intrusion is required; (j–l) just prior to debond. Patient treated by, and data reproduced with the kind permission of Jag Prabhu.

12.4 Posterior open bite

Posterior open bite occurs more rarely than anterior open bite and the aetiology is less well understood. In some cases an increase in the vertical skeletal proportions is a factor, although this is more commonly associated with an anterior open bite which also extends posteriorly. A lateral open bite is occasionally seen in association with early extraction of first permanent molars (Fig. 12.12), possibly occurring as a result of lateral tongue spread.

Posterior open bite is also seen in cases with eruption disturbances. Primary failure of eruption is a condition which almost exclusively affects molar teeth and has recently been linked to a specific gene. Affected teeth may erupt and then cease to keep pace with vertical development becoming relatively submerged or may fail to erupt at all (Fig. 12.13). Although these teeth are not ankylosed they do not respond normally to orthodontic force and indeed usually become ankylosed if traction is applied. Extraction is the only treatment alternative.

More rarely, posterior open bite is seen in association with unilateral condylar hyperplasia, which also results in facial asymmetry. If this problem is suspected, a bone scan will be required. If the scan indicates excessive cell division in the condylar head region, a condylectomy alone, or in combination with surgery to correct the resultant deformity, may be required.

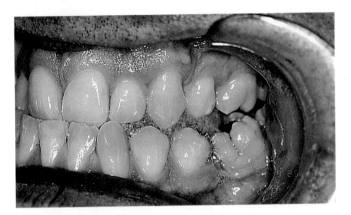

Fig. 12.12 Posterior open bite in a patient who had all four first permanent molars extracted in the mixed dentition.

Relevant Cochrane reviews:

Orthodontic and orthopaedic treatment for anterior open bite in children
Lentine-Oliveira, D.A. *et al.* (2008).
http://onlinelibrary.wiley.com/doi/10.1002/14651858.
CD005515.pub2/abstract
Authors concluded that recommendations for clinical practice could not be made based on the results of the review.

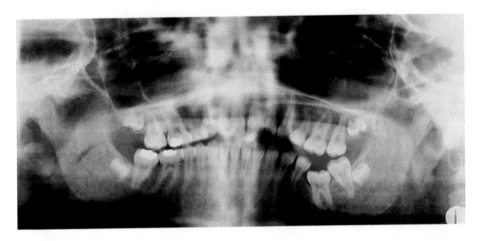

Fig. 12.13 OPT radiographs showing failure of eruption of the lower left first permanent molar.

Principal sources and further reading

Baek, M-S., Choi, Y-J., Yu, H-S., Lee, K-L., Kwak, J., and Park, Y.C. (2010). Long-term stability of anterior open-bite treatment by intrusion of maxillary posterior teeth. *American Journal of Orthodontics and Dentofacial Orthopedics*, **138**, 396–8.
A short online article with an interesting Q&A section with the lead author and the journal's editor.

Chate, R. A. C. (1994). The burden of proof: a critical review of orthodontic claims made by some general practitioners. *American Journal of Orthodontics and Dentofacial Orthopedics*, **106**, 96–105.
An excellent discussion of the evidence on the postulated and actual effects of mouth breathing upon the dentition, plus much other information. Highly recommended.

Dung, D. J. and Smith, R. J. (1998). Cephalometric and clinical diagnoses of open bite tendency. *American Journal of Orthodontics and Dentofacial Orthopedics*, **94**, 484–90.

The authors also look at predictors of successful treatment.

Greenlee, G.M., Huang, G.J. Chen, S. S-H., Chen, J., Koepsell, T., and Hujoel, P. (2010). Stability of treatment for anterior open-bite malocclusion: A meta-analysis. *American Journal of Orthodontics and Dentofacial Orthopedics*, **139**, 154–9.

Unfortunately the authors were only able to find case series types of studies that satisfied the inclusion criteria, therefore their findings must be viewed with caution.

Kim, Y.H. (1987). Anterior open bite and its treatment with multi-loop edgewise archwire. *Angle Orthodontist*, **57**, 290–321.

Linder-Aronson, S. (1970). Adenoids: their effect on mode of breathing and nasal airflow and their relationship to characteristics of the facial skeleton and dentition. *Acta Otolaryngologica (Supplement)*, **265**, 1.

Lopez-Gavito, G., Wallen, T. R., Little, R. M., and Joondeph, D. R. (1985). Anterior open-bite malocclusion: a longitudinal 10-year postretention evaluation of orthodontically treated patients. *American Journal of Orthodontics*, **87**, 175–86.

Mizrahi, E. (1978). A review of anterior open bite. *British Journal of Orthodontics*, **5**, 21–7.

A worthy review.

Orton, H. S. (1990). *Functional Appliances in Orthodontic Treatment*. Quintessence Books, London.

A beautifully illustrated and informative book. The maxillary and buccal intrusion splints are described.

Vaden, J. L. (1998). Non-surgical treatment of the patient with vertical discrepancy. *American Journal of Orthodontics and Dentofacial Orthopedics*, **113**, 567–82.

 References for this chapter can also be found at www.oxfordtextbooks.co.uk/orc/mitchell4e/. Where possible, these are presented as active links which direct you to the electronic version of the work, to help facilitate onward study. If you are a subscriber to that work (either individually or through an institution), and depending on your level of access, you may be able to peruse an abstract or the full article if available.

13

Crossbites

Chapter contents

13.1 Definitions

- **Crossbite:** a discrepancy in the buccolingual relationship of the upper and lower teeth. By convention the transverse relationship of the arches is described in terms of the position of the lower teeth relative to the upper teeth.

- **Buccal crossbite:** the buccal cusps of the lower teeth occlude buccal to the buccal cusps of the upper teeth (Fig. 13.1).

- **Lingual crossbite:** the buccal cusps of the lower teeth occlude lingual to the lingual cusps of the upper teeth. This is also known as a scissors bite (Fig. 13.2).

- **Displacement:** on closing from the rest position the mandible encounters a deflecting contact(s) and is displaced to the left or the right, and/or anteriorly, into maximum interdigitation (Fig. 13.3).

13.2 Aetiology

A variety of factors acting either singly or in combination can lead to the development of a crossbite.

13.2.1 Local causes

The most common local cause is crowding where one or two teeth are displaced from the arch. For example, a crossbite of an upper lateral incisor often arises owing to lack of space between the upper central incisor and the deciduous canine, which forces the lateral incisor to erupt palatally and in linguo-occlusion with the opposing teeth. Posteriorly, early loss of a second deciduous molar in a crowded mouth may result in forward movement of the upper first permanent molar, forcing the second premolar to erupt palatally. Also, retention of a primary tooth can deflect the eruption of the permanent successor leading to a crossbite.

13.2.2 Skeletal

Generally, the greater the number of teeth in crossbite, the greater is the skeletal component of the aetiology. A crossbite of the buccal segments may be due purely to a mismatch in the relative width of the arches, or to an anteroposterior discrepancy, which results in a wider part of one arch occluding with a narrower part of the opposing jaw. For this reason buccal crossbites of an entire buccal segment are most commonly associated with Class III malocclusions (Fig. 13.4), and lingual crossbites are associated with Class II malocclusions. Anterior crossbites are associated with Class III skeletal patterns. Crossbites can also be associated with true skeletal asymmetry and/or asymmetric mandibular growth.

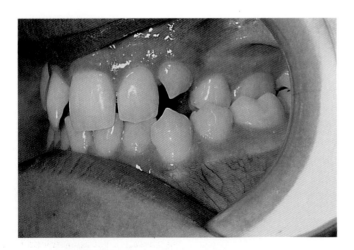

Fig. 13.1 A buccal crossbite.

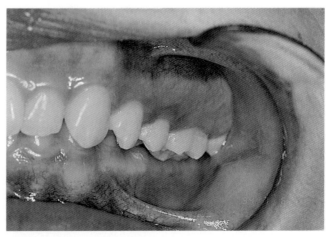

Fig. 13.2 A lingual (scissors) crossbite.

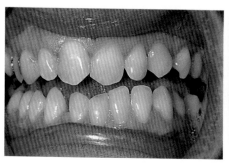 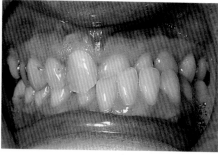

Fig. 13.3 Displacement on closure into crossbite.

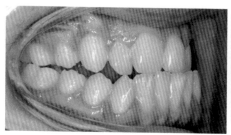 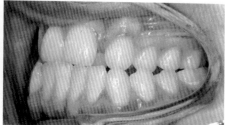

Fig. 13.4 A Class III malocclusion with buccal crossbite.

13.2.3 Soft tissues

A posterior crossbite is often associated with a digit-sucking habit, as the position of the tongue is lowered and a negative pressure is generated intra-orally.

13.2.4 Rarer causes

These include cleft lip and palate, where growth in the width of the upper arch is restrained by the scar tissue of the cleft repair. Trauma to, or pathology of, the temporomandibular joints can lead to restriction of growth of the mandible on one side, leading to asymmetry.

13.3 Types of crossbite

13.3.1 Anterior crossbite

An anterior crossbite is present when one or more of the upper incisors is in linguo-occlusion (i.e. in reverse overjet) relative to the lower arch (Fig. 13.5). Anterior crossbites involving only one or two incisors are considered in this chapter, whereas management of more than two incisors in crossbite is covered in Chapter 11 (Class III malocclusions).

Anterior crossbites are frequently associated with displacement on closure (see Fig. 13.3).

13.3.2 Posterior crossbites

Crossbites of the premolar and molar region involving one or two teeth or an entire buccal segment can be subdivided as follows.

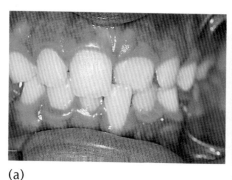 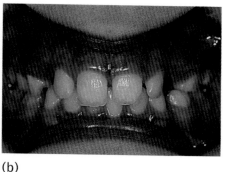

(a)   (b)

Fig. 13.5 Correction of an anterior crossbite, using a removable appliance: (a) pre-treatment (note the gingival recession of the lower incisor in crossbite); (b) post-treatment.

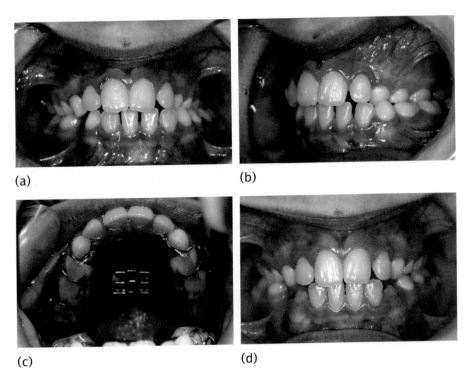

(a)

(b)

(c)

(d)

Fig. 13.6 (a, b) A patient in the mixed dentition with an unilateral crossbite with mandibular displacement and associated centreline shift; (c) URA used to expand upper arch to correct crossbite; (d) occlusion following expansion showing correction of centrelines due to elimination of mandibular displacement.

Unilateral buccal crossbite with displacement

This type of crossbite can affect only one or two teeth per quadrant, or the whole of the buccal segment. When a single tooth is affected, the problem usually arises because of the displacement of one tooth from the arch, plus or minus the opposing tooth, leading to a deflecting contact on closure into the crossbite.

When the whole of the buccal segment is involved, the underlying aetiology is usually that the maxillary arch is of a similar width to the mandibular arch (i.e. it is too narrow) with the result that on closure from the rest position the buccal segment teeth meet cusp to cusp. In order to achieve a more comfortable and efficient intercuspation, the patient displaces their mandible to the left or right (see Section 5.5.3 Fig. 5.13). It is often difficult to detect this displacement on closure as the patient soon learns to close straight into the position of maximal interdigitation. This type of crossbite may be associated with a centreline shift in the lower arch in the direction of the mandibular displacement (Fig. 13.6).

Unilateral buccal crossbite with no displacement

This category of crossbite is less common. It can arise as a result of deflection of two (or more) opposing teeth during eruption, but the greater the number of teeth in a segment that are involved, the greater the likelihood that there is an underlying skeletal asymmetry.

Bilateral buccal crossbite

Bilateral crossbites (Fig. 13.7) are more likely to be associated with a skeletal discrepancy, either in the anteroposterior or transverse dimension, or in both.

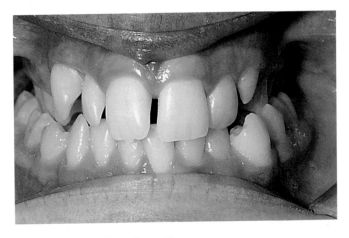

Fig. 13.7 A bilateral buccal crossbite.

Unilateral lingual crossbite

This type of crossbite is most commonly due to displacement of an individual tooth as a result of crowding or retention of the deciduous predecessor.

Bilateral lingual crossbite (scissors bite)

Again, this crossbite is typically associated with an underlying skeletal discrepancy, often a Class II malocclusion with the upper arch further forward relative to the lower so that the lower buccal teeth occlude with a wider segment of the upper arch.

13.4 Management

13.4.1 Rationale for treatment

There is some evidence that displacing contacts *may* predispose towards temporomandibular joint dysfunction syndrome in a *susceptible* individual (see Chapter 1, Section 1.7). Recent work has also suggested that unilateral crossbites associated with mandibular displacement result in asymmetric mandibular growth. Therefore some argue that a crossbite associated with a displacement is a functional indication for orthodontic treatment. However, treatment for a bilateral crossbite without displacement should be approached with caution, as partial relapse may result in a unilateral crossbite with displacement. In addition, a bilateral crossbite is probably as efficient for chewing as the normal buccolingual relationship of the teeth. However, the same cannot be said of a lingual crossbite where the cusps of affected teeth do not meet together at all.

Anterior crossbites, as well as being frequently associated with displacement, can lead to movement of a lower incisor labially through the labial supporting tissues, resulting in gingival recession. In this case early treatment is advisable (see Fig. 13.5).

13.4.2 Treatment of anterior crossbite

The following factors should be considered.

- What type of movement is required? If bodily or apical movement is required then fixed appliances are indicated; however, if in the mixed dentition tipping movements will suffice, a removable appliance can be considered.

- How much overbite is expected at the end of treatment? For treatment to be successful there must be some overbite present to retain the corrected incisor position. However, when planning treatment it should be remembered that proclination of an upper incisor will result in a reduction of overbite compared with the pre-treatment position (Fig. 11.10).

- Is there space available within the arch to accommodate the tooth/teeth to be moved? If not, are extractions required and if so which teeth?

- Is reciprocal movement of the opposing tooth/teeth required?

In the mixed dentition, provided that there is sufficient overbite and tilting movements will suffice, treatment can often be accomplished more readily with a removable appliance. The appliance should incorporate good anterior retention to counteract the displacing effect of the active element (where two or more teeth are to be proclined, a screw appliance may circumvent this problem) and buccal capping just thick enough to free the occlusion with the opposing arch (see Chapter 17). Otherwise it may be advisable to wait until the permanent dentition is established and comprehensive fixed appliance treatment can be carried out (Fig. 13.8). If there will be insufficient overbite to retain the corrected incisor(s), then consideration should be given to moving the lower incisors lingually within the confines of the soft tissue envelope in order to try and increase overbite.

If the upper arch is crowded, the upper lateral incisor often erupts in a palatal position relative to the arch. If the lateral incisor is markedly bodily displaced, relief of crowding by extraction of the displaced tooth itself may sometimes be an option, but it is wise to seek a specialist opinion before taking this step.

13.4.3 Treatment of posterior crossbite

It is important to consider the aetiology of this feature before embarking on treatment. For example, is the crossbite due to displacement of one tooth from the arch, in which case correction will involve aligning this tooth, or is reciprocal movement of two or more opposing teeth required? Also, if there is a skeletal component, will it be possible to compensate for this by tooth movement? The inclination of the affected teeth should also be evaluated. Upper arch expansion is more likely to be stable if the teeth to be moved were initially tilted palatally.

Even when fixed appliances are used, expansion of the upper buccal segment teeth will result in some tipping down of the palatal cusps (Fig. 13.9). This has the effect of hinging the mandible downwards leading to an increase in lower face height, which may be undesirable in patients who already have an increased lower facial height and/or reduced overbite. If expansion is indicated in these patients, fixed appliances are required to apply buccal root torque to the buccal segment teeth in order to try and resist this tendency, perhaps with high-pull headgear as well.

Recent work has indicated that transverse problems which are amenable to orthodontic correction are best treated in the pre-pubertal growth spurt. But the actual timing of treatment will depend upon other features of the malocclusion.

As expansion will create additional space, it may be advisable to defer a decision regarding extractions until after the expansion phase has been completed.

Where a crossbite is due to skeletal asymmetry then a thorough assessment is required to determine the aetiology and contribution of both the maxilla and mandible to the presenting features. Correction will require a combined approach involving orthognathic surgery (see Chapter 21) once growth has slowed to adult levels.

Interestingly, a Cochrane review on this topic reported that due to a paucity of good quality evidence the authors were not able to make recommendations regarding treatment of crossbite in the mixed and permanent dentitions. However, they did find that removal of premature contacts in the deciduous dentition was effective in preventing posterior crossbites being perpetuated into mixed/permanent dentition. Furthermore, when grinding alone was not effective an URA could be used to expand the upper arch to reduce the risk of the crossbite persisting.

Unilateral buccal crossbite

Where this problem has arisen owing to the displacement of one tooth from the arch, for example an upper premolar tooth which has been crowded palatally, treatment will involve movement of the displaced tooth into the line of the arch, relieving crowding where and if necessary. If the displacement is marked, consideration can be given to extracting the displaced tooth itself.

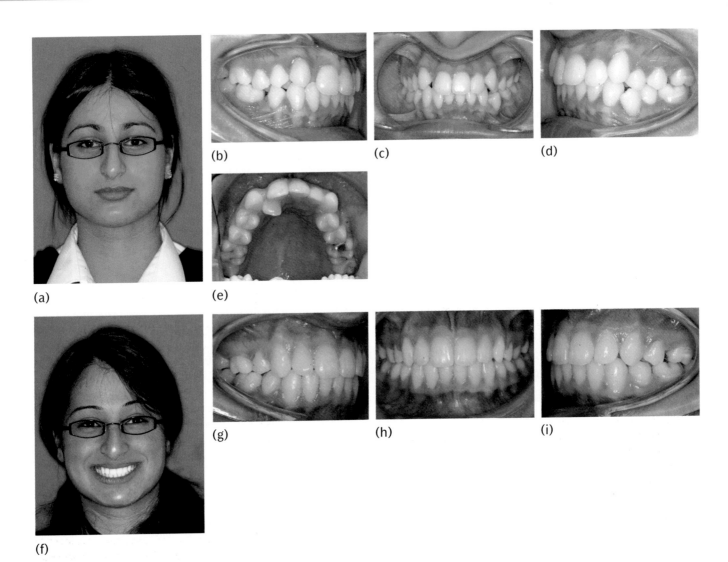

Fig. 13.8 A patient with a crossbite of the upper right lateral incisor who was treated by extraction of all four second premolars and fixed appliances: (a–e) pre-treatment; (f–i) post-treatment.

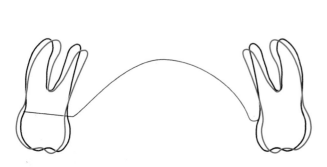

Fig. 13.9 Expansion of the upper arch results in the palatal cusps of the buccal segment teeth swinging down occlusally.

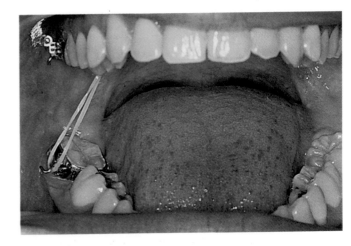

Fig. 13.10 Cross elastics.

If correction of a crossbite requires movement of the opposing teeth in opposite directions, this can be achieved by the use of cross elastics (Fig. 13.10) attached to bands or bonded brackets on the teeth involved. If this is the only feature of a malocclusion requiring treatment, it is wise to leave the attachments *in situ* following correction, stopping the elastics for a month to review whether the corrected position is stable. If the crossbite relapses, the cross elastics can be re-instituted and an alternative means of retention or more comprehensive treatment considered.

A unilateral crossbite involving all the teeth in the buccal segment is usually associated with a displacement, and treatment is directed towards expanding the upper arch so that it fits around the lower arch at the end of treatment. If the upper buccal teeth are tilted palatally, this can be accomplished with an upper removable appliance incorporating a midline screw and buccal capping (see Fig. 13.6). More commonly a quadhelix appliance (see Section 13.4.4) can be used, particularly if comprehensive fixed appliance treatment is indicated. As a degree of relapse can be anticipated, some slight overexpansion of the upper arch is advisable, but it is wise to remember that stability is aided by good cuspal interdigitation. It is important to avoid too much over-expansion as a lingual crossbite or fenestration of the buccal periodontal support may result.

Bilateral buccal crossbite

Unless the upper buccal segment teeth are tilted palatally to a significant degree, bilateral buccal crossbites are often accepted. Rapid maxillary expansion (see Section 13.4.5) can be used to try and expand the maxillary basal bone, but even with this technique a degree of relapse in the buccopalatal tooth position occurs following treatment, with the risk of development of a unilateral crossbite with displacement. Surgically assisted RME can also be considered (see Section 13.4.5).

Bilateral buccal crossbites are common in patients with a repaired cleft of the palate. Expansion of the upper arch by stretching of the scar tissue is often indicated in these cases (see Chapter 22) and is readily achieved using a quadhelix appliance (Fig. 13.11).

Lingual crossbite

If a single tooth is affected, this is often the result of displacement due to crowding. If extraction of the displaced tooth itself is not indicated to relieve crowding, then fixed appliances can be used to move the affected upper tooth palatally. More severe cases with a greater skeletal element usually need a combination of buccal movement of the affected lower teeth and palatal movement of the upper teeth with fixed appliances. Treatment is not straightforward and should only be tackled by the experienced orthodontist, particularly as a scissors bite will often dislodge fixed attachments on the buccal aspect of the lower teeth until the crossbite is eliminated.

13.4.4 The quadhelix appliance

The quadhelix is a very efficient fixed slow expansion appliance (Fig. 13.12). The quadhelix appliance can also be adjusted to give more expansion anteriorly or posteriorly as required and can also be used to de-rotate rotated molar teeth. When active expansion is complete it can be made passive to aid retention of the expansion.

A quadhelix is fabricated in 1 mm stainless steel wire and attached to the teeth by bands cemented to a molar tooth on each side. Preformed types are available which slot into palatal attachments welded onto bands on the molars and can be readily removed by the operator for adjustment. However, the appliance can also be custom-made in a laboratory. The usual activation is about half a tooth width each side. Over-expansion can occur readily if the appliance is overactivated, and therefore its use should be limited to those who are experienced with fixed appliances (see also Fig. 18.22).

A tri-helix has only one anterior coil and is therefore less efficient. Its use is limited to cases with narrow and/or high palatal vaults, for example in cleft lip and palate patients.

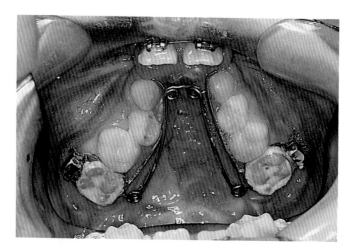

Fig. 13.11 Expansion of a repaired cleft maxilla with a quadhelix appliance.

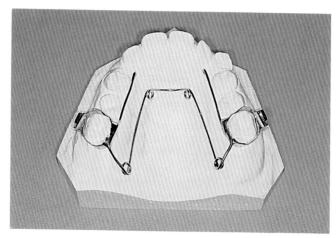

Fig. 13.12 A quadhelix appliance.

13.4.5 Rapid maxillary expansion (RME)

This upper appliance incorporates a Hyrax screw (similar to the type used for expansion in removable appliances) soldered to bands, usually to both a premolar and molar tooth on both sides. The screw is turned twice daily, resulting in expansion of the order of 0.2–0.5 mm/day, usually over an active treatment period of 2 weeks (Fig. 13.13). The large force generated is designed to open the midline suture and expand the upper arch by skeletal expansion rather than by movement of the teeth. For this reason some advocate limiting this approach to patients in their early teens before the suture fuses, or cleft palate patients where it can be utilized to expand the cleft seg-ments by stretching the scar tissue. If considering this approach it is advisable to check that there is adequate buccal supporting bone and soft tissues.

Once expansion is complete the appliance is left *in situ* as a retain-er, usually for several months. Bony infill of the expanded suture has been demonstrated but on removing the appliance approximately 50 per cent of the expansion gained is lost, and for this reason some over-expansion is indicated. This appliance should only be used by the expe-rienced clinician.

Surgically assisted RME (SARPE) is gaining acceptance, however claims of reduced periodontal support loss (compared with conven-tional expansion) and improved nasal airflow are unsubstantiated. This approach involves surgically cutting the mid-palatal suture prior to expansion (see Section 21.7.1).

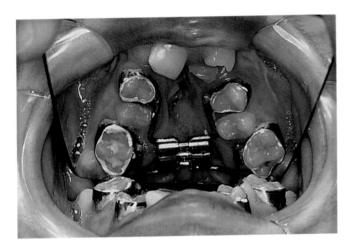

Fig. 13.13 A rapid maxillary expansion appliance being used to expand a repaired cleft maxilla.

> **Relevant Cochrane reviews:**
>
> Orthodontic treatment for posterior crossbites
> Harrison, J. *et al.* (2001).
> http://onlinelibrary.wiley.com/doi/10.1002/14651858.
> CD000979/abstract;jsessionid=8458FEEE3D8AD35875FE62D8C
> 4E0BF0F.d01t02
>
> The authors concluded that there is some evidence which suggests that removal of premature contacts in the deciduous dentition is effective in preventing a posterior crossbite from being perpetu-ated to the mixed dentition. When grinding alone is not effective, using an upper removable appliance to expand the upper arch will decrease the risk of a posterior crossbite from being perpetuated to the permanent dentition.

Principal sources and further reading

Birnie, D. J. and McNamara, T. G. (1980). The quadhelix appliance. *British Journal of Orthodontics*, **7**, 115–20.

The fabrication, manageme nt, and modifications of the quadhelix appliance are described in this paper.

Hermanson, H., Kurol, J., and Ronnerman, A. (1985). Treatment of unilateral posterior crossbites with quadhelix and removable plates. A retrospective study. *European Journal of Orthodontics*, **7**, 97–102.

In this study it was found that the clinical results achieved were similar with the two types of appliance. However, the number of visits and chairside time were greater for the removable appliance. The authors calculated that the mean cost of treatment was 40 per cent greater for the removable appliance compared with the quadhelix.

Herold, J. S. (1989). Maxillary expansion: a retrospective study of three methods of expansion and their long-term sequelae. *British Journal of Orthodontics*, **16**, 195–200.

Kilic, N., Kiki, A., and Oktay, H. (2008). Condylar asymmetry in unilateral posterior crossbite patients. *American Journal of Orthodontics and Dentofacial Orthopedics*, **133**, 382–7.

Lagravere, M. O., Major, P. W., and Flores-Mir, C. (2005). Long-term dental arch changes after rapid maxillary expansion treatment: a systematic review. *Angle Orthodontist*, **75**, 151–7.

Unfortunately only four studies satisfied the inclusion criteria and due to their design no meaningful conclusions could be drawn.

Lagravere, M. O., Major, P. W., and Flores-Mir, C. (2005). Long-term dental arch changes after rapid maxillary expansion treatment: a systematic review. *Angle Orthodontist*, **75**, 833–9.

Only three articles satisfied the inclusion criteria and due to the paucity of strong evidence no meaningful conclusions could be drawn.

Lee, R. (1999). Arch width and form: a review. *American Journal of Orthodontics and Dentofacial Orthopedics*, **115**, 305–13.

Linder-Aronson, S. and Lindgren, J. (1979). The skeletal and dental effects of rapid maxillary expansion. *British Journal of Orthodontics*, **6**, 25–9.

Marshall, S.D. *et al.* (2008). Ask us – Long term stability of maxillary expansion. *American Journal of Orthodontics and Dentofacial Orthopedics*, **133**, 780–1.

References for this chapter can also be found at www.oxfordtextbooks.co.uk/orc/mitchell4e/. Where possible, these are presented as active links which direct you to the electronic version of the work, to help facilitate onward study. If you are a subscriber to that work (either individually or through an institution), and depending on your level of access, you may be able to peruse an abstract or the full article if available.

14

Canines

Learning objectives for this chapter

- Be aware of normal development of the maxillary permanent canine and the importance of the early detection of displacement
- Gain an appreciation of the different methods for localizing the position of an unerupted maxillary permanent canine
- Gain an understanding of the treatment options for buccally and palatally displaced maxillary canines

14.1 Facts and figures

Development of the upper and lower canines commences between 4 and 5 months of age. The upper canines erupt, on average, at 11–12 years of age. The lower canines erupt, on average, at 10–11 years of age.

In a Caucasian population (Gorlin *et al.* 1990): congenital absence of upper canines, 0.3 per cent; congenital absence of lower canines, 0.1

per cent; impaction of upper canines, 1–2 per cent, of which 8 per cent are bilateral; impaction of lower canines, 0.35 per cent; resorption of upper incisors due to impacted canine, 0.7 per cent of 10–13-year-olds. A recent meta-analysis found a prevalence of transposition of 0.33 per cent.

14.2 Normal development

The development of the maxillary canine commences around 4 to 5 months of age, high in the maxilla. Crown calcification is complete around 6 to 7 years of age. The permanent canine then migrates forwards and downwards to lie buccal and mesial to the apex of the deciduous canine before erupting down the distal aspect of the root of the

upper lateral incisor. Pressure from the unerupted canine on the root of the lateral incisor, leads to flaring of the incisor crowns, which resolves as the canine erupts. In normal development the maxillary canines should be palpable in the labial sulcus by age 11 years.

14.3 Aetiology of maxillary canine displacement

Canine displacement is generally classified into buccal or palatal displacement. More rarely, canines can be found lying horizontally above the apices of the teeth of the upper arch (Fig. 14.1) or displaced high adjacent to the nose (Fig. 14.2).

The aetiology of canine displacement is still not fully understood (see also Box 14.1). The following have been suggested as possible causative factors.

- **Displacement of the crypt.** This is the probable aetiology behind the more marked displacements such as those shown in Figs 14.1 and 14.2.

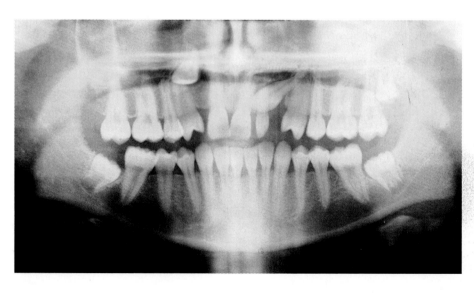

Fig. 14.1 Ectopic upper maxillary canines – with the upper right being significantly displaced. NB. absent upper right lateral incisor, a peg-shaped upper left lateral incisor.

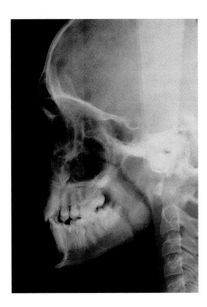

Fig. 14.2 Severely displaced maxillary canine.

- **Long path of eruption.**
- **Short-rooted or absent upper lateral incisor.** A 2.4-fold increase in the incidence of palatally displaced canines in patients with absent or short-rooted lateral incisors has been reported (Becker *et al.* 1981) (Fig. 14.1). It has been suggested that a lack of guidance during eruption is the reason behind this association. Because of the association of palatal displacement of an upper canine with missing or peg-shaped lateral incisors it is important to be particularly observant in patients with this anomaly.
- **Crowding.** Jacoby (1983) found that 85 per cent of buccally displaced canines were associated with crowding, whereas 83 per cent of palatal displacements had sufficient space for eruption. If the upper arch is crowded, this often manifests as insufficient space for the canine, which is the last tooth anterior to the molar to erupt. In normal development the canine comes to lie buccal to the arch and in the presence of crowding will be deflected buccally.

> **Box 14.1 Aetiology of canine displacements**
>
> *Palatal*: polygenic
>   multifactorial
> *Buccal*: crowding

> **Box 14.2 Dental anomalies associated with palatally displaced canines**
>
> - Hypodontia
> - Tooth size reduction including peg-shaped lateral incisors
> - Transposition
> - Impacted upper first permanent molars
> - Ectopic position of other teeth
> - Infra-occluded deciduous molars

- **Retention of the primary deciduous canine.** This usually results in mild displacement of the permanent tooth buccally. However, if the permanent canine itself is displaced, normal resorption of the deciduous canine will not occur. In this situation the retained deciduous tooth is an indicator, rather than the cause, of displacement.
- **Genetic factors.** It has been suggested that palatal displacement of the maxillary canine is an inherited trait with a pattern that suggests polygenic inheritance. The evidence cited for this includes:

  (a) the prevalence varies in different populations with a greater prevalence in Europeans than other racial groups;
  (b) affects females more commonly than males;
  (c) familial occurrence;
  (d) occurs bilaterally with a greater than expected frequency;
  (e) occurs in association with other dental anomalies (Figs 14.1 and 14.3; Box 14.2).

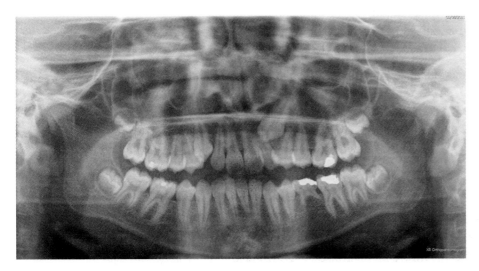

Fig. 14.3 OPT radiograph of patient with a displaced upper left canine and absent lower second premolars.

14.4 Interception of displaced canines

Because management of ectopic canines is difficult and early detection of an abnormal eruption path gives the opportunity, if appropriate, for interceptive measures, it is essential to routinely palpate for unerupted canines when examining any child aged 10 years and older. It is also important to locate the position of the canines before undertaking the extraction of other permanent teeth.

Canines, which are palpable in the normal developmental position, which is buccal and slightly distal to the upper lateral incisor root, have a good prognosis for eruption. Clinically, if a definite hollow and/or asymmetry is found on palpation, further investigation is warranted. On occasion, routine panoramic radiographic examination may demonstrate asymmetry in the position and development of the canines.

A number of studies have investigated the widely held belief that extraction of the deciduous canine facilitates an improvement in the position of a palatally displaced canine (Fig. 14.4) where the unerupted tooth is not markedly ectopic. However, a recent Cochrane Review concluded that there were deficiencies in the design and reporting of these studies and that there is currently no robust evidence to support this practice. It must be borne in mind that this is not to say that extracting the deciduous canine does not favour improvement, rather that there is currently no data from controlled trials upon which to base this approach. If a palatally displaced canine is detected in the mixed dentition then the orthodontist should discuss with the patient and their parent/guardian:

- the evidence base (i.e. clinical experience)
- the potential benefits (i.e. successful eruption of the permanent canine or improvement in its position)
- the negative aspects (i.e. an extraction and the commitment to proceed to exposure and orthodontic alignment if the hoped for improvement in position does not occur)

14.5 Assessing maxillary canine position

The position of an unerupted canine should initially be assessed clinically, followed by radiographic examination if displacement is suspected.

14.5.1 Clinically

It is usually possible to obtain a good estimate of the likely location of an unerupted maxillary canine by palpation (in the buccal sulcus and palatally) and by the inclination of the lateral incisor (Fig. 14.5).

14.5.2 Radiographically

The views commonly used for assessing ectopic canines (Box 14.3) include the following.

- **Dental panoramic tomogram** (OPT, OPG or DPT). This film gives a good overall assessment of the development of the dentition and canine position. However, this view suggests that the canine is further

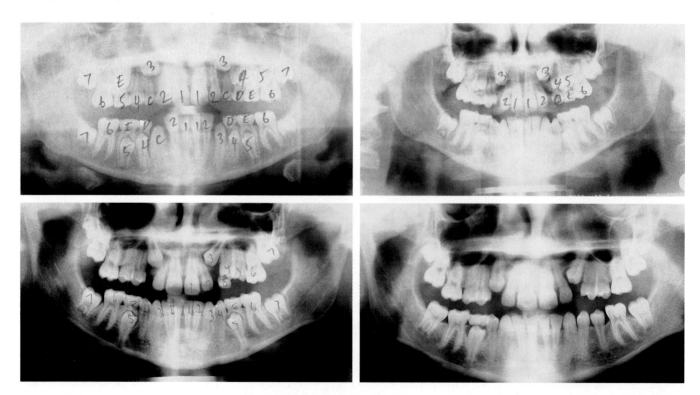

Fig. 14.4 DPT radiographs of a patient whose displaced maxillary permanent canines improved following the extraction of the upper deciduous canines.

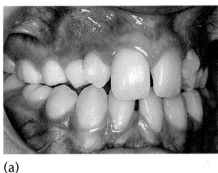

(a)

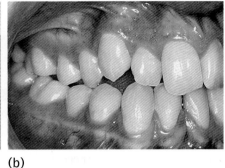

(b)

Fig. 14.5 (a) Patient aged 9 years showing distal inclination of the upper lateral incisor caused by the position of the unerupted canine; (b) the same patient aged 13 years showing the improvement that has occurred in the inclination of the lateral incisor following eruption of the permanent canine.

away from the midline and at a slightly less acute angle to the occlusal plane, i.e. more favourably positioned for alignment, than is actually the case (Fig. 14.6a). This view should be supplemented with an intra-oral view.

- **Periapical.** This view is useful for assessing the prognosis of a retained deciduous canine and for detecting resorption (Fig. 14.6b).

- **Upper anterior occlusal.** To facilitate the use of vertical parallax in conjunction with an OPT radiograph the angle of the tube should be increased to 70–75° (rather than the customary 60–65°).

- **Lateral cephalometric.** For accurate localization this view should be combined with an anteroposterior view (e.g. an OPT) (Fig. 14.6c).

- **Cone beam computerized tomography (CBCT).** Due to the increased radiographic dose, most orthodontists restrict CBCT to those ectopic canines where accurate localization has not been possible with conventional views and/or root resorption of adjacent teeth is suspected (see Fig. 5.17).

The principle of parallax can be used to determine the position of an unerupted tooth relative to its neighbours. To use parallax two radiographs are required with a change in the position of the X-ray tube

> **Box 14.3 The radiographic assessment of a displaced canine should include the following:**
>
> - location of the position of both the canine crown and the root apex relative to adjacent teeth and the arch;
> - the prognosis of adjacent teeth and the deciduous canine, if present;
> - the presence of resorption, particularly of the adjacent central and/or lateral incisors.

between them. The object furthest away from the X-ray beam will appear to move in the same direction as the tube shift. Therefore, if the canine is more palatally positioned than the incisor roots it will move with the tube shift (Fig. 14.6b). Conversely, if it is buccal it will move in the opposite direction to the tube shift. Examples of combinations of radiographs which can be used for parallax include two periapical radiographs (horizontal parallax) and an OPT and an upper anterior occlusal (vertical parallax).

14.6 Management of buccal displacement

NB the width of the maxillary canine is greater than that of the first premolar which in turn is greater than that of the deciduous canine.

Buccal displacement is usually associated with crowding, and therefore relief of crowding prior to eruption of the canine will usually effect some spontaneous improvement (Fig. 14.7). Buccal displacements are more likely to erupt than palatal displacements because of the thinner buccal mucosa and bone. Erupted, buccally displaced canines are managed by relief of crowding, if indicated, and alignment—usually with a fixed appliance.

In severely crowded cases where the upper lateral incisor and first premolar are in contact and no additional space exists to accommodate the wider canine tooth, extraction of the canine itself may be indicated.

In some patients the canine is so severely displaced that a good result is unlikely, necessitating removal of the canine tooth and the use of fixed appliances to close any residual spacing.

More rarely a buccally displaced canine tooth does not erupt or its eruption is so delayed that treatment for other aspects of the malocclusion is compromised. In these situations exposure of the impacted tooth may be indicated. To ensure an adequate width of attached gingiva either an apically repositioned or, preferably, a replaced flap should be used. In the latter case, in order to be able to apply traction to align the canine, an attachment can be bonded to the tooth at the time of surgery. A gold chain or a stainless steel ligature can be attached to the bond or band and used to apply traction.

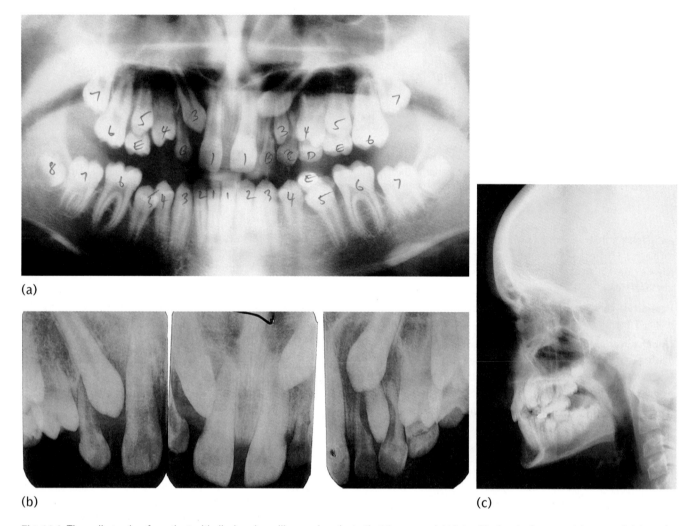

(a)

(b)

(c)

Fig. 14.6 The radiographs of a patient with displaced maxillary canines (note that the upper right lateral incisor is absent and the upper left lateral incisor is peg-shaped): (a) OPT radiograph; (b) periapical radiographs (note that both maxillary canines are palatally positioned as their position changes in the same direction as the tube shift); (c) lateral cephalometric radiograph.

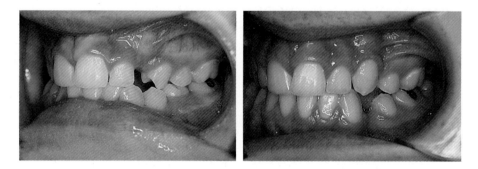

Fig. 14.7 Mildly buccally displaced maxillary canine which erupted spontaneously into a satisfactory position following relief of crowding.

14.7 Management of palatal displacement

The treatment options available are as follows (see also Box 14.4).

Box 14.4 Factors affecting treatment decision

- Patient's opinion of appearance and motivation towards orthodontic treatment
- Malocclusion
- Position of displaced canine: is it within range of orthodontic alignment?
- Presence of spacing/crowding
- Condition of retained deciduous canine, if present
- Condition of adjacent teeth

14.7.1 Surgical removal of canine

This option can be considered under the following conditions:

- The retained deciduous canine has an acceptable appearance and the patient is happy with the aesthetics and/or reluctant to embark on more complicated treatment (Fig. 14.8). The clinician must ensure that the patient understands that the primary canine will be lost eventually and a prosthetic replacement required. However, if the occlusion is unfavourable, for example a deep and increased overbite is present, this may affect the feasibility of bridgework later, necessitating the exploration of alternative options.
- The upper arch is very crowded and the upper first premolar is adjacent to the upper lateral incisor. Provided that the first premolar is not mesiopalatally rotated, the aesthetic result can be acceptable (Fig. 14.9).
- The canine is severely displaced. Depending upon the presence of crowding and the patient's wishes, either any residual spacing can be closed by forward movement of the upper buccal segments with fixed appliances, or a prosthetic replacement can be considered.

If space closure is not planned, it may be preferable to keep the unerupted canine under biannual radiographic observation until the fate of the third molars is decided. However, if any pathology, for example resorption of adjacent teeth or cyst formation, intervenes, removal should be arranged as soon as possible.

14.7.2 Surgical exposure and orthodontic alignment

Indications are as follows:

- well-motivated patient
- well-cared-for dentition
- favourable canine position
- space available (or can be created)

Whether orthodontic alignment is feasible or not depends upon the three-dimensional position of the unerupted canine:

- **Height:** the higher a canine is positioned relative to the occlusal plane the poorer the prognosis. In addition, the access for surgical exposure will be more restricted. If the crown tip is at or above the apical third of the incisor roots, orthodontic alignment will be very difficult.
- **Anteroposterior position:** the nearer the canine crown is to the midline, the more difficult alignment will be. Most operators regard canines, which are more than halfway across the upper central incisor to be outside the limits of orthodontics.
- **Position of the apex:** the further away the canine apex is from normal, the poorer the prognosis for successful alignment. If it is distal to the second premolar, other options should be considered.
- **Inclination:** the smaller the angle with the occlusal plane the greater the need for traction.

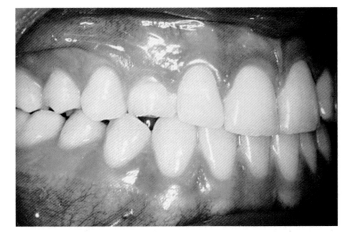

Fig. 14.8 This patient decided that the appearance of her retained deciduous canine was satisfactory and elected to have her unerupted displaced maxillary canine removed.

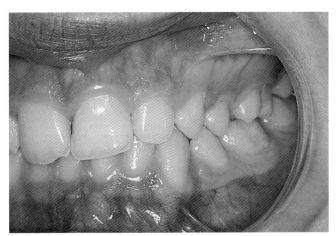

Fig. 14.9 Aesthetic result following removal of the displaced upper left permanent canine.

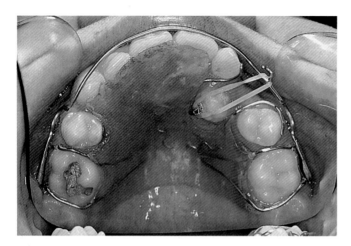

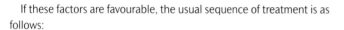

Fig. 14.10 Traction applied to an exposed canine using a removable appliance.

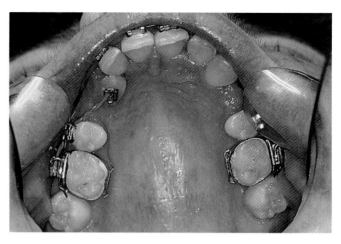

Fig. 14.11 A fixed appliance being used to move an exposed canine towards the line of the arch.

If these factors are favourable, the usual sequence of treatment is as follows:

(1) Make space available (although some operators are reluctant to embark on permanent extractions until after the tooth has been exposed and traction successfully started).

(2) Arrange exposure.

(3) Allow the tooth to erupt for 2 to 3 months.

(4) Commence traction.

With deeply buried canines there is a danger that the gingivae may cover the tooth again. If this is likely to be a problem, either an attachment plus the means of traction (for example a wire ligature or gold chain) can be bonded to the tooth at the time of exposure or about 2 days after pack removal.

Traction can be applied using either a removable appliance (Fig. 14.10) or a fixed appliance (Fig. 14.11). To complete alignment a fixed appliance is necessary, as movement of the root apex buccally is required to complete positioning of the canine into a functional relationship with the lower arch.

14.7.3 Transplantation

In the past the long-term results of transplantation have been disappointing. Recent work has highlighted the importance of timing, in view of the stage of root development of the canine and careful surgical technique. Transplantation should be carried out when the canine root is two-thirds to three-quarters of its final length; unfortunately, by the time most ectopic canines are diagnosed root development is further advanced.

If transplantation is to be attempted, it must be possible to remove the canine intact and there must be space available to accommodate the canine within the arch and occlusion. In some cases this will mean that some orthodontic treatment will be required prior to transplantation.

The main causes of failure of transplanted canines are replacement resorption and inflammatory resorption. Replacement resorption, or ankylosis, occurs when the root surface is damaged during the surgical procedure and is promoted by rigid splinting of the transplanted tooth, which encourages healing by bony rather than fibrous union. A more recent study has indicated that a careful surgical technique is essential to prevent damage to the root surface and the transplanted canine should be positioned out of occlusion and splinted with a sectional archwire for 6 weeks.

Inflammatory resorption follows death of the pulpal tissues, and therefore the vitality of the transplanted tooth must be carefully monitored.

14.8 Resorption

Unerupted and impacted canines can cause resorption of adjacent lateral incisor roots and may sometimes progress to cause resorption of the central incisor. The increasing use of CBCT has shown that the prevalence of root resorption is greater than previously thought. A recent study indicated that two-thirds of upper lateral incisors associated with ectopic canines showed signs of resorption. This sequelae is more common in females than males.

Swift intervention is essential, as resorption often proceeds at a rapid rate. If it is discovered on radiographic examination, specialist advice should be sought quickly. Extraction of the canine may be necessary to halt the resorption. However, if the resorption is severe it may be wiser to extract the affected incisor(s), thus allowing the canine to erupt (Fig. 14.12).

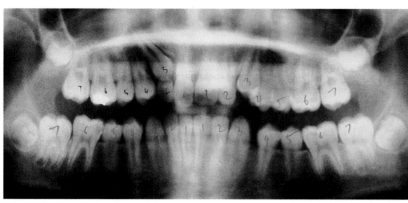

(a)

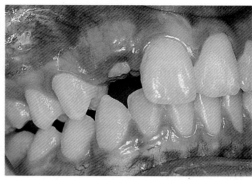

(b)

Fig. 14.12 (a) Resorption of the upper right lateral incisor by an unerupted maxillary canine; (b) following extraction of the lateral incisor the canine erupted adjacent to the central incisor.

14.9 Transposition

Transposition is the term used to describe interchange in the position of two teeth. This anomaly is comparatively rare, but almost always affects the canine tooth. It affects males and females equally and is more common in the maxilla. In the upper arch the canine and the first premolar are most commonly involved; however, transposition of the canine and lateral incisor is also seen (Fig. 14.13). In the mandible the canine and lateral incisor appear to be almost exclusively affected (Fig 14.14). The aetiology of this condition is not understood.

Management depends upon whether the transposition is complete (i.e. the apices of the affected teeth are transposed); or partial; the malocclusion; and the presence or absence of crowding. Possible treatment options include acceptance (particularly if transposition is complete), extraction of the most displaced tooth if the arch is crowded, or orthodontic alignment. In the last case, the relative positions of the root apices will be a major factor in deciding whether the affected teeth are corrected or aligned in their transposed arrangement.

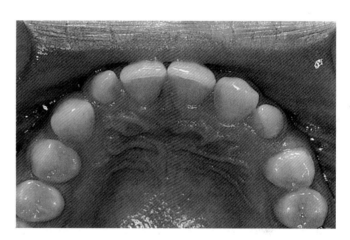

Fig. 14.13 Transposition of the upper left maxillary canine and lateral incisor.

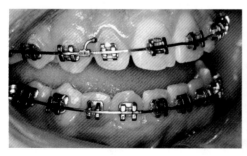

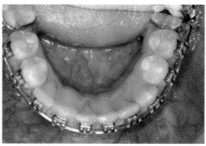

Fig. 14.14 Patient with transposition of lower left canine and lateral incisor.

Key points

- It is important that the position of the maxillary canine is assessed from age 10 years onwards and if displacement is suspected further investigation instigated
- Palatal displacement is associated with a number of common dental anomalies therefore it is especially important to check the position of the canine in affected patients

Relevant Cochrane reviews:

Extraction of primary (baby) teeth for unerupted palatally displaced permanent canine teeth in children
Parkin, N. *et al*. (2009)
http://onlinelibrary.wiley.com/doi/10.1002/14651858.CD004621.pub2/abstract
(see Section 14.4)
Open versus closed surgical exposure of canine teeth that are displaced in the roof of the mouth
Parkin, N. *et al*. (2008)
http://onlinelibrary.wiley.com/doi/10.1002/14651858.CD006966.pub2/abstract
This review concluded that currently, there is no evidence to support one surgical technique over the other in terms of dental health, aesthetics, economics and patient factors

Principal sources and further reading

Armstrong, C., Johnstone, C., Burden, D., and Stevenson, M. (2003). Localising ectopic maxillary canines – horizontal or vertical parallax. *European Journal of Orthodontics*, **25**, 585–9.

Becker, A., Smith, P., and Behar, R. (1981). The incidence of anomalous maxillary lateral incisors in relation to palatally-displaced cuspids. *Angle Orthodontist*, **51**, 24–9.

Brough, E., Donaldson, A.N., and Naini, F.B. (2010). Canine substitution for missing maxillary lateral incisors: The influence of canine morphology, size, and shade on perceptions of smile attractiveness. *American Journal of Orthodontics and Dentofacial Orthopedics*, **138**, 705–7.

An interesting question and answer exchange between the editor of the journal and the authors.

Fleming, P.S., Sharma, P.K., and DiBiase, A.T. (2010). How to . . . mechanically erupt a palatal canine. *Journal of Orthodontics*, **37**, 262–71.

A well-illustrated paper that describes the practical steps in aligning a palatal canine following exposure.

Gorlin, R. J., Cohen, M. M., and Levin, L. S. (1990). *Syndromes of the Head and Neck* (3rd edn). Oxford University Press, Oxford.

This excellent reference book includes, amongst a wealth of other information, data on the development and incidence of canine anomalies.

Hussain, J., Burden, D., and McSherry, P. (2010). Management of the palatally ectopic maxillary canine. *Faculty of Dental Surgery of the Royal College of Surgeons of England* ((http://www.rcseng.ac.uk/fds/publications-clinical-guidelines/clinical_guidelines/index.html).

This review evaluates the evidence relating to the management of palatally displaced canines.

Jacobs, S. G. (1999). Localisation of the unerupted maxillary canine: how to and when to. *American Journal of Orthodontics and Dentofacial Orthopedics*, **115**, 314–22.

An interesting discussion of different radiographic approaches to localizing unerupted maxillary canines.

Leonardi, M., Armi, P., Franchi, L., and Baccetti, T. (2004). Two interceptive approaches to palatally displaced canines: A prospective longitudinal study. *Angle Orthodontist*, **74**, 581–6.

McSherry, P. F. and Richardson, A. (1999). Ectopic eruption of the maxillary canine quantified in three dimensions on cephalometric radiographs between the ages of 5 and 15 years. *European Journal of Orthodontics*, **21**, 41–8.

This interesting study found that differences in the eruption pattern of palatally ectopic canines was evident from as early as 5 years of age.

Parkin, N. and Benson, P. (2011). Current ideas on the management of palatally displaced canines. *Faculty Dental Journal*, **2**, 24–9.

An excellent article by the authors of the two Cochrane reviews putting their findings into context.

Peck, S. M., Peck, L., and Kataja, M. (1994). The palatally displaced canine as a dental anomaly of genetic origin. *Angle Orthodontist*, **64**, 249–56.

References for this chapter can also be found at www.oxfordtextbooks.co.uk/orc/mitchell4e/. Where possible, these are presented as active links which direct you to the electronic version of the work, to help facilitate onward study. If you are a subscriber to that work (either individually or through an institution), and depending on your level of access, you may be able to peruse an abstract or the full article if available.

15

Anchorage planning

F. Dyer

Chapter contents

15.1 Introduction

Anchorage is defined as the resistance to unwanted tooth movement.

Tooth movement is achieved through the forces generated by an orthodontic appliance. However, the force generated has an equal and opposite reactionary force, as described by Newton's Third Law, which will in turn be spread over the teeth that are contacted by the appliance. It is the anchorage support that resists these reactionary forces and prevents unwanted tooth movement. The aim of anchorage is to minimize the unwanted tooth movement and maximize the desired tooth movements.

An analogy which may help to simplify this difficult concept is that of ice skating. Imagine that you are standing on the ice and push against the barrier of the rink. You will move backwards and the barrier will remain stationary. The barrier in this instance is analogous to absolute anchorage (see Section 15.3) for example an ankylosed tooth or osseintegrated implant.

If two skaters push against each other equally, and they themselves are of similar size, both will move backwards by an equal amount. This is an equal and opposite reaction. If one skater is larger than the other, the smaller skater will be pushed away, whereas the larger skater will only move slightly, or not at all. However, if the larger skater now pushes against two smaller skaters then the larger skater will move. This can be considered similar to pitting one larger tooth

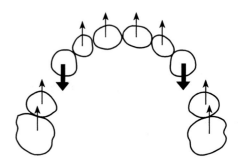

Fig. 15.1 Diagram showing the effect upon the anchor teeth of retracting upper canines with a fixed appliance.

against another smaller tooth, or against two smaller teeth. The more teeth you try to move the more likely your anchorage unit will move as well.

A clinical scenario is the retraction of upper canines using a fixed appliance, with all the available teeth involved in the appliance. An equal and opposite force to that being generated by retracting canines will also be acting on the remaining upper arch teeth to move them anteriorly, which can comprise the anchorage unit causing unwanted tooth movement of the rest of the dentition (Fig. 15.1).

15.2 Assessing anchorage requirements

Anchorage requirements should be considered in three dimensions, anteroposteriorly, vertically and transversely. Planning anchorage is a fundamental part of treatment planning and should be considered as part of managing space requirements. When considering anchorage management it is important to assess the following:

15.2.1 Space requirements

The amount of crowding or spacing should be assessed as part of treatment planning. This can be done using visual assessment or more formally using a space analysis (Section 7.7).

Maximum anchorage support is required when all or most of the space created, most commonly through tooth extraction, is required in order to achieve the desired tooth movements.

15.2.2 The type of tooth movement to be achieved

There are six different types of tooth movement: tipping, bodily movement, rotation, torquing, intrusion and extrusion. Tipping occurs when the crown of a tooth moves in one direction and the root moves by a lesser amount in the opposite direction (Fig. 15.2). Bodily movement occurs when both the crown and the root move in the same direction equally (Fig. 15.3). Rotation movement occurs when a force is applied mesially or distally to the labial aspect of a tooth.

Teeth have a centre of resistance around which movement occurs. If force is applied to the centre of resistance then the tooth will move bodily, however, the centre of resistance lies within the root and hence a force cannot be applied directly. A simple force applied to the crown of a

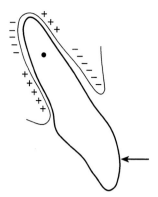

Fig. 15.2 Diagram showing the effect of a tipping force applied to the crown of a tooth (+ = pressure; - = tension).

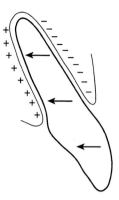

Fig. 15.3 Diagram showing the distribution of the applied force with bodily movement (+ = pressure; - = tension).

tooth will cause the tooth to tip, however with a fixed appliance in place, the built-in program of the bracket interacting with the orthodontic wire causes the force to act as a couple, which can be used to change the inclination of teeth or to produce bodily movement.

Bodily movement requires more force than tipping movements and is therefore more anchorage demanding.

15.2.3 The number of teeth to be moved

As the number of teeth to be moved increases so does the anchorage demand. If the anchorage requirements of treatment are high then consideration should be given to, for example, moving a single tooth in stages or only a few teeth at a time to conserve anchorage.

15.2.4 The distance of the movement required

The greater the distance the teeth are to be moved, the greater the strain on the anchorage, and the greater the risk of unwanted tooth movement.

15.2.5 Aims of treatment

The fewer teeth that need to be moved to achieve the aims of treatment then the lesser anchorage demand, however, if treatment is complex and multiple teeth are to be moved there will be a greater anchorage demand. The aims of treatment should be clear. In cases with a Class II molar relationship, anchorage needs will be greater if a Class I molar (and canine) relationship is to be achieved rather than a Class II molar (and Class I canine) relationship (Fig. 15.4). The need to achieve a Class I canine relationship is essential for the success of all treatment, anchorage planning should therefore focus not only on the intended molar movements but also importantly on the required movements of the canines to achieve this goal (Fig. 15.5).

15.2.6 Root surface area of the teeth to be moved

The size of the root surface area of the tooth or teeth to be moved influences the anchorage requirements – the larger the root surface area the greater the demand (Fig. 15.6). For tooth movement to occur, a threshold of force must be achieved. This applies equally to the teeth in the

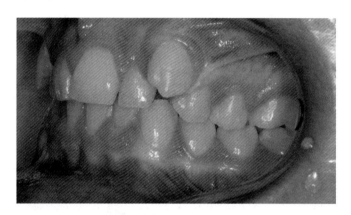

Fig. 15.4 Anchorage requirements will alter dramatically in this patient depending on whether you aim to treat to Class I or Class II molars. For both, however, anchorage reinforcement is required as the molars are already a full unit Class II. No mesial movement at all is allowable and so this case has a high anchorage need.

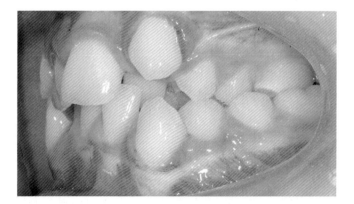

Fig. 15.5 This case demonstrates significant upper and lower arch crowding. Extractions will therefore be required in both arches and so the lower canines will move distally during treatment. In order to achieve a Class I canine relationship the upper canines will require significant distal movement and anchorage reinforcement for example with headgear is indicated.

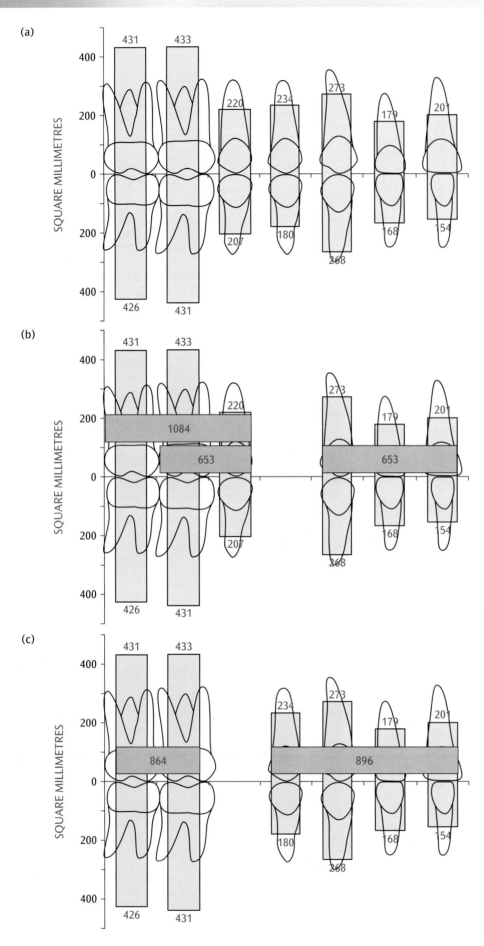

Fig. 15.6 Diagrammatic representation of the relative root surface areas of the permanent dentition and the effect on anchorage requirements. (a) Root surface areas for the permanent dentition (excluding third molars). (b) Anchorage balance following the extraction of all four first premolars. If the second molars are not included then space closure will occur equally from the posterior teeth moving mesially and the anterior teeth moving distally, due to the similar root surface areas of the anterior teeth, and the second premolar and first permanent molar. However, if the second permanent molar is included in the appliance then the anchorage balance will be shifted to favour distal movement of the anterior teeth. (c) Anchorage balance following removal of second premolars. If the second permanent molars are not included in the appliance, most of the space closure will occur by the first permanent molars moving mesially (adapted from Jepson, 1963).

anchorage unit and if the threshold is exceeded unwanted movement of the anchor teeth will occur and anchorage will be lost. Therefore the forces applied to achieve the desired tooth movements must be carefully selected to try and ensure they remain below the threshold of the teeth acting as the anchorage unit. Increasing the number of teeth acting in an anchorage unit (for example including the second molars in a fixed appliance) is one method of increasing this threshold.

15.2.7 Growth rotation and skeletal pattern

An increased rate of tooth movement has been associated with patients who have an increased vertical dimension or backward growth rotation. It has been suggested that space closure or anchorage loss may occur more rapidly in these high angled cases. Conversely in a patient with reduced vertical dimensions or a forward growth rotation, space loss or anchorage loss may be slower. A possible explanation that has been proposed for this observation is the relative strength of the facial muscles, with reduced vertical dimensions having a stronger musculature.

15.3 Classification of anchorage

- **Simple anchorage** – one tooth against another.
- **Intramaxillary compound anchorage** – multiple teeth are used in an anchorage unit in the same arch, for example using a molar and a second premolar as an anchorage unit for retraction of a canine.
- **Intermaxillary compound anchorage** – multiple teeth in opposing arches, for example intermaxillary elastics.

15.4 Intra-oral anchorage

Anchorage reinforcement can be achieved by utilizing the teeth, soft tissues and skeletal structures intra-orally.

15.4.1 Increasing the number of teeth in the anchorage unit

Incorporating as many teeth as possible into an anchorage unit will aid in reducing anchorage loss, and if the anchorage demand is high then consideration should be given to moving one tooth at a time to prevent strain of the anchorage unit (conserving anchorage).

15.4.2 Differential extraction pattern

The extraction pattern planned for the patient can influence the anchorage balance of a case. Extracting teeth closer to the site of crowding reduces the amount of tooth movement required and thus the risk of anchorage loss. Also by selection of the teeth to be extracted the number of teeth in the anchorage unit can be increased, thus making it more resistant to unwanted movement (Fig.15.6).

A differential extraction pattern, between arches, can aid in anchorage management. One such example is the treatment of Class II division

15.2.8 Occlusal interdigitation and occlusal interferences

Occlusal interdigitation or occlusal interferences can prevent or slow tooth movement, this in turn can increase the anchorage demand and, if severe, may prevent the desired tooth movement and increase the likelihood of unwanted tooth movement. It has been suggested that if teeth in the anchorage unit have a good interdigitation this may increase the anchorage by reducing mesial movement of the anchorage unit.

15.2.9 Bone quality

Maxillary bone is less dense than mandibular bone so the threshold for tooth movement in the maxillary teeth is lower than that in the mandibular teeth. Teeth move more readily through cancellous bone than cortical bone and anchorage can be increased by moving the roots of teeth closer to the cortical plate, however this may put them at increased risk of root resorption so should be done with care.

- **Reciprocal anchorage** – two groups of teeth of equal size or equivalent anchorage value are pitted against each other, resulting in movement of both units. For example, a quadhelix used to expand the maxillary arch. (Fig. 15.7) or applying power chain on an upper fixed appliance to two central incisors across a diastema.
- **Stationary/absolute anchorage** – this can only be achieved when using an osseintegrated implant or ankylosed tooth as an anchorage unit.

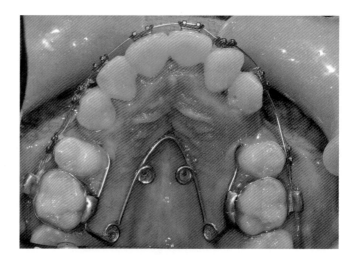

Fig. 15.7 Quadhelix fixed appliance to expand the upper arch.

I cases where the upper first premolars are extracted to aid reduction of an overjet and correction of the canine relationship to Class I. This becomes possible as the anchorage unit is greater posteriorly in the maxilla with the upper first molars and second premolars on board. In the lower arch the extraction of the lower second premolars will prevent retraction of the lower labial segment but also work favourably for molar correction with the lower molars more likely to move mesially. This extraction pattern can be reversed in the treatment of Class III cases with extraction of lower first premolars and upper second premolars. This differential extraction pattern will aid the camouflage of the reverse overjet with retroclination of the lower labial segment.

15.4.3 Care with initial intra-arch orthodontic mechanics

Engagement of severely displaced teeth in the early stages of alignment may increase anchorage demands. Anchorage loss will also occur if there is friction in the system as a greater force needs to be exerted to overcome friction and achieve the planned tooth movement. As a result of the higher forces applied, the reactionary force is higher and may result in unwanted tooth movement of the anchorage unit.

15.4.4 Bodily movement of teeth

Bodily movement requires more force than tipping movements and is therefore more anchorage demanding. Use of large rectangular stainless steel archwires will ensure bodily movement occurs rather than tipping, as the archwire will fill more of the bracket slot (see Fig. 18.6).

15.4.5 Transpalatal and lingual arches

Both a transpalatal arch (usually connecting the upper first molars) and a lower lingual arch (usually connecting lower first molars) can be used to reinforce anchorage by linking contralateral molar teeth (Figs 15.8 and 15.9). The teeth are joined with an arch bar, usually 1 mm diameter stainless steel, which connects across the vault of the palate or around the lingual aspect of the lower arch. This linking of teeth helps to prevent or reduce unwanted mesial molar movement. Anchorage can potentially be further increased by adding an acrylic button or Nance button, which lightly contacts the anterior palatal mucosa (Fig. 15.10). Caution should be taken with all these appliances as if anchorage is lost (that is, the molars move mesially) the lingual arch can cause proclination of the lower labial segment, or the U-loop of the transpalatal arch or acrylic of the Nance button may become engaged in the palatal mucosa. With this in mind the palatal loop of the transpalatal arch would normally face distally.

15.4.6 Intermaxillary anchorage

Anchorage from one arch can be used to reinforce anchorage in the other. This is typically the outcome when using intermaxillary elastic traction (see Section 18.3.4). Intra-oral elastics are available in a variety of sizes and strengths. Class II elastics will be run anteriorly in the upper arch to posteriorly in the lower. Class III elastics are the reverse, anteriorly in the lower to posteriorly in the upper (Figs 15.11 and 15.12).

As with any force applied there can be unwanted effects, and intermaxillary traction is not without this problem. Class II or Class III elastics

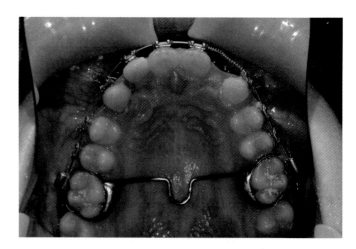

Fig. 15.8 Transpalatal arch (NB. U-loop facing distally).

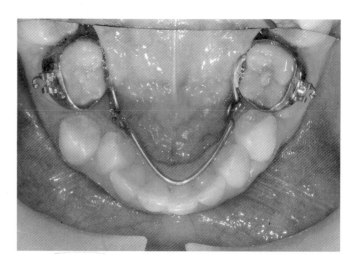

Fig. 15.9 Lingual arch.

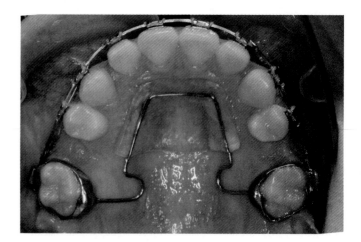

Fig. 15.10 Transpalatal arch with Nance button. The anterior palatal vault is used as additional anchorage with the addition of an acrylic button.

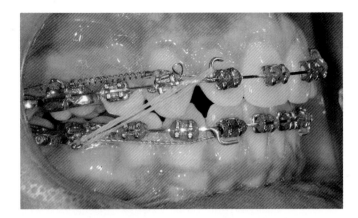

Fig. 15.11 Class II intermaxillary traction (elastics).

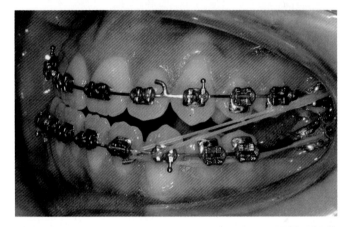

Fig. 15.12 Class III intermaxillary traction (elastics).

can lead to extrusion of the molars, which will in turn reduce the overbite and also cause an increase in the face height, this might be beneficial in a few patients but for the majority these movements would be unwanted. In an unspaced lower arch then use of Class II elastics can result in proclination of the lower labial segment.

15.4.7 Removable and functional appliances

Removable appliances can be used alone or to reinforce anchorage in conjunction with a fixed appliance (Fig. 15.13). By virtue of their palatal coverage they increase anchorage. Other design features which reinforce anchorage include:

- Anteroposteriorly – by colleting around the posterior teeth with acrylic; inclined bite-blocks, palatal bows or the use of incisor capping.

- Transversely – the pitting of one side of the arch against the other can reinforce transverse anchorage, typically seen where an expansion screw or coffin screw is used for increasing the palatal transverse dimension (Fig. 15.14).

- Vertically – by either reducing the vertical dimensions during treatment of a high angle patient by intruding the posterior teeth, or increasing the vertical dimension by allowing differential eruption with the use of an anterior bite-plane.

All of these three dimensional features can be incorporated into functional appliances, which additionally can be used to gain anchorage in the anteroposterior direction to aid in the treatment of a Class II malocclusion.

15.4.8 Temporary anchorage devices (TADs)

The use of TADs, also known as orthodontic bone anchorage devices, is becoming increasingly popular in contemporary orthodontics (Fig. 15.15). They first became popular in the 1990s and were developed from the dental implants used in restorative dentistry and maxillofacial bone plates. There are three distinct types (Box 15.1):

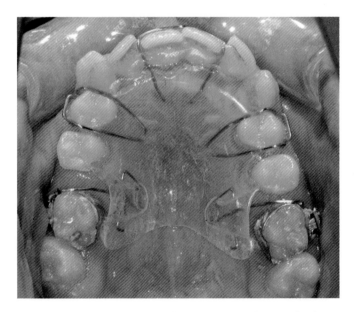

Fig. 15.13 Nudger removable appliance used as an adjunct to fixed appliance treatment. The nudger is worn full time, holding the distal movement achieved during the part-time (12–14 hours) headgear wear.

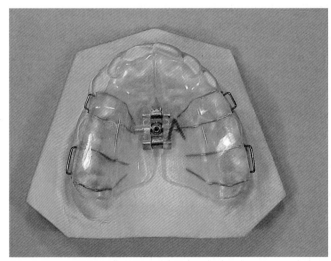

Fig. 15.14 Upper removable appliance with midline expansion screw – demonstrates reciprocal anchorage.

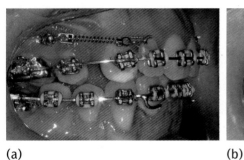

(a)

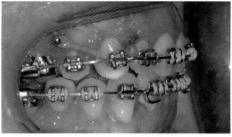

(b)

Fig 15.15 Temporary Anchorage Device to conserve anchorage in maximum anchorage case: (a) at commencement of space closure; (b) 3 months later.

- Osseointegrated implants

These were modified from dental implants, making them shorter, with a wider diameter than those used in restorative dentistry. Osseointegrated implants can be used to provide maximum anchorage, and are useful if large or difficult tooth movements are required. A randomized controlled trial compared this type of implant placed in the mid-palatal region and attached to a palatal arch with conventional headgear (Fig. 15.16). The authors concluded that mid-palatal implants are an acceptable technique for reinforcement of anchorage.

They have three principle disadvantages:

(1) They need to be left for 3 months after placement to allow osseointegration

(2) Due to their size they are restricted to being used in edentulous areas

(3) Since the implant osseointegrates it requires a complex surgical procedure together with bone removal at the completion of treatment and some patients may find this unacceptable.

- Miniplate systems

These are based on maxillofacial bone plates, with a transmucosal portion projecting into the mouth to allow connection to the fixed appliance. They can provide reliable anchorage, but require a surgical procedure to place them and remove them.

- Miniscrews

These were developed from the screws of maxillofacial plating systems. No osseointegration is required (or desired) and they are small in size (typically 6 to 12 mm long and 1.5 to 2 mm in diameter). The

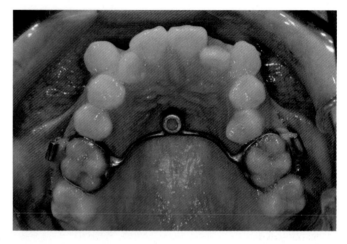

Fig 15.16 Osseointegrated midpalatal implant used in conjunction with transpalatal arch to achieve absolute anchorage.

head and neck configuration has been adapted to facilitate placement of auxiliaries to the fixed appliance (see Fig. 12.11).

Due to their ease of use – for both the patient and the orthodontist – the miniscrew approach is now the most popular. They can be placed under local anaesthesia, and can usually be removed at the end of treatment without requiring any anaesthetic.

Bone anchorage devices have the ability to provide anchorage in three dimensions: anteroposteriorly, vertically and transversely. They can provide anchorage either directly or indirectly:

Direct anchorage is achieved when forces are applied directly to the TAD.

Indirect anchorage is achieved when the TAD is linked to the anchorage teeth, and then the orthodontic forces are applied to this anchorage unit.

The use of TADs is allowing different approaches to anchorage, as well as possibly altering the scope of what was previously thought possible with fixed appliances.

Box 15.1 Classification of TADs

Mechanical retention
 –Screw design
 –Plate design
Osseointegration

15.5 Extra-oral anchorage

15.5.1 General principles

Headgear can be used for:

- Extra-oral traction or
- Extra-oral anchorage

Extra-oral anchorage holds the posterior teeth in position, preventing unwanted mesial movement of the anchorage unit.

Extra-oral traction applies a distal force to the posterior teeth to achieve tooth movement usually in a distal direction. Traction is also used to attempt to restrict the growth of the maxilla forwards and downwards (an orthopaedic effect). In simple terms traction requires greater forces for longer periods of time.

There are three directions of pull that can be achieved with headgear and should be considered at the time of treatment planning (Box 15.2):

- **High or occipital-pull headgear** which helps to control the vertical as well as anteroposterior anchorage and is typically used in cases with increased vertical proportions (Fig. 15.17).

- **Straight or combi-pull headgear** which controls the anteroposterior and is typically used in cases with average vertical proportions (Fig. 15.18).

- **Low or cervical-pull headgear** which aid in the control of anteroposterior anchorage but is also used to increase the vertical dimension by having an extrusive effect on the molars in cases of reduced vertical proportions (Fig. 15.19). Care should be taken with low pull headgear in a Class II skeletal pattern as extrusion of the maxillary molars may lead to a clockwise rotation of the mandible making the class II skeletal pattern worse as the mandible rotates downwards and backwards.

The amount of force applied to the headgear is controlled by adjusting the attachment straps and can and should be carefully monitored at each visit. For orthodontic change is it normal to apply 250–350 g to achieve anchorage reinforcement, for extra-oral traction the force is increased to 400–450 g. For orthopaedic change, termed maxillary restraint, the forces are increased to 500 g.

The duration of force also varies according to the purpose. Extra-oral anchorage requires a minimum of 10 hours per day, usually best achieved at bedtime. Extra-oral traction requires increased duration and a minimum of 12 hours of wear per day is required though most operators ask for 14 hours. For orthopaedic changes the wear requested is normally also 14 hours, but the length of treatment with the headgear appliance is longer when compared to extra-oral traction (which may be achieved, in a co-operative patient, within 6–9 months).

The effect of a force depends on where it is applied in relation to the centre of resistance. If the force passes directly through the centre of resistance then pure translation will occur. If not then tipping will arise.

The centre of resistance for forces applied to the upper first molars is felt to be at the trifurcation of their roots. The centre of resistance for the maxilla, as a whole however, is further forward, and is suggested to be between the premolar roots. Adjustment of the direction of force applied by the headgear relative to the centre of resistance of the first molar will influence how the molar will move.

In theory intrusion of the upper incisors can be attempted by applying headgear to the anterior labial segment of a working archwire,

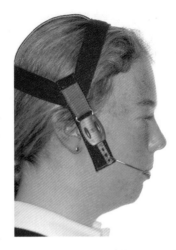

Fig. 15.17 High-pull headgear attached to face-bow with snap-away design.

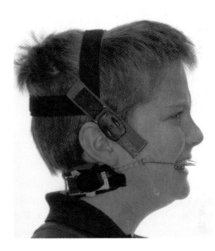

Fig 15.18 Combination headgear using high-pull and cervical pull together.

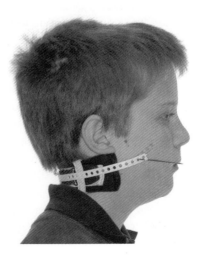

Fig. 15.19 Cervical pull headgear with neck strap.

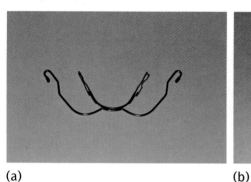
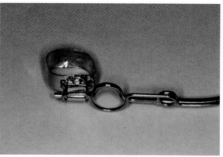

(a)   (b)

Fig. 15.20 NiTom locking face-bow: (a) the left side is closed and the right side open; (b) shows face-bow inserted into headgear tube on molar band.

though the forces used must be light to avoid possible root resorption of the upper incisors. Due to concerns over safety this technique is now largely abandoned.

Headgear can be added to a removable appliance or a functional appliance, such as a Twin Block. In this case the forces are kept above the occlusal plane, not only to control the vertical dimension but also to prevent dislodging the appliance.

15.5.2 Components of headgear

The components of headgear have been modified dramatically in the last 10 years to improve safety (see Section 15.5.3). Where headgear is to be used in conjunction with a fixed appliance, patients first need to be fitted with upper molar orthodontic bands with buccal headgear tubes. Where headgear is being used with a removable or functional appliance then either tubes need to be added to the molar clasps or headgear tubes incorporated into the acrylic (see Fig. 17.7).

- Face-bow. The face-bow slots into the headgear tubes. Currently the face-bow of choice is a NiTom locking face-bow produced with a specialized safety catch (Fig. 15.20). However, a less complex safety version is the Hamill face-bow with a reverse loop attachment (Fig. 15.21).

- Headcap or strap. A headcap or neck strap can be used independently or together to achieve the direction of pull required.

Cervical pull: use of neck strap alone (Fig. 15.19). The force will be downwards and backwards with an extrusive element. Useful in patients with deep bites and low mandibular plane angles as this direction will tend to extrude the molars resulting in an increase in the lower face height and reduction of the overbite.

Headcap (Fig. 15.17): this produces intrusive forces and will affect the vertical element by intrusion of the molars. This approach is useful where no increase in the vertical proportions can be tolerated during treatment. The forces will also prevent further eruption of the molars.

Combination pull (Fig. 15.18): uses the headcap and neck strap together. In this situation it is anticipated that the movements of the molars will be more translational with no intrusive or extrusive effects. Greater forces are applied with the headcap (250–300 g) than the neck strap (100–150 g).

- Spring mechanism or strap. This element connects the face-bow to the headcap or neck strap. Adjustment to this allows for an increase in the magnitude of the force applied. Elastics are rarely used due to their tendency to break.

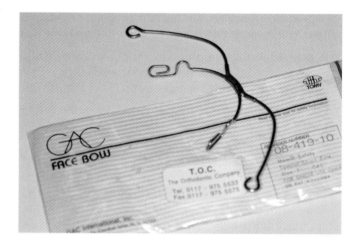

Fig. 15.21 Hamill safety face-bow with reverse loop attachment.

15.5.3 Headgear safety

Injuries associated with headgear have been reported in the past. Most notably these include serious ocular injuries which reportedly resulted in blindness. This is as a result of the ends of the face-bow coming out of the mouth and causing direct trauma to the eyes. This can occur if the face-bow is pulled out of the mouth and recoils back into the face, but has also been reported after spontaneous disengagement at night.

Therefore when fitting headgear it is essential that safety features are incorporated to prevent injuries. The British Orthodontic Society recommends that at least two safety features are incorporated into the headgear. These can take several forms including a snap-away safety release mechanism, rigid neck strap, locking face-bow or safety face-bow (Figs 15.22 and 15.23).

The simplest safety element is the Masel strap (Fig. 15.23), which resists dislodgement of the face-bow. However evidence suggests that this is not a foolproof method as head posture will affect the fit of the strap and still allow detachment of the face-bow (Fig. 15.24).

15.5.4 Reverse headgear

A face-mask or reverse headgear has two uses.

- Tooth movement: moving the posterior maxillary teeth mesially, thereby closing up excess space typically found in hypodontia cases, however this use has diminished due to the increasing use of TADs.

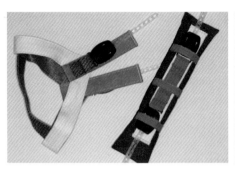

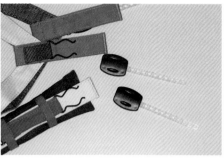

Fig. 15.22 Safety release headgear with a snap-away spring mechanism which breaks apart when excessive force is applied.

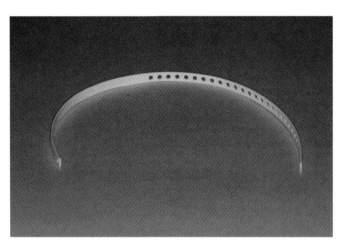

Fig 15.23 Rigid Masel safety strap.

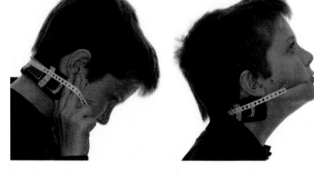

Fig. 15.24 Masel safety strap in use demonstrating how head extension can alter its effectiveness.

- Skeletal changes: advancement of the maxilla can be achieved in patients, where a face-mask is fitted and worn a minimum of 14 hours per day (Fig. 15.25). This approach is discussed further in Chapter 11.

15.6 Monitoring anchorage during treatment

15.6.1 Single-arch treatments

In the situation of an upper removable appliance alone, the lower arch can be used as a guide to monitor anchorage during treatment, in this way the lower arch acts as a reference guide. This would be the same situation in a single-arch fixed case, commonly where the upper arch is being expanded with a quadhelix prior to placement of comprehensive fixed appliances. In both cases a record at each visit of the molar and canine relationships bilaterally should be made, together with overjet changes. In this way any adverse tooth movements can be identified and dealt with.

15.6.2 Definitive orthodontic treatment with upper and lower fixed appliances

In this situation, tooth movements are occurring in both arches simultaneously making assessment more complex. Careful recording of

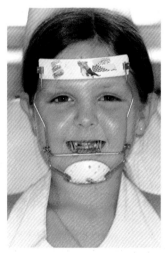

Fig 15.25 Reverse headgear/face-mask.

molar and canine relationships, together with overjet and overbite and space, is essential for these cases. Once alignment has been achieved and prior to starting space closure, anchorage requirements should be re-assessed. In many cases anchorage can be reinforced using either Class II or Class III elastic traction between the arches. Failure to assess the case correctly at this stage may compromise achieving the aims of treatment. Some clinicians advocate taking a lateral cephalogram at this stage to enable comparison with the pre-treatment cephalogram, however this is certainly not required for all patients and in view of the radiation dose should be prescribed with care.

15.7 Common problems with anchorage

Anchorage problems arise when the following occurs:

- Failure to correctly plan anchorage requirements at the start of treatment.
- Poor patient compliance: repeated breakages or failure to wear intermaxillary elastics as instructed will have deleterious effects on the treatment. Lack of headgear wear will necessitate finding alternative methods of anchorage reinforcement, perhaps with the use of TADs or resorting to extractions in a previously non-extraction case.

There is no harm in being over-cautious with anchorage requirements at the start of treatment. A transpalatal arch can be easily removed when the canines are Class I, headgear wear can be reduced. However, to tell a patient that headgear is needed some 6 months into treatment or extractions are now required, when not previously discussed, makes a compromise more likely.

15.8 Summary

Anchorage is the balance between the tooth movements desired to achieve correction of a malocclusion and the undesirable movement of any other teeth. The type of tooth movement carried out will determine the strain applied in turn to the anchorage unit. Anchorage can be increased by maximizing the number of teeth (and surface area of roots) resisting the active tooth movement, either within the same arch (intra maxillary anchorage) or in the opposing arch (intermaxillary anchorage). Extra-oral forces with headgear can also be used, although there is an increasing use in temporary anchorage devices which importantly reduce the need for patient compliance.

Relevant Cochrane reviews:

Skeggs RM, Benson PE, Dyer F (2007). Reinforcement of anchorage during orthodontic brace treatment with implants or other surgical methods. Cochrane Database Syst Rev.Jul 18;(3):CD005098. http://onlinelibrary.wiley.com/o/cochrane/clsysrev/articles/CD005098/frame.html

Key points

- Anchorage is resistance to unwanted movement
- Goals of anchorage management: maximize desired tooth movement and minimize unwanted tooth movement
- Anchorage is not just an anteroposterior phenomenon, unwanted tooth movements occur in the vertical and transverse dimensions also

Principal sources and further reading

Bowden, D. E. J. (1978). Theoretical considerations of headgear therapy; a literature review. *British Journal of Orthodontics*, **5**, 145–52.

Bowden, D. E. J. (1978). Theoretical considerations of headgear therapy: a literature review. Clinical response and usage. *British Journal of Orthodontics*, **5**, 173–81.

These two papers provide an authoritative review of the principles of headgear.

Cousley, R. (2005) Critical aspects in the use of orthodontics palatal implants. *American Journal of Orthodontics and Dentofacial Orthopaedics*, **127**, 723–9.

Crismani, A.G., Berti, M.H., Celar, A.G., Bantleton, H.P., and Burstone, C.J. (2010) Mini-screws in orthodontic treatment: review and analysis of published clinical trials. *American Journal of Orthodontics and Dentofacial Orthopedic*, **137**, 108–13.

This review indicated that mini-screws (TADs) can be used to reinforce anchorage with a failure rate of less than one in five.

Firouz, M., Zernik, J., and Nanda, R. (1992). Dental and orthopaedic effects of high-pull headgear in treatment of Class II, division 1 malocclusion. *American Journal of Orthodontics and Dentofacial Orthopedics*, **102**, 197–205.

Papadopoulos, M. A., Papageorgiou, S. N., and Zogakis, I. P. (2011) Clinical effectiveness of orthodontics miniscrew implants: a meta – analysis. *Journal of Dental Research*, **90,** 969–76. Epub 2011 May 18.

Postlethwaite, K. (1989) The range and effectiveness of safety products. *European Journal of Orthdontics*, **11,** 228–34.

Prahbu, J. and Cousley, R. R. J. (2006). Current products and practice: Bone anchorage devices in Orthodontics. *Journal of Orthodontics*, **33,** 288–307.

This paper is an overview of currently available bone anchorage devices.

Proffit, W. R., Fields, H. R., and Sarver, D. M. (2007). *Contemporary Orthodontics*, 4th edn, Mosby, St Louis.

Reynders, R., Ronchi, L., and Bipat, S. (2009). Mini-implants in orthodontics: a systematic review of the literature. *American Journal of Orthodontics and Dentofacial Orthopaedics*, **135,** 564.e1–564.e19.

Sandler, J., Benson, P. E., Doyle, P., Majumder, A., O'Dwyer, J., Speight, P., Thiruvenkatachari, B., and Tinsley, D. (2008) Palatal implants are a good alternative to headgear: a randomised trial. *American Journal of Orthodontics and Dentofacial Orthopedics*, **133,** 51–7.

Randomised clinical trial to compare headgear wear with mid-palatal implants. Using clinical and radiographic interpretation the mid-palatal implant was found to be very effective.

Stivaros, N., Lowe, C., Dandy, N., Doherty, B., and Mandall, N. A. (2009) A randomized clinical trial to compare the Goshgarian and Nance palatal arch. *European Journal of Orthodontic*, **32,** 171–6. Epub 2009 Dec 3.

Samuels, R. H. (1996). A review of orthodontic face-bow injuries and safety equipment. *American Journal of Orthodontics and Dentofacial Orthopedics*, **110,** 269–72.

Samuels, R. H. (1997). A new locking face-bow. *Journal of Clinical Orthdontics*, **31,** 24–7.

Upadhyay, M., Yadav, S., Nagaraj, K., and Patil, S. (2008) Treatment effects of mini-implants for en-masse retraction of anterior teeth in bialveolar dental protrusion patients: a randomized controlled trial. *American Journal of Orthodontics Dentofacial Orthopaedics*, **134,** 18–29.

Upadhyay, M., Yadav, S., Nagaraj, K., Uribe, F., and Nanda , R. (2011). Mini-implants vs fixed functional appliances for treatment of young adult Class II female patients. *The Angle Orthodontist*, epub Aug 2011.

Zablocki, H. L., McNamara, J. A. Jr., Franchi, L., and Baccetti, T. (2008) Effect of the transpalatal arch during extraction treatment. *American Journal Orthodontics and Dentofacial Orthopaedics*, **133,** 852–60.

References for this chapter can also be found at www.oxfordtextbooks.co.uk/orc/mitchell4e/. Where possible, these are presented as active links which direct you to the electronic version of the work, to help facilitate onward study. If you are a subscriber to that work (either individually or through an institution), and depending on your level of access, you may be able to peruse an abstract or the full article if available.

16

Retention

S. J. Littlewood

Chapter contents

16.1 Introduction

One of the commonest risks of orthodontic treatment is relapse. Orthodontists use orthodontic retention to try and minimize this relapse. Orthodontic retention needs to be planned and discussed with the patient as part of the initial treatment plan.

16.2 Definition of relapse

Relapse is officially defined by the British Standards Institute as the return, following correction, of the features of the original malocclusion. However, for patients, relapse is perhaps better described as any change from the final tooth position at the end of treatment. This may be a return towards the original malocclusion, but may also be movement caused by age changes and unrelated to the orthodontic treatment.

16.3 Aetiology of relapse

The exact causes of relapse are difficult to identify, but four broad areas have been suggested as possible reasons for relapse (Fig 16.1):

- Gingival and periodontal factors
- Occlusal factors
- Soft tissues factors
- Growth factors

These factors are discussed below, including some suggestions as to how these problems may be overcome.

16.3.1 Gingival and periodontal factors

When teeth are moved the periodontal ligament and associated alveolar bone remodels. Until the periodontium adapts to the new position, there is a tendency for the stretched periodontal fibres to pull the tooth back to its original position. Different parts of the periodontal ligament complex remodel at different rates (Fig. 16.2). The alveolar bone remodels within a month, the principal fibres rearrange in 3–4 months and the collagen fibres in the gingivae re-organize after 4–6 months. However, elastic fibres in the dento-gingival and interdental fibres can take more than 8 months to remodel. Until the fibres have remodelled there is a tendency for the tooth to be pulled back to its original position. This is particularly true when teeth are rotated.

In practice this means that teeth need to be held long enough to allow the periodontal fibres to remodel to their new position. As mentioned, this is important for rotated teeth, which are particularly prone to relapse due to the gingival fibres. By correcting any rotated teeth early, this ensures that they are held in the correct position for longer by the fixed appliance. An alternative approach is to actively cut the fibres above the alveolar bone (the interdental and dento-gingival fibres). This process is known as pericision (see Box 16.1).

16.3.2 Occlusal factors

The way the teeth occlude at the end of treatment may affect stability. It has been suggested that if the teeth interdigitate well at the end

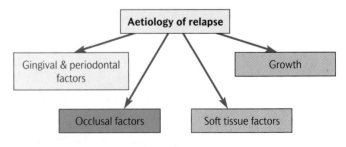

Fig. 16.1 Aetiology of relapse.

of treatment then the result is likely to be more stable. While theoretically this sounds sensible, this has not yet been proved clinically. However, there are a number of situations where occlusal factors do affect stability.

When a deep overbite is corrected it has been shown that stability is increased if the lower incisor edge lies 0–2 mm anterior to the mid-point of the root axis of the upper incisor, known as the centroid (Fig. 16.3). It is also desirable to have a favourable inter-incisal angle close to 135°, to produce a strong occlusal stop and prevent the incisors erupting past each other (Fig. 16.4).

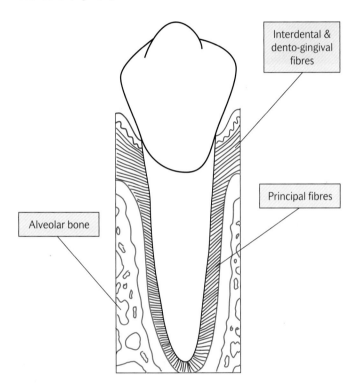

Fig. 16.2 Gingival and periodontal fibres.

One of the few occasions when no retainers are required at all is when a labial crossbite is corrected and the result is maintained by the overbite.

16.3.3 Soft tissues

The teeth lie in an area of balance between the tongue on the lingual aspect and the cheeks and lips on the buccal and labial aspect. This area of balance is sometimes referred to as the neutral zone. Although the forces from the tongue are stronger, the activity of a healthy periodontium will resist proclination of the teeth. However, the further teeth are moved out of this zone of stability, the more unstable they are likely to be. This is particularly true for the lower labial segment. If this is either proclined or retroclined excessively, relapse is more likely. In the same way, if the archform (overall shape of the arch) is markedly changed it is more likely to relapse due to soft tissue pressures. Changes in a patient's intercanine width are more unstable than changes in the intermolar width, which in turn are more unstable than changes in the interpremolar width. Where possible the original lower archform is therefore maintained throughout treatment, and the upper archform is then planned around the lower (Fig. 16.5).

Although the theory about placing the teeth in the neutral zone is useful, practically there are two major problems for the clinician. Firstly, we do not know exactly where the neutral zone is and how big it is. Secondly, it is likely that due to changes in muscle tone with age, the neutral zone will change as the patient gets older.

16.3.4 Growth

Although the majority of a patient's growth is complete by the end of puberty, it is now known that small age changes may be occurring throughout life. Subtle changes in the relative positions of the maxilla and the mandible mean that the oral environment and therefore the pressures on the dentition are constantly changing. If the pressures on the teeth are always changing, then it is perhaps not surprising that there is a risk of relapse of the teeth as the patient gets older. These late,

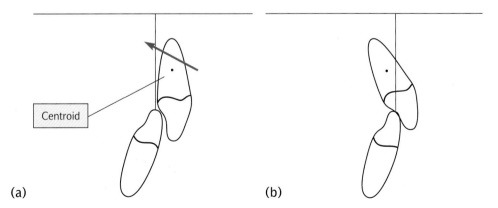

(a)   (b)

Fig. 16.3 Relapse of overbite reduction and the edge–centroid relationship. (a) This diagram demonstrates an increased overbite. The overbite reduction will be more stable if the upper incisor centroid (the mid-point of the root axis) lies palatal to the lower incisor edge. Ideally this is achieved by moving the upper root palatally, but in severe cases the alveolar bone may not be thick enough to allow full correction. In these circumstances some advancement of the lower incisor edges may be required, but stability of the lower labial segment is then compromised. (b) A stable reduction of the overbite, with correction of the edge–centroid relationship.

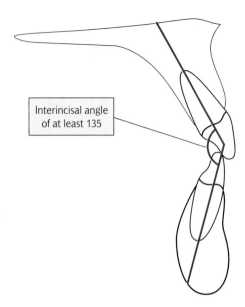

Interincisal angle
of at least 135

Fig. 16.4 Inter-incisal angle after overbite reduction.

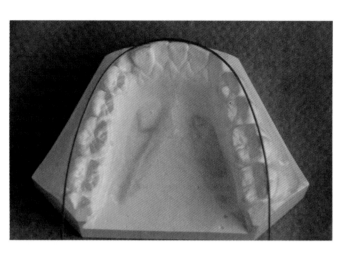

Fig. 16.5 Maintaining the original lower archform to reduce relapse. The most stable archform (shape of the arch) is thought to be the patient's original archform. Where possible this should be maintained in the lower arch, particularly the intercanine width. This figure shows a lower stainless steel archwire being shaped to maintain the existing archform.

small growth changes may at least partly explain the late lower incisor crowding that is seen in patients who have had, but also in those that have not had, orthodontic treatment.

16.3.5 Can the orthodontist prevent relapse in the long term?

If a patient has a healthy periodontium the orthodontist can influence periodontal risk factors for relapse by maintaining the teeth in position for long enough to allow fibres to remodel, or by cutting the supra-crestal fibres in a process known as pericision (see Section 16.7.1). Occlusal

risk factors can also be minimized by the orthodontist, who has the ability to position teeth in the correct occlusal relationships.

The orthodontist however cannot prevent long-term growth and soft tissue changes, which perhaps should be regarded as normal age changes. At the present time we are unable to predict the nature of these late changes, which remain an unpredictable risk for relapse throughout life. These late changes may have little or nothing to do with the orthodontic treatment, but patients may attribute the unwanted relapse to this orthodontic treatment. During the consent process for orthodontic treatment it is important that patients are informed about the risk of these unpredictable late age changes, and how they can be minimized.

16.4 How common is relapse?

Long-term studies of relapse following fixed appliances have shown that 10 years after retainers are stopped, up to 70 per cent of patients may need re-treatment due to relapse. This relapse continues to get worse over the next decade.

Relapse is unpredictable and it has been difficult to identify factors that may predict a patient's risk of relapse. Some patients who forget or refuse to wear retainers can have no relapse, while others have considerable relapse. At the present time we are not able to identify which

patients will relapse and which will not. This is perhaps not surprising, as although the orthodontist has control of gingival and periodontal factors, occlusal factors, and some soft tissue factors, it is not possible to control age changes that can contribute to relapse. Consequently the current approach is that all patients should be treated as if they have the potential to relapse. This information must be passed onto the patient as part of the informed consent process.

16.5 Informed consent and relapse

Relapse and retention should be discussed with the patient before treatment. It must form part of the informed consent process, as it requires a commitment from the patient after the active treatment is complete. At the present time we are unable to identify which patients will remain relatively stable and which will relapse. Consequently every

patient needs to be informed that they have the potential to relapse. The only way to overcome this is to continue some form of retention indefinitely. The clinician's role is to position the teeth in as stable position as possible, inform the patient of the long-term risk of relapse and provide them with some form of retention, including clear instructions on how to prevent any unwanted side-effects of wearing retainers long term. It is then up to the patient to decide whether they will continue wearing the retainers long term, or whether to accept the risk of some relapse. The responsibility for retention is the patient's and they must be made aware of this. If they are wearing removable retainers, they are responsible for complying with the regimen advised, and if they have bonded retainers, they must have them checked regularly by a general dental practitioner or orthodontist.

16.6 Retainers

Retainers are used to help reduce relapse. The clinician is faced with a multitude of different options when choosing which retainer to use and for how many hours per day the patient should wear it. When choosing the retention regimen, the following factors should be considered:

- Likely stability of the result
- Initial malocclusion
- Type of appliances used
- Oral hygiene
- Quality of the result (is any settling-in of the occlusion required?)
- Compliance of patient
- Patient expectations
- Patient preference

Retainers can either be removable or fixed. The potential advantages and disadvantages of these will be considered, followed by a detailed look at the most popular retainers in current use.

16.6.1 Removable or fixed retainers?

There are potential advantages to both fixed and removable retainers. The benefits of removable retainers are that they are:

- easier for oral hygiene (they can be removed by the patient for cleaning)
- capable of being worn part-time if required
- the responsibility of the patient, not the orthodontist

As retainers are now often recommended for long-term use, it is unrealistic for the orthodontist to keep reviewing all patients that are wearing retainers forever. With removable retainers it is the patient's responsibility to wear them, and if they choose not to, and the teeth relapse, they must accept these consequences. However, if the patient is wearing fixed retainers and they come loose, the orthodontist carries some of the responsibility.

The potential advantages of fixed retainers include the fact that:

- patients do not need to remember to wear them
- they are useful when the result is very unstable

There are certain cases where the final result will be extremely unstable. In these cases it is essential that a retainer is *in situ* full-time, otherwise relapse could occur. In these cases a fixed retainer is recommended (see Box 16.1).

16.6.2 Introduction to removable retainers

There are many different types of removable retainers, including Hawley (Fig.16.6a), vacuum-formed (Fig.16.6b), Jensen (Fig.16.6c), Begg, and Barrer. The positioner is sometimes also included as a type of removable retainer, but it is really an active appliance made of an elastomeric material. They are used in cases where the occlusion is not well intercuspated at the end of treatment. The teeth are cut off the cast and repositioned and the positioner is then made over this corrected cast. As the patient clenches on the positioner the teeth can be guided into a better occlusion. Positioners are rarely used as they are expensive to construct and patient compliance can be a problem.

The most popular types of removable retainers are the Hawley and vacuum-formed and these will be considered in more detail, but initially we will determine how often removable retainers should be worn.

16.6.3 How often should removable retainers be worn?

We have already mentioned that due to the unpredictable nature of relapse, long-term wear is advisable. However, how many hours per day should patients wear removable retainers? Recent high-quality research suggests that both Hawley and vacuum-formed retainers only need to be worn at night. This of course excludes cases with a high risk of relapse, when full-time wear using a bonded retainer is indicated (see Box 16.1).

16.6.4 Hawley retainer

The Hawley retainer is the original removable retainer. It is a simple and robust appliance made from an acrylic baseplate with a metal labial bow (Fig. 16.7). It was originally designed as an active removable appliance, but it became clear that it could be used as a retainer to maintain the teeth in the correct position after treatment. It has the advantages of

---

Box 16.1 High risk relapse cases where a full-time (bonded) retainer is advisable

- closure of spaced dentition (including median diastema)
- following correction of severely rotated teeth
- where there has been substantial movement of the lower labial segment, either excessive proclination or retroclination, or a significant change in the intercanine width
- where an overjet has been reduced, but the lips are still incompetent
- combined periodontal and orthodontic cases, where reduced periodontal support makes relapse more likely (see Chapter 20, Section 20.4.1)

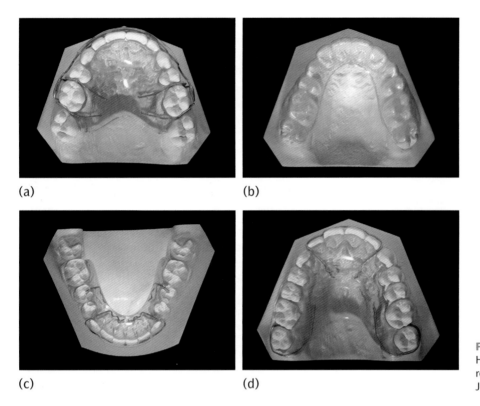

Fig. 16.6 Removable retainers. (a) Upper Hawley retainer; (b) upper vacuum-formed retainer; (c) lower Jensen and (d) upper Jensen retainers.

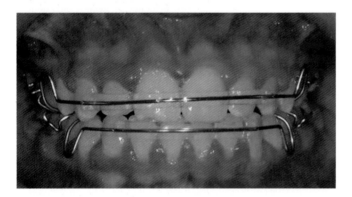

Fig. 16.7 Hawley retainers. These upper and lower Hawley retainers have an acrylic facing added to the labial bow. This acrylic provides increased contact with the teeth and is designed to reduce relapse, particularly with rotated teeth.

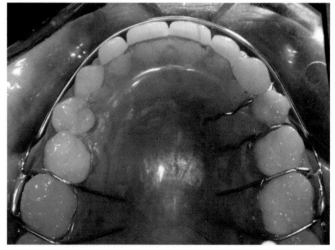

Fig. 16.8 Prosthetic tooth added to Hawley retainer. This patient presented with missing upper left first premolar and both upper second premolars. It was decided to maintain the second deciduous molars which had good roots. A space was localized in the area of the upper first premolar, and this Hawley was fitted with a prosthetic tooth in that region. Note the presence of the mesial and distal stops either side of the prosthetic tooth to reduce the relapse potential.

being simple to construct, reasonably robust, rigid enough to maintain transverse corrections and it is easy to add a prosthetic tooth. When replacing missing teeth it is important to put rigid stops on the retainer mesial and distal to any prosthetic tooth, to prevent relapse (Fig. 16.8). Hawley retainers also allow more rapid vertical settling of teeth than vacuum-formed retainers, due to the lack of complete occlusal coverage.

Various adaptations are possible, depending on the case:

- Acrylic facing can be added to the labial bow to help control rotations.

- A reverse U-loop can be used to control the canine position.

- A passive bite-plane can be added to maintain corrections of deep overbites.

- The labial bow can be soldered to the cribs, so there are fewer wires to cross the occlusal surfaces and interfere with the occlusion.

16.6.5 Vacuum-formed retainers

Vacuum-formed retainers (Fig. 16.9) offer a number of potential advantages over Hawley retainers:

- Superior aesthetics
- Less interference with speech
- More economical and quicker to make
- Less likely to break
- Ease of fabrication (Fig. 16.10)
- Superior retention of the lower incisors

Both Hawley and vacuum-formed retainers are equally successful in the upper arch, but the vacuum-formed retainers are better at preventing relapse in the lower arch.

Vacuum-formed retainers only need to be worn at night, every night. It is important that the patient is instructed never to drink with the vacuum-formed retainer *in situ*, particularly cariogenic drinks (Fig. 16.11). The retainer can act like a reservoir, holding the cariogenic drink in contact with the incisal edges and cuspal tips and leading to decalcification.

Vacuum-formed retainers are contraindicated in patients with poor oral hygiene. This is because these types of retainers are retained by the plastic engaging the undercut gingival to the contact point. If the oral hygiene is poor, then hyperplastic gingivae can obliterate these areas of undercut.

16.6.6 Fixed retainers

Fixed or bonded retainers are usually attached to the palatal aspect of the upper or lower labial segment, using normal acid-etch composite bonding. There are different types of bonded retainers:

- Multistrand retainers bonded to each tooth (Fig. 16.12)
- Rigid canine and canine retainers, which are only bonded to the canine teeth
- Reinforced fibres

The multistrand wire type, bonded to each tooth in the labial segment, is the bonded retainer of choice. Those retainers bonded only to the canine teeth often result in relapse of the incisors; and the reinforced fibre retainers tend to fracture more frequently.

Bonding retainers is a very technique-sensitive process. The tooth surface should be thoroughly cleaned before bonding, in particular removing any calculus lingual to the lower labial segment (etching alone is often not sufficient). A dry field is maintained and the wire held passively in position while bonding with a composite resin using the acid-etch technique. If the bonded retainer is not passive when it is bonded it can cause minor unwanted tooth movement.

As mentioned earlier one of the potential problems of bonded retainers is localized relapse if there is partial debond of the retainer. To overcome this, some clinicians use dual retention – using a bonded retainer, backed up with a removable retainer at night. This 'belt and braces' approach ensures that if a bonded retainer partially debonds, the teeth can be maintained in position until it can be repaired (Fig. 16.13).

16.6.7 Care of retainers

In the past, patients were asked to wear retainers for only 1–2 years. However, now that we have a better understanding of the risk of relapse, we need to ask our patients to wear them for longer. It is therefore essential that the patients have a clear understanding of how to look after the retainers.

Removable retainers are easier to care for, as they can be removed to allow oral hygiene intra-orally, in addition to easier cleaning of the

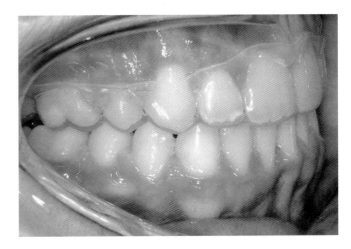

Fig. 16.9 Upper vacuum-formed retainer. The upper vacuum-formed retainer has been trimmed to finish 1–2 mm above the gingival margin. The exception is the area cut away over the canine to make it simpler for the patient to remove the retainer.

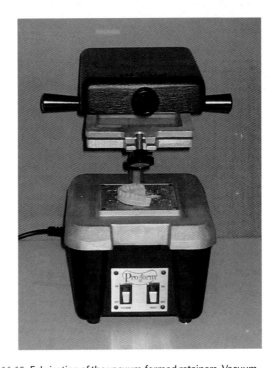

Fig. 16.10 Fabrication of the vacuum-formed retainers. Vacuum-formed retainers can be made on-site, as the fabrication is a relatively straightforward procedure using simple equipment. If retainers do not have to be sent to a laboratory this can reduce costs and allow fitting of the retainers on the same day that the appliances are removed, if required.

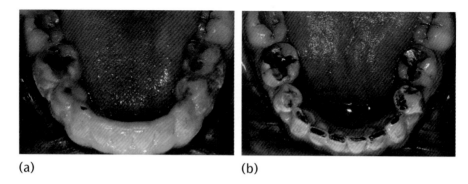

(a)   (b)

Fig. 16.11 Cariogenic drinks and vacuum-formed retainers. It is vital that patients are instructed not to wear vacuum-formed retainers when eating or drinking. This patient wore a vacuum-formed retainer full-time (a), while regularly drinking fizzy drinks, leading to substantial tooth surface loss and caries (b). (Figures reproduced with permission from Simon Littlewood, 'Stability and retention' in *Orthodontics: Principles and Practice*, D.S. Gill and F.B. Naini (Eds), Wiley-Blackwell).

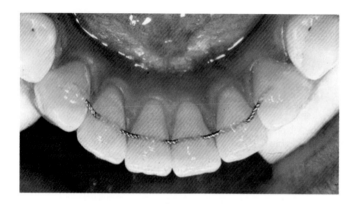

Fig. 16.12 Multistrand bonded retainer. This multistrand stainless steel retainer is bonded to each tooth from lower canine to lower canine, using composite resin. The diameter of the round wire is 0.0195 inches which allows some flexibility between the teeth. This flexibility allows the teeth to move very slightly in function.

retainers themselves. Although toothpaste can be used to clean acrylic-based retainers, like the Hawley retainer, many vacuum-formed retainers need to be cleaned with special cleaning materials that do not degrade the plastic. Some clinicians provide a spare retainer for each arch, in case the original is lost. This is particularly the case with vacuum-formed retainers, which are cheaper to fabricate. Figure 16.14 shows an example of a patient information sheet for vacuum-formed retainers.

Fixed retainers have the potential to cause both periodontal disease and caries unless they are well maintained. Fixed retainers can be used safely in the long term, provided patients are properly instructed how to look after them. They should be shown how to clean interdentally – either by using floss that can be threaded under the wire, or by the gentle use of small interdental brushes (Fig. 16.15). Fixed retainers need to be reviewed on a regular basis by the orthodontist or dental practitioner to check for any bond failure.

It is the orthodontist's responsibility to ensure that the patient is fully informed on how to look after their retainers in the long term to avoid any adverse effects.

16.7 Adjunctive techniques used to reduce relapse

Adjunctive techniques are additional soft and hard tissue procedures, usually used in addition to retainers, to help enhance stability:

- Pericision
- Interdental stripping

16.7.1 Pericision

This is also known as circumferential supracrestal fiberotomy. The principle is to cut the interdental and dento-gingival fibres above the level of the alveolar bone (Fig. 16.2). The elastic fibres within the interdental and dento-gingival fibres have a tendency to pull the teeth back towards their original position. This is particularly true with teeth that have been derotated.

Pericision is a simple procedure undertaken under local anaesthetic and requires no periodontal dressing after the cuts are made. The cuts are made vertically into the periodontal pocket, severing the supra-alveolar fibres around the neck of the teeth, but taking care not to touch the alveolar bone. The technique has been shown to reduce rotational relapse by up to 30 per cent and is most effective in the maxilla. There are no adverse effects on the periodontal health, provided there is no evidence of inflammation or periodontal disease before the pericision.

16.7.2 Enamel interproximal stripping

This is also known as reproximation (see Section 7.7.5). The removal of small amounts of enamel mesio-distally has been used to reshape teeth and to create small amounts of space (Fig. 7.7). It is not clear why this process can reduce relapse. It has been suggested that by flattening the interdental contacts, this will increase the stability between adjacent teeth. It may also be the case that by removing small amounts of tooth tissue any minor crowding is relieved, avoiding possible proclination of the lower labial segment and increase in the intercanine width, both of which are potentially unstable movements.

16.8 Conclusions about retention

Retention is an important part of almost every case of orthodontic treatment. This is because relapse is an unpredictable risk for every patient. Relapse can be due to orthodontic factors, but it can also be due to factors out of the control of the orthodontist, such as further mild growth and changes in soft tissues. The patient needs to be made aware of the long-term risk of relapse and informed of ways of reducing the risk of this relapse. This should be discussed before treatment.

Reducing relapse usually means the patient wearing a retainer. The choice of retainer is affected by the likely stability of the result, the original presenting malocclusion, patient compliance, patient expectations and the quality of the result.

The patient must be given information about the implications of relapse and how to look after the retainers, so that the patient can take responsibility for the retention phase of treatment.

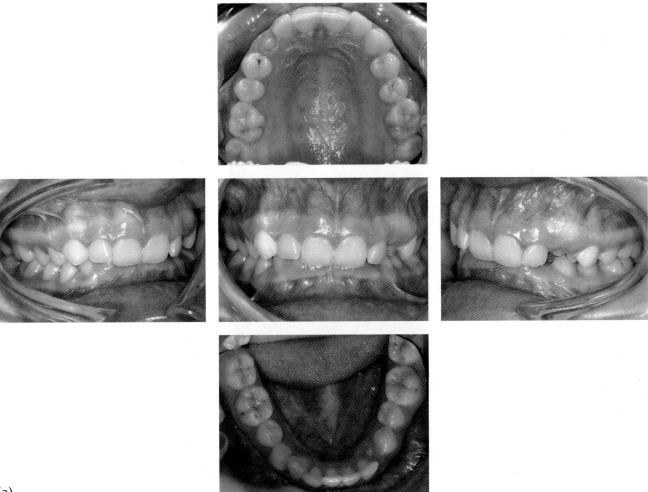

(a)

Fig. 16.13 (a) Initial presentation. This patient presented with a Class II division 2 incisor relationship. It was decided to treat the case as non-extraction, using some enamel stripping in the lower arch and accepting some proclination of the lower labial segment. This would help to reduce the overbite, but would increase the risk of instability. The patient was therefore informed that she would require permanent retention of the lower labial segment at the end of treatment.

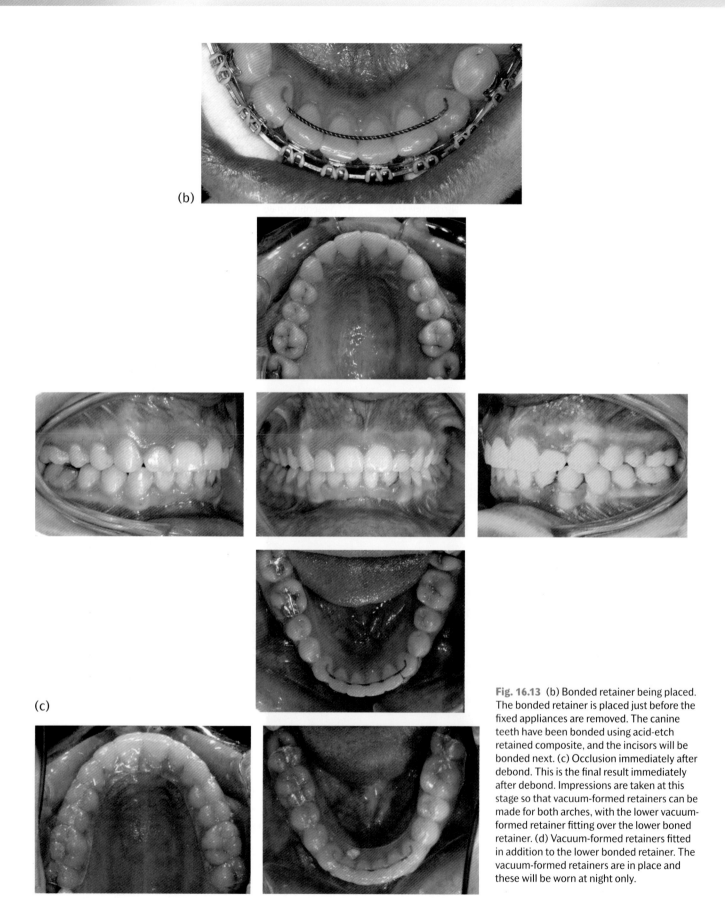

(b)

(c)

(d)

Fig. 16.13 (b) Bonded retainer being placed. The bonded retainer is placed just before the fixed appliances are removed. The canine teeth have been bonded using acid-etch retained composite, and the incisors will be bonded next. (c) Occlusion immediately after debond. This is the final result immediately after debond. Impressions are taken at this stage so that vacuum-formed retainers can be made for both arches, with the lower vacuum-formed retainer fitting over the lower boned retainer. (d) Vacuum-formed retainers fitted in addition to the lower bonded retainer. The vacuum-formed retainers are in place and these will be worn at night only.

Patient Information Sheet about Vacuum-formed Retainers

1. **Your retainers are as important as your braces.**
   If you do not wear your retainers as instructed your teeth will move back towards how they were before treatment. If you cannot wear your retainers, please contact.

2. **How often do I wear them?**
   You should wear the retainers at night, <u>every</u> night.

3. **How long do I have to wear them?**
   The best way to reduce the risk of teeth going crooked is to continue wearing the retainers at night. This is because we now know that teeth move all through our life.

4. **How do I keep them clean?**
   Clean your retainers with a toothbrush and water but do <u>not use toothpaste</u> on the retainer. Toothpaste will discolour and degrade the retainer. Your orthodontist may recommend using a special retainer cleaner.

5. **Do not eat or drink with the retainer in.**
   You should never eat or drink when you are wearing the retainer.

6. **Keep the retainer safe**
   When you are not wearing the retainer keep it safely in a protective box.

7. **What do I do if I miss wearing it for a night?**
   You must try and wear the retainers every night. If you do forget, then wear the retainer full-time except meals for 2 days. This is often enough to squeeze the teeth back into place.

8. **What do I do if I lose a retainer?**
   If you lose a retainer, wear the spare we have provided. Then contact the department and if you bring the models back in we will be able to make another spare for you. There will be a small charge to make the replacement.

9. **What do I do if the retainer rubs?**
   If the retainer rubs you can smooth it with an emery board used to file nails. If this doesn't work, then contact us.

10. **Bring your retainers to every appointment**
    It is important that you bring your retainers to every appointment, so that we can check and adjust them if needed.

Fig. 16.14 Patient information sheet on vacuum-formed retainers. This information can be given to patients who are prescribed vacuum-formed retainers. This sheet can be downloaded from www.oxfordtextbooks.co.uk/orc/mitchell4e/.

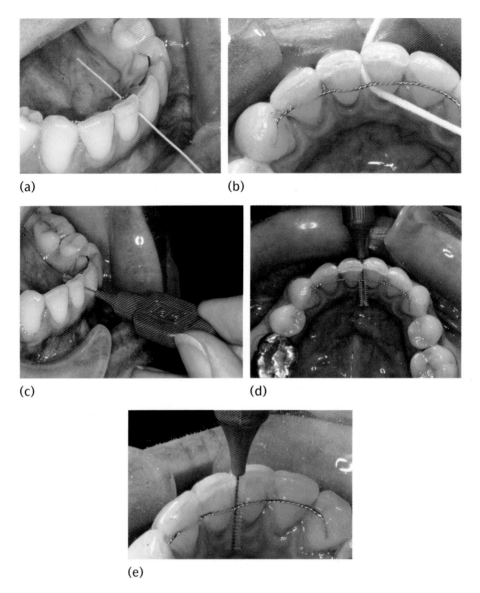

(a)　　　　　　　　　　　　(b)

(c)　　　　　　　　　　　　(d)

(e)

Fig. 16.15 Care of bonded retainers. Patients are educated about how to maintain excellent oral hygiene in the presence of a bonded retainer. Techniques are demonstrated to the patient before placing the appliance. (a) This shows 'superfloss' being threaded through the contact point so that it emerges below the bonded retainer wire. (b) This shows the superfloss under the bonded retainer wire being used to clean interdentally. (c) Here the interdental brush is being inserted above the papilla, and below the contact point and below the bonded retainer wire. (d) Interdental brush being used to clean below the wire and interdentally. (e) Interdental brush being used to clean behind the bonded retainer wire.

Key points about retention

- Relapse is an unpredictable risk for every orthodontic patient
- Relapse can be due to orthodontic factors, but can also be due to age changes out of the orthodontist's control
- As part of the informed consent process the patient needs to be aware of the long-term risk of relapse and informed of ways of reducing this risk
- Removable and fixed retainers can be used to reduce relapse, in addition to adjunctive techniques such as pericision
- Removable retainers only need to be worn at night
- The patient must recognize their responsibilities in the retention phase of treatment

Principal sources and further reading

Houston, W. J. B. (1989). Incisor edge–centroid relationships and overbite depth. *European Journal of Orthodontics*, **11**, 139–43.

Overbite stability is discussed in the paper.

Little, R. M., Wallen, T. R., and Riedel, R. A. (1981). Stability and relapse of mandibular alignment – first four premolar extraction cases treated by traditional edgewise orthodontics. *American Journal of Orthodontics and Dentofacial Orthopedics*, **80**, 349–65.

A classic paper that demonstrates the high risk of relapse after orthodontic treatment.

Littlewood, S. J., Millett, D. T., Bearn, D. R., Doubleday, B., and Worthington, H. V. (2011). Chapter 12 Retention in *Evidence-based Orthodontics* edited by Huang G.J., Richmond S. & Vig, K.W.L., Wiley-Blackwell.

This chapter provides a contemporary look at the high quality evidence on orthodontic retention.

Melrose, C. and Millet, D. T. (1998). Toward a perspective on orthodontic retention? *American Journal of Orthodontics and Dentofacial Orthopedics*, **113**, 507–14.

This considers the problems of orthodontic retention, with a particularly good review of the possible aetiological factors behind relapse.

Rowland, H., Hichens, L., Williams, A., Hills, D., Killingback, N., Ewings, P., Clark, S., Ireland, A.J., and Sandy, J.R (2007). The effectiveness of Hawley and vacuum-formed retainers: A single-center randomized controlled trial. *American Journal of Orthodontics and Dentofacial Orthopedics*, **132**, 730–7.

Hichens, L., Rowland, H., Williams, A., Hollinghurst, S., Ewings, P., Clark, S., Ireland, A.J., and Sandy, J.R. (2007). Cost-effectiveness and patient satisfaction: Hawley and vacuum-formed retainers. *European Journal of Orthodontics*, **29**, 372–8.

These two papers describe a well-designed RCT comparing Hawley retainers and vacuum-formed retainers.

References for this chapter can also be found at www.oxfordtextbooks.co.uk/orc/mitchell4e/. Where possible, these are presented as active links which direct you to the electronic version of the work, to help facilitate onward study. If you are a subscriber to that work (either individually or through an institution), and depending on your level of access, you may be able to peruse an abstract or the full article if available.

17

Removable appliances

Medical Devices Directive 93/42/EEC
In the UK all removable appliances (including removable functional appliances and retainers) are classified as custom made devices and therefore must comply with the above directive.
http://www.mhra.gov.uk/Howweregulate/Devices/MedicalDevicesDirective/index.htm

Learning objectives for this chapter

- Gain an understanding of the limitations of removable appliances
- Gain an appreciation of contemporary use of removable appliances
- Gain an understanding of the design, insertion and adjustment of removable appliances

This chapter concerns those appliances that are fabricated mainly in acrylic and wire, and can be removed from the mouth by the patient. Functional appliances are made of the same materials, but work primarily by exerting intermaxillary traction and so are considered separately in Chapter 19. Clear orthodontic aligners are considered in Section 20.5.2.

17.1 Mode of action of removable appliances

Removable appliances are capable of the following types of tooth movement:

- Tipping movements – because a removable appliance applies a single-point contact force to the crown of a tooth, the tooth tilts around a fulcrum, which in a single-rooted tooth is approximately 40 per cent of the root length from the apex.
- Movements of blocks of teeth – because removable appliances are connected by a baseplate (see Section 17.5) they are more efficient at moving blocks of teeth than fixed appliances.
- Influencing the eruption of opposing teeth – this can be achieved either by use of:
  (1) a flat anterior bite-plane, which frees the occlusion of the lower incisors allowing their eruption. This is useful in overbite reduction (see Section 17.5.2)
  (2) buccal capping, which frees the contact between the buccal segment teeth (see Section 17.5.3). This may also be of value when intrusion of the buccal segments is required (see Chapter 12, Section 12.3.1)

17.1.1 Indications for the use of removable appliances

Although widely utilized in the past as the sole appliance to treat a malocclusion, with the increasing availability and acceptance of fixed appliances the limitations of the removable appliance have become more apparent. The removable appliance is only capable of producing tilting movements of individual teeth (see Figs 4.19 and 15.4), which can be used to advantage where simple tipping movements are required, but can lead to a compromise result if employed where more complex tooth movements are indicated. As a result the role of the removable appliance has changed and it is now widely used as an adjunct to fixed appliance treatment.

Removable appliances provide a useful means of applying extra-oral traction to segments of teeth, or an entire arch, to help achieve intrusion and/or distal movement. The maxillary segment intrusion splint discussed in Chapter 12 is an example of this type of appliance. Removable appliances are also employed for arch expansion, which is another example of their usefulness in moving blocks of teeth. Removable appliances are particularly helpful where a flat anterior bite-plane or buccal capping is required to influence development of the buccal segment teeth and/or to free the occlusion with the lower arch.

Removable appliances are also utilized in a passive role as space maintainers following permanent tooth extractions and also as retaining appliances following fixed appliance treatment, as wear can be reduced, allowing the occlusion to 'settle in' and making prolonged retention practicable.

The advantages and disadvantages of removable appliances are summarized in Table 17.1.

Lower removable appliances are generally less well tolerated by patients. This is due in part to their encroachment upon tongue space, but also the lingual tilt of the lower molars makes retentive clasping difficult.

Although less likely to cause iatrogenic damage, for example, root resorption or decalcification, removable appliances can be detrimental to the patient if used inappropriately. Skill is required to judge the situations where their use is applicable and to carry out tooth movement effectively.

17.2 Designing removable appliances

17.2.1 General principles

The design of an appliance should never be delegated to a laboratory as they are only able to utilize the information provided by the plaster casts. Success depends upon designing an appliance that is easy for the patient to insert and wear, and is relevant to the occlusal aims of treatment.

Table 17.1 Advantages and disadvantages of removable appliances

Advantages	Disadvantages
Can be removed for tooth-brushing	Appliance can be left out
Palatal coverage increases anchorage	Only tilting movements possible
Easy to adjust	Good technician required
Less risk of iatrogenic damage (e.g. root resorption) than with fixed appliances	Affects speech
Acrylic can be thickened to form flat anterior bite-plane or buccal capping	Intermaxillary traction not practicable
Useful as passive retainer or space maintainer	Lower removable appliances are difficult to tolerate
Can be used to transmit forces to blocks of teeth	Inefficient for multiple individual tooth movements

17.2.2 Steps in designing a removable appliance

Four components need to be considered for every removable appliance:

- Active component(s)
- Retaining the appliance
- Anchorage
- Baseplate

A detailed consideration of each of these components is given in the sections below.

Generally, extractions should be deferred until after an appliance is fitted. The rationale for this is two-fold:

(1) If the extractions are carried out first, there is a real risk that the teeth posterior to the extraction site will drift forward, resulting in an appliance that does not fit well or even does not fit at all. This is most noticeable when upper first permanent molars have been extracted or there is a conspicuous delay before the appliance is fitted.

(2) Occasionally a patient decides after an appliance is fitted that they do not wish to continue wearing it and therefore decide against continuing with treatment. It is obviously preferable if this change of mind occurs before any extractions have been undertaken.

Rarely, it is necessary to carry out extractions first, for example when a displaced tooth will interfere with the design of the appliance. However, even in these cases it is preferable to take impressions for the fabrication of the appliance before the extractions and to instruct the technician to remove the tooth concerned from the model. The appliance should then be fitted as soon as practicable after the tooth, or teeth are extracted.

17.3 Active components

17.3.1 Springs

Springs are the most commonly used active component. Their design can readily be adapted to the needs of a particular clinical situation and they are inexpensive. However, a skilled technician is required to fabricate a spring that works efficiently with the minimum of adjustment on fitting.

The expression for the force F exerted by an orthodontic spring is one of only a few formulae remembered by the author and on this basis is recommended to the reader as being worthwhile:

$$F \propto \frac{dr^4}{\beta}$$

where d is the deflection of the spring on activation, r is the radius of the wire and l is the length of the spring.

Thus even small changes in the diameter or length of wire used in the construction of a spring will have a profound impact upon the force delivered, for example, doubling the radius of the wire increases the force by a factor of 16. It is obviously desirable to deliver a light (physiological) force (Chapter 4) over a long activation range, but there are practical restrictions upon the length and diameter of wire used to construct a spring. The span of a spring is usually constrained by the size of the arch or the depth of the sulcus. However, incorporating a coil into the design of a spring increases the length of wire and therefore results in the application of a smaller force for a given deflection. A spring with a coil will work more efficiently if it is activated in the direction that the wire has been wound so that the coil unwinds as the tooth moves.

In practice the smallest diameter of wire that can be used for spring construction is 0.5 mm. However, wire of this diameter is liable to distortion or breakage and therefore some designs are protected by acrylic e.g. the palatal finger spring (Fig. 17.1) or strengthened by being sleeved in tubing (Fig. 17.2).

It is essential that a spring is adjusted to ensure that the point of application will give the desired direction of movement. The further the spring is from the centre of resistance of the tooth the greater the degree of tilting. Therefore a spring should be adjusted so that it is as near the gingival margin as possible without causing gingival trauma. If the spring is over-activated this increases the force on the tooth and has the effect of moving the centre of resistance more apically (therefore more tipping occurs).

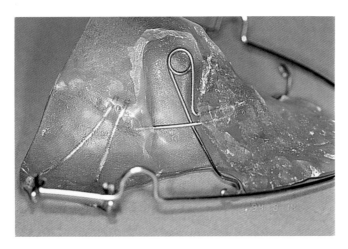

Fig. 17.1 Palatal finger spring. Note that the spring is boxed in with acrylic and a guard wire is present to help prevent distortion.

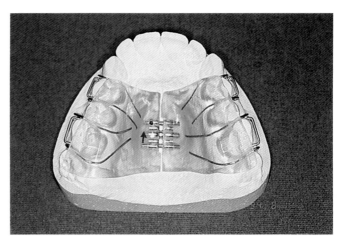

Fig. 17.3 Screw appliance to expand the upper arch.

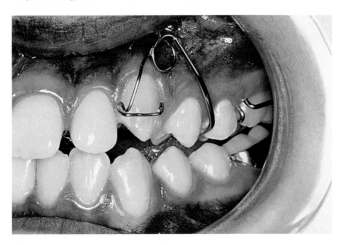

Fig. 17.2 Buccal canine retractor (distal section sleeved in tubing).

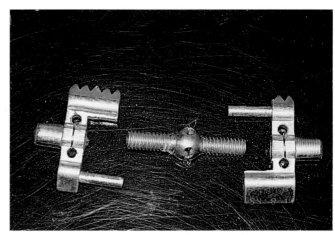

Fig. 17.4 Components of a screw.

17.3.2 Screws

Screws are less versatile than springs, as the direction of tooth movement is determined by the position of the screw in the appliance. They are also bulky and more expensive. However, a screw appliance may be useful when it is desirable to utilize the teeth to be moved for additional clasping to retain the appliance. This is helpful when a number of teeth are to be moved together (for example in an appliance to expand the upper arch (Fig. 17.3) or in the mixed dentition where retaining an appliance is always difficult.

The most commonly used type of screw consists of two halves on a threaded central cylinder (Fig. 17.4) turned by means of a key which separates the two halves by a predetermined distance, usually about 0.25 mm for each quarter turn.

Activation of a screw is limited by the width of the periodontal ligament, as to exceed this would result in crushing the ligament cells and cessation of tooth movement (see Chapter 4). One quarter-turn opens the two sections of the appliance by 0.25 mm.

17.3.3 Elastics

Special intra-oral elastics are manufactured for orthodontic use (see Chapter 18, Fig. 18.20). These elastics are usually classified by their size, ranging from 1/8 inch to 3/4 inch, and the force that they are designed to deliver, usually 2, 3.5 or 4.5 ounces. Selection of the appropriate size and force is based upon the root surface area of the teeth to be moved and the distance over which the elastic is to be stretched. The elastics should be changed every day. Latex-free alternatives are now widely available.

17.4 Retaining the appliance

17.4.1 Adams clasp

This crib was designed to engage the undercuts present on a fully erupted first permanent molar at the junctions of the mesial and distal surfaces with the buccal aspect of the tooth (Fig. 17.5). The crib is usually fabricated in hard 0.7 mm stainless steel wire and should engage about 1 mm of undercut. In practice this means that in children the

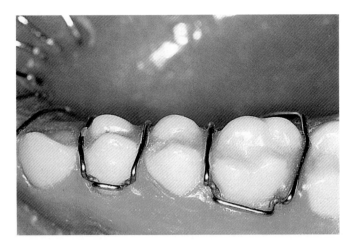

Fig. 17.5 Adams clasp.

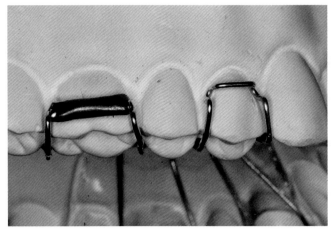

Fig. 17.7 A tube for an extra-oral face-bow has been soldered onto the bridge of this Adams crib.

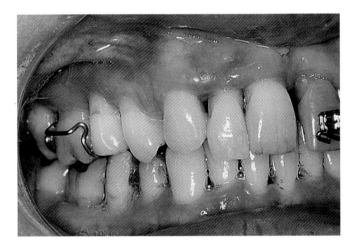

Fig. 17.6 Ideally the Adams clasp should engage about 1 mm of undercut. Therefore in adults with some gingival recession the arrowheads will probably lie part way down the crown of the tooth.

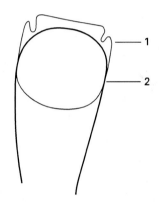

1 Arrowhead moves horizontally in towards tooth

2 Arrowhead moves in towards tooth and also vertically towards gingival crevice

Fig. 17.8 Adjustment of an Adams clasp.

arrowheads will lie at or just below the gingival margin. However, in adults with some gingival recession the arrowheads should lie part way down the crown of the tooth (Fig. 17.6).

This crib can also be used for retention on premolars, canines, central incisors, and deciduous molars. However, it is advisable to use 0.6 mm wire for these teeth. When second permanent molars have to be utilized for retention soon after their eruption, it is wise to omit the distobuccal arrowhead, as little undercut exists and if included it may irritate the cheek.

The reason for the popularity of the Adams crib is its versatility as it can be easily adapted:

- Extra-oral traction tubes, labial bows, or buccal springs can be soldered onto the bridge of the clasp (Fig. 17.7).
- Hooks or coils can be fabricated in the bridge of the clasp during construction.
- Double cribs can be constructed which straddle two teeth.

Adjustment: the crib can be adjusted in two places. Bends in the middle of the flyover will move the arrowhead down and in towards the tooth. Adjustments near the arrowhead will result in more movement towards the tooth and will have less effect in the vertical plane (Fig. 17.8).

17.4.2 Other methods of retention

Southend clasp

This clasp (Fig. 17.9) is designed to utilize the undercut beneath the contact point between two incisors. It is usually fabricated in 0.7 mm hard stainless steel wire.

Adjustment: retention is increased by bending the arrowhead in towards the teeth.

Ball-ended clasps

These clasps are designed to engage the undercut interproximally. This design affords minimal retention and can have the effect of prising the teeth apart.

Adjustment: the ball is bent in towards the contact point between the teeth.

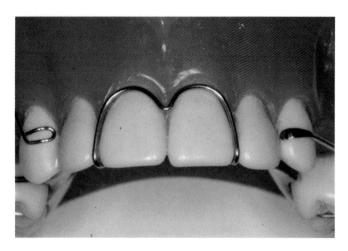

Fig. 17.9 Southend clasp.

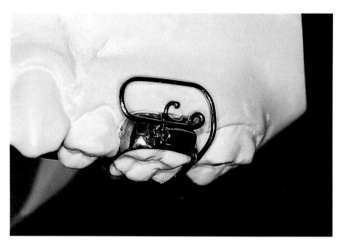

Fig. 17.10 Plint clasp.

Plint clasp

This clasp (Fig. 17.10) is used to engage under the tube assembly on a molar band.

Adjustment: by moving the clasp under the molar tube.

Labial bows

A labial bow (Fig. 17.11) is useful for anterior retention, particularly if mesial or distal tooth movement is planned, as it will help to guide tooth movement along the arch and prevent buccal flaring. Acrylic may be added to the labial bow to provide additional retention and is often used in Hawley retainers following fixed appliance treatment.

Adjustment: this will depend upon the exact design of an individual bow. However, the most commonly used type with U-loops is adjusted by squeezing together the legs of the U-loop and then adjusting the height of the labial bow by a bend at the anterior leg to compensate (Fig. 17.12).

17.5 Baseplate

The other individual components of a removable appliance are connected by means of an acrylic baseplate, which can be a passive or active component of the appliance.

17.5.1 Self-cure or heat-cure acrylic

Heat-curing of polymethylmethacrylate increases the degree of polymerization of the material and optimizes its properties, but is technically more demanding to produce. It is common practice to make the majority of appliances in self-cure acrylic, retaining heat-cure acrylic for those situations where additional strength is desirable, for example some functional appliances.

17.5.2 Anterior bite-plane

Increasing the thickness of acrylic behind the upper incisors forms a bite-plane onto which the lower incisors occlude. A bite-plane is prescribed when either the overbite needs to be reduced by eruption of the lower buccal segment teeth or elimination of possible occlusal interferences is necessary to allow tooth movement to occur.

Anterior bite-planes are usually flat. Inclined bite-planes may lead to proclination or retroclination of the lower incisors, depending upon their angulation.

When prescribing a flat anterior bite-plane the following information needs to be given to the technician:

- How far posteriorly the bite-plane should extend. This is most easily conveyed by noting the overjet.
- The depth of the bite-plane. To increase the likelihood that the patient will wear the appliance, the bite-plane should result in a separation of only 1–2 mm between the upper and lower molars. The depth is prescribed in terms of the height of the bite-plane against the upper incisors, for example '$1/2$ height of the upper incisor'.

In a proportion of cases more than 1–2 mm of overbite reduction is required, and therefore it will be necessary to make additions to the depth of the bite-plane during treatment.

17.5.3 Buccal capping

Buccal capping is prescribed when occlusal interferences need to be eliminated to allow tooth movement to be accomplished and reduction of the overbite is undesirable. Buccal capping is produced by carrying the acrylic over the occlusal surface of the buccal segment teeth (Fig. 17.13) and has the effect of propping the incisors apart. The acrylic should be as thin as practicably possible to aid patient tolerance. During treatment it is not uncommon for the capping to fracture and it is wise to warn patients of this, advising them to return if a sharp edge results. However, if as a result a tooth is left free of the acrylic and is liable to over-erupt, a new appliance will be necessary (as additions to buccal capping are rarely successful).

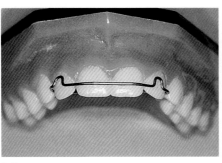

(a)

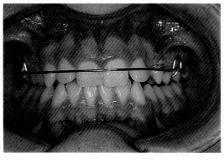

(b)

Fig. 17.11 Two types of labial bow.

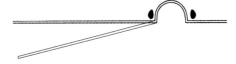

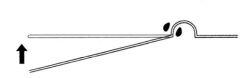

Fig. 17.12 Diagram illustrating how to tighten a labial bow. The first adjustment is to squeeze together the two legs of the U-loop. This causes the anterior section of the bow to move occlusally and therefore a second adjustment is required to lift it back to the desired horizontal position.

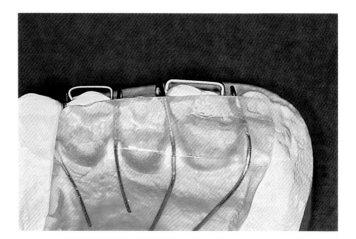

Fig. 17.13 Buccal capping.

17.6 Commonly used removable appliances

17.6.1 To correct anterior crossbite in mixed dentition

See Section 3.5.

Movement labially of upper incisors in the mixed dentition can be accomplished either using a spring or screw design depending upon the number of incisors to be moved. To move a single incisor buccally a Z-spring is commonly used (Fig. 17.14). This design is also known as a double-cantilever spring when it is used for moving more than one tooth. A Z-spring for a single tooth should be fabricated in 0.5 mm wire, but for longer spans 0.6 or 0.7 mm is advisable. Good anterior retention is required to resist the displacing effect of this spring.

Activation is by pulling the spring about 1–2 mm away from the baseplate at an angle of approximately 45° in the direction of desired movement (so that the spring is not caught on the incisal edge(s) as the appliance is inserted).

A screw design is often used where three or all of the upper incisors need to be moved labially as then the teeth to be moved can be used for retention of the appliance (Fig. 17.15). However the disadvantage is that this results in a much bulkier appliance anteriorly.

Buccal capping is usually incorporated into this appliance to free the occlusion with the lower arch.

17.6.2 Screw appliance to expand upper arch

As mentioned above a design incorporating a screw is useful for moving blocks of teeth and has the additional advantage that the teeth being moved can also be clasped for retention. Again buccal capping is also used to free occlusion with the lower arch (Fig. 17.13).

Activation: this is by means of turning the screw a one-quarter turn. One quarter-turn opens the two sections of the appliance by 0.25 mm. For active movement the patient should turn the screw twice a week (for example on a Wednesday and a Saturday). If opened too far, the screw will come apart; therefore patients should be warned that if the screw portion becomes loose they should turn it back one turn and not advance the screw again.

17.6.3 Nudger appliance

This appliance is used in conjunction with headgear to bands on the first molar teeth (Fig. 17.16). It is usually used to achieve distal movement of the molar teeth when it is intended to go onto fixed appliances to complete alignment. The appliance incorporates palatal finger springs (in 0.5 mm wire) to retract the first permanent molars. The appliance is worn full-time and the patient asked to wear the headgear for 12 to 16 hours per day. The palatal finger springs are only lightly activated with the aim of minimizing forward movement of the molar when the headgear is not worn. This appliance is also very useful if unilateral distal movement is

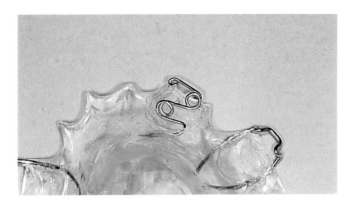

Fig. 17.14 Z-spring.

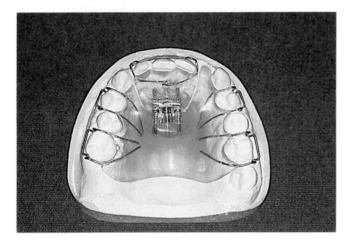

Fig. 17.15 Screw appliance for proclination of the incisors.

Box 17.1 Instruments which are useful for fitting and adjusting removable appliances

- Adams pliers (no. 64)
- Spring-forming pliers (no. 65)
- Maun's wire cutters
- Pair of autoclavable dividers
- Steel rule
- A straight handpiece and an acrylic bur (preferably tungsten carbide)
- A pair of robust hollow-chop pliers is a useful addition, but not essential

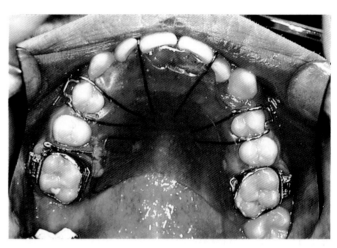

Fig. 17.16 Nudger appliance for unilateral movement of the upper right first permanent molar.

required. In this case the contralateral molar can be clasped to aid retention. If overbite reduction is required then a bite-plane can be included in the appliance. It is advisable to fit the bands on the molar teeth and then take an impression to fabricate the appliance.

17.6.4 Expansion and Labial Segment Alignment Appliance (ELSAA)

This appliance is used in Class II division 2 malocclusions prior to functional appliance therapy to correct an anteroposterior discrepancy (see Section 10.3.2 and Fig. 10.20).

17.6.5 Hawley retainer

This passive appliance is used for retention (see chapter 16) following active orthodontic treatment. See section 16.6.4 for further details and pictures

17.7 Fitting a removable appliance

It is always useful to explain again to the patient (and their parent/guardian) the overall treatment plan and the role of the appliance that is to be fitted. It is also prudent to delay any permanent extractions until after an appliance has been fitted and the patient's ability to achieve full-time wear has been demonstrated.

Fitting an appliance can be approached in the following way (see also Box 17.1):

(1) Check that you have the correct appliance for the patient in the chair and that your prescription has been followed.

(2) Show the appliance to the patient and explain how it works.

(3) Check the fitting surface for any roughness.

(4) Try in the appliance. If it does not fit check the following:

- Have any teeth erupted since the impression was taken? If wnecessary, adjust the acrylic.

- Have any teeth moved since the impression was recorded? This usually occurs if any extractions have been recently carried out.

- Has there been a significant delay between taking the impression and fitting the appliance?

(5) Adjust the retention until the appliance just clicks into place.

(6) If the appliance has a bite-plane or buccal capping, this will need to be trimmed so that it is active but not too bulky.

(7) The active element(s) should be gently activated, provided that extractions are not required to make space available into which the teeth are to be moved.

(8) Give the patient a mirror and demonstrate how to insert and remove the appliance. Then let the patient practice.

(9) Go through the instructions with the patient (and parent or guardian), stressing the importance of full-time wear. A sheet outlining the important points and containing details of what to do in the event of problems is advisable. Medicolegally, it is prudent to note in the patient's records if instructions have been given.

(10) Arrange the next appointment.

If a working model is available, it is wise to store this with the patient's study models as it may prove helpful if the appliance has to be repaired.

17.8 Monitoring progress

Ideally, patients wearing active removable appliances should be seen around every 4 weeks. Passive appliances can be seen less frequently, but it is advisable to check, and if necessary adjust, the retention of the clasps every 3 months.

During active treatment it is important to establish that the patient is wearing the appliance as instructed. Indications of a lack of compliance include the following:

- the appliance shows little evidence of wear and tear;
- the patient lisps (ask the patient to count from 65 to 70 with, and without, their appliance);
- no marks in the patient's mouth around the gingival margins palatally or across the palate;
- frequent breakages.

If wear is satisfactory the following should be considered:

- Check the treatment plan (and progress onto the next step if indicated).
- The patient's oral hygiene.
- Record the molar relationship, overjet and overbite.
- Re-assess anchorage.
- Tooth movement since the last visit.
- Retention of the appliance (see Section 17.4).
- Whether the active elements of the appliance need adjustment.
- Whether the bite-plane or buccal capping need to be increased and/or adjusted.
- Record what action needs to be undertaken at the next visit.

17.8.1 Common problems during treatment
Slow rate of tooth movement

Normally tooth movement should proceed at approximately 1 mm per month in children, and slightly less in adults. If progress is slow, check the following:

- Is the patient wearing the appliance full-time? If the appliance is not being worn as much as required, the implications of this need to be discussed with the patient (and if applicable, the parent). If poor co-operation continues, resulting in a lack of progress, consideration will have to be given to abandoning treatment.

- If the active element is a spring – is this correctly positioned and optimally activated?

- If the active element is a screw – is the patient adjusting this correctly, at the frequency requested?

- Is tooth movement obstructed by the acrylic or wires of the appliance? If this is the case, these should be removed or adjusted.

- Is tooth movement prevented by occlusion with the opposing arch? It may be necessary to increase the bite-plane or buccal capping to free the occlusion.

Frequent breakage of the appliance

The main reasons for this are as follows:

- The appliance is not being worn full-time.
- The patient has a habit of clicking the appliance in and out (this habit also results in an appliance that rapidly becomes loose).
- The patient is eating inappropriate foods whilst wearing the appliance. Success lies in dissuading the patient from eating hard and/or sticky foods altogether. Partial success is a patient who removes their appliance to eat hard or sticky foods!

Anchorage loss

This can be increased by the following:

- Part-time appliance wear, thus allowing the anchor teeth to drift forwards.
- The forces being applied by the active elements exceed the anchorage resistance of the appliance. Care is required to ensure that the springs, etc. are not being overactivated or that too much active tooth movement is being attempted at a time.

If anchorage loss is a problem see Chapter 15.

Palatal inflammation

This can occur for two reasons:

(1) Poor oral hygiene. In the majority of cases the extent of the inflammation exactly matches the coverage of the appliance and is

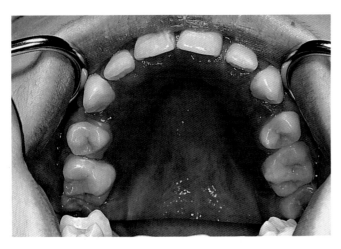

Fig. 17.17 Inflammation of the palate corresponding to the coverage of a removable appliance.

caused by a mixed fungal and bacterial infection (Fig. 17.17). This may occur in conjunction with angular cheilitis. Management of this condition must address the underlying problem, which is usually poor oral hygiene. However, in marked cases it may be wise to supplement this with an antifungal agent (e.g. nystatin, amphotericin, or miconazole gel) which is applied to the fitting surface of the appliance four times daily. If associated with angular cheilitis, miconazole cream may be helpful.

(2) Entrapment of the gingivae between the acrylic and the tooth/teeth being moved.

17.9 Appliance repairs

Before arranging for a removable appliance to be repaired the following should be considered:

- How was the appliance broken? If a breakage has been caused by the patient failing to follow instructions, it is important to be sure any co-operation problems have been overcome before proceeding with the repair.
- Would it be more cost-effective to make a new appliance?
- Occasionally it is possible to adapt what remains of the spring or another component of the appliance to continue the desired movement.

- Is the working model available, or is an up-to-date impression required to facilitate the repair?
- How will the tooth movements which have been achieved be retained while the repair is being carried out? Often there is no alternative but to try and carry out the repair in the shortest possible time.

See also Chapter 23.

Key points

Removable appliances are:

- Only capable of tipping movements of individual teeth
- Useful for moving blocks of teeth
- Useful for freeing the occlusion with the opposing arch
- Useful as passive appliances (e.g. for retention)
- More commonly used nowadays as an adjunct to fixed appliances (rather than the sole appliance to correct a malocclusion)

Principal sources and further reading

Houston, W. J. B. and Isaacson, K. G. (1980). *Orthodontic Treatment with Removable Appliances* (2nd edn). Wright, Bristol.

Isaacson, K. G., Muir, J. D., and Reed, R. T. (2002). *Removable Orthodontic Appliances*. Wright, Oxford.

Kerr, W. J. S., Buchanan, I. B., and McNair, F. I. (1993). Factors influencing the outcome and duration of removable appliance treatment. *European Journal of Orthodontics*, **16**, 181–6.

Littlewood, S. J., Tait, A. G., Mandall, N. A., and Lewis, D. H. (2001). The role of removable appliances in contemporary orthodontics. *British Dental Journal*, **191**, 304–10.

A readable and well-illustrated article.

Lloyd, T. G. and Stephens, C. D. (1979). Spontaneous changes in molar occlusion after extraction of all first premolars: a study of Class II division 1 cases treated with removable appliances. *British Journal of Orthodontics*, **6**, 91–4.

Richmond, S., Andrew, M., and Roberts, C. T. (1993). The provision of orthodontic care in the General Dental Services of England and Wales: extraction patterns, treatment duration, appliance types and standards. *British Journal of Orthodontics*, **20**, 345–50.

Evidence that fixed appliances produce superior results to those achieved with removable appliances in the GDS in the UK.

Ward, S. and Read, M. J. F. (2004). The contemporary use of removable appliances. *Dental Update*, **May**, 215–7.

Yettram, A. L., Wright, K. W., and Houston, W. J. (1977). Centre of rotation of a maxillary central incisor under orthodontic loading. *British Journal of Orthodontics*, **4**, 23–7.

References for this chapter can also be found at www.oxfordtextbooks.co.uk/orc/mitchell4e/. Where possible, these are presented as active links which direct you to the electronic version of the work, to help facilitate onward study. If you are a subscriber to that work (either individually or through an institution), and depending on your level of access, you may be able to peruse an abstract or the full article if available.

18

Fixed appliances

Chapter contents

18.1 Principles of fixed appliances

Fixed appliances are attached to the teeth and are thus capable of a greater range of tooth movements than is possible with a removable appliance. Not only does the attachment on the tooth surface (called a bracket) allow the tooth to be moved vertically or tilted, but also a force couple can be generated by the interaction between the bracket and an archwire running through the bracket (Fig. 18.1). Thus rotational and apical movements are also possible. The interplay between the archwire and the bracket slot determines the type and direction of movement achieved. A bewildering variety of different types of bracket are now manufactured, and the choice of archwire materials and configurations is extensive. Although historical, to aid understanding of the principles of fixed appliances we shall consider the edgewise type of bracket (Fig. 18.2) in this section; other bracket systems are described in Section 18.6.

The edgewise bracket is rectangular in shape and is typically described by the width of the bracket slot, usually 0.018 or 0.022 inch. The depth of the slot is commonly between 0.025 and 0.032 inch. Modifying the shape of the bracket can affect tooth movement. For example, a narrow bracket (Fig. 18.3) results in a greater span of archwire between the brackets which increases the flexibility of the archwire. In contrast, a wider bracket reduces the interbracket archwire span, but is more efficient for de-rotation and mesiodistal control. Nowadays a wide variety of bracket designs is available. In most modern appliance systems each bracket is a different width corresponding to the type of tooth for which it is intended; for example, lower incisors have the narrowest brackets (see photographs of fixed appliances shown later in the chapter).

A round wire in a rectangular edgewise type of slot will give a degree of control of mesiodistal tilt, vertical height, and rotational position. The closer the fit of the archwire in the bracket, the greater the control gained. However, with a round wire only tipping movements in a buccolingual direction are possible (Fig. 18.4). When a rectangular wire is used in a rectangular slot, a force couple can be generated by the interaction between the walls of the slot and the sides of the archwire and buccolingual apical movement is produced (Fig. 18.5). However, some tipping movements will take place before the rectangular wires engage the sides of the bracket slot, with the degree of 'slop' depending on the differences between the dimensions of the archwire and the bracket slot (Fig. 18.6).

Thus fixed appliances can be used in conjunction with rectangular archwires to achieve tooth movement in all three spatial planes. In orthodontics these are described by the types of bend that are required in an archwire to produce each type of movement (Fig. 18.7):

• First-order bends are made in the plane of the archwire to compensate for differing tooth widths and buccolingual position.

• Second-order bends are made in the vertical plane to achieve correct mesiodistal angulation or tilt of the tooth.

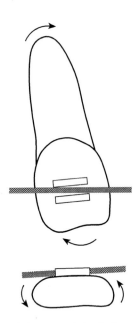

Fig. 18.1 Generation of a force couple by the interaction between the bracket slot and the archwire.

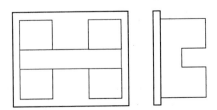

Fig. 18.2 Diagrammatic representation of an edgewise bracket.

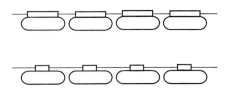

Fig. 18.3 Narrower brackets increase the span of wire between brackets, thus increasing the flexibility of the archwire. However, wider brackets allow greater rotational and mesiodistal control, as the force couple generated has a greater moment.

- Third-order bends are applicable to rectangular archwires only. They are made by twisting the plane of the wire so that when it is inserted into the rectangular bracket slot a buccolingual force is exerted on the tooth apex. This type of movement is also known as torque.

In the original edgewise appliance (see below) these bends were placed in the archwire during treatment so that the teeth were moved into their correct positions. Modern bracket systems have average values for tip (Fig. 18.8) and torque built into the bracket slot itself, and the bracket bases are of differing thicknesses to produce an average buccolingual crown position (known ingeniously as in–out). These 'pre-adjusted' systems have the advantage that the amount of wire bending required is reduced. However, they do not eliminate the need for archwire adjustments because average values do not always suffice. The disadvantage to the pre-adjusted appliance is that a larger inventory of brackets is required as each individual tooth has different requirements in terms of tip, in–out, and torque. Pre-adjusted systems are discussed in more detail in Section 18.6.

Whilst it is possible to achieve a more sophisticated range of tooth movement with fixed appliances than with removable appliances, the opportunity for problems to arise is increased. Fixed appliances are also more demanding of anchorage, and therefore adequate training should be obtained before embarking on treatment with fixed appliances.

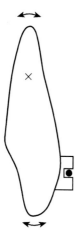

Fig. 18.4 When a round wire is used in a rectangular slot, buccolingual forces tip the tooth around a fulcrum in the root.

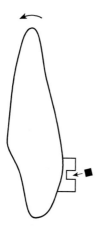

Fig. 18.5 When a rectangular wire is used with a rectangular slot more control of buccolingual root movement is achieved, allowing bodily and torquing movements to be accomplished.

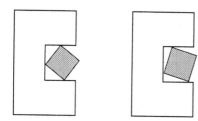

Fig. 18.6 When an archwire closely fits the dimensions of the bracket slot there is less latitude before it binds and therefore interacts with the bracket. With a smaller rectangular archwire, more tilting and rotation can occur before it binds with the walls of the bracket slot. This latitude is known as 'slop'.

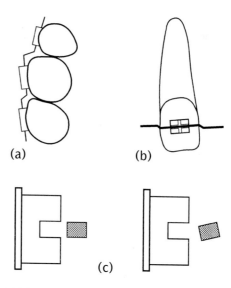

Fig. 18.7 (a) A first-order bend; (b) a second-order bend; (c) a third-order bend.

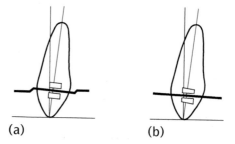

Fig. 18.8 Diagram (a) to show an edgewise bracket with a second-order bend placed in the archwire to achieve the desired amount of tip. Diagram (b) to show a pre-adjusted bracket with tip built into the bracket slot.

18.2 Indications for the use of fixed appliances

Fixed appliances are indicated when precise tooth movements are required.

- Correction of mild to moderate skeletal discrepancies: as fixed appliances can be used to achieve bodily movement it is possible, within limits, to compensate for skeletal discrepancies and treat a greater range of malocclusions.
- Intrusion/extrusion of teeth: vertical movement of individual teeth, or tooth segments, requires some form of attachment onto the tooth surface on which the force can act.
- Correction of rotations.
- Overbite reduction by intrusion of incisors.
- Multiple tooth movements required in one arch.
- Active closure of extraction spaces, or spaces due to hypodontia: fixed appliances can be used to achieve bodily space closure and ensure a good contact point between the teeth.

Fixed appliances are not as effective at moving blocks of teeth as are removable or functional appliances.

Fixed appliances are *not* indicated as an alternative to poor co-operation with removable appliances. Indeed, if a successful result is to be achieved with the minimum of deleterious side-effects, treatment with fixed appliances should only be embarked upon in patients who are willing to:

- maintain a high level of oral hygiene;
- avoid hard or sticky foods and restrict the consumption of sugar-containing foodstuffs between meals;
- co-operate fully with wearing headgear or elastic traction, if required;
- attend regularly to have the appliance adjusted.

In essence, the patient must want treatment sufficiently to be able to work with the orthodontist to achieve the desired final result. If patient compliance is suspect then it is usually wiser to defer treatment.

18.3 Components of fixed appliances

Tooth movement with fixed appliances is achieved by the interaction between the attachment or bracket on the tooth surface and the archwire which is tied into the bracket. Brackets can be carried on a band which is cemented to the tooth or attached directly to the tooth surface by means of an adhesive (known colloquially as bonds).

18.3.1 Bands

These are rings encircling the tooth to which buccal, and as required, lingual, attachments are soldered or welded (Fig. 18.9). Prior to the introduction of the acid-etch technique, bands were the only means of attaching a bracket to a tooth. With the development of modern bonding

techniques, directly bonded attachments became popular. However, many operators still use bands for molar teeth, particularly for the upper molars when headgear or a cemented palatal arch is to be used.

Bands can be used on teeth other than molars, most commonly following the failure of a bonded attachment, but for aesthetic reasons bonds are preferred (Fig. 18.10).

Prior to placement of a band it may be necessary to separate the adjacent tooth contacts. The most widely used method involves placing a small elastic doughnut around the contact point (Fig. 18.11), which is left *in situ* for 2 to 7 days and removed prior to band placement. These separating elastics are inserted by being stretched, with

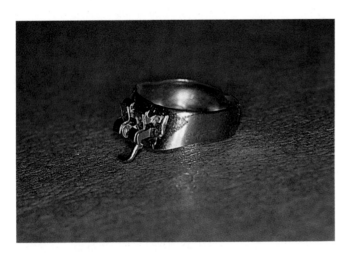

Fig. 18.9 A lower first permanent molar band. Note the gingivally positioned hook, which is useful for applying elastic traction.

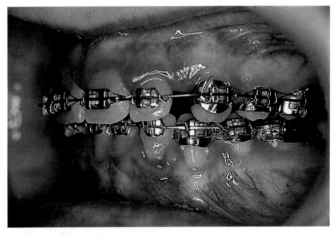

Fig. 18.10 Fixed appliance case where bands have been used for the canines, premolars and molar teeth. The impact of bands upon the aesthetics of the appliance can be readily appreciated.

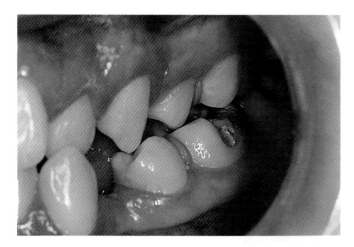

Fig. 18.11 Separating elastics have been placed between the contact points of the second premolars and first permanent molars prior to placement of bands on the latter.

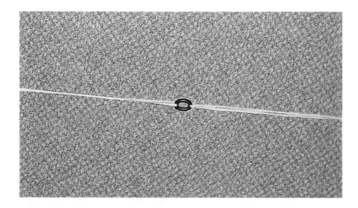

Fig. 18.12 A separating elastic being stretched between two pieces of floss. One side of the elastic is then worked through the contact point so that it encircles the contact point.

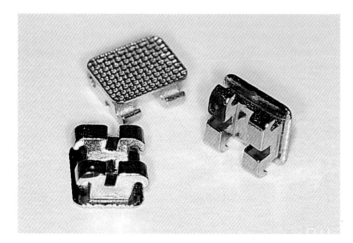

Fig. 18.13 Brackets for bonding showing a mesh base which increases the surface area for mechanical attachment of the composite.

either special pliers or floss (Fig. 18.12), and working one side through the contact point.

Band selection is aided by trying to guess the approximate size of the tooth from the patient's study models. A snug fit is essential to help prevent the band from becoming loose during treatment. The edges of the band should be flush with the marginal ridges with the bracket in the midpoint of the clinical crown at 90° to the long axis of the tooth (or crown, depending upon the type of bracket). Most orthodontists use glass ionomer cement for band cementation.

18.3.2 Bonds

Bonded attachments were introduced with the advent of the acid-etch technique and the modern composite (see Fig. 18.14 and Section 18.3.3). Adhesion to the base of metal brackets is gained by mechanical interlock (Fig. 18.13). A variety of approaches have been used to try and make fixed appliances more aesthetic (see Chapter 20, Section 20.5) including the introduction of ceramic brackets (Fig. 20.6). A number of disadvantages have limited the applicability of ceramic brackets (see Box 18.1 and Chapter 20, Section 20.5.1).

Brackets are subdivided according to the width of the bracket slot in inches. Two systems are widely used, 0.018 and 0.022. The depth of the slot varies between 0.025 and 0.032 inches.

18.3.3 Orthodontic adhesives

The most popular cement for cementing bands is glass ionomer, mainly because of its fluoride-releasing potential and affinity to stainless steel and enamel. Glass ionomers can also be used for retaining bonded attachments, but unfortunately the bracket failure rate with this material is not clinically acceptable. Much current research work is directed towards hybrid compomer materials which it is hoped will combine the advantages of composites and glass ionomer adhesives.

Use of the acid-etch technique with a composite produces clinically acceptable bonded attachment failure rates of the order of 5–10 per cent for both self- and light-cured materials. Although conventional self-cured composites can be used for bonding, a modification has been manufactured specifically for orthodontics which does not require mixing to circumvent the problem of air bubbles, which would obviously compromise bond retention. A recent development has been the introduction of the self-etching primer (Fig. 18.15). This acidulated phosphoric ester effectively combines the etching and primer into one step and eliminates the need to wash away the etchant, thereby saving time. Research suggests that slightly increased bond failure rates are seen compared with the conventional

---

Box 18.1 Problems with ceramic brackets

- Attachment to bonding adhesive (chemical bond too strong, mechanical interlock difficult)
- Frictional resistance is high – limiting sliding mechanics
- Brittle
- Can cause tooth wear if opposing tooth in contact
- Problems with debonding

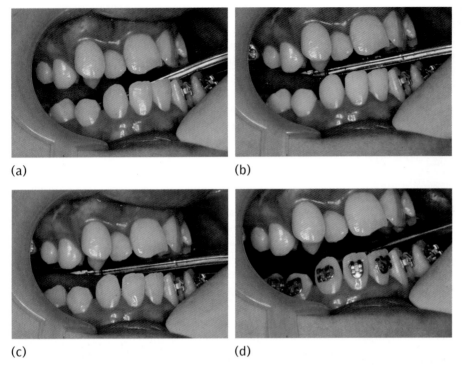

(a)

(b)

(c)

(d)

Fig. 18.14 Stages in the placement of bonded attachments: (a) isolation (b) following etching for 15 seconds the teeth are washed and dried (note the frosted appearance of the etched enamel) (c) bonding adhesive is applied to the etched enamel prior to (d) placement of the pre-coated bonded attachments and light-curing.

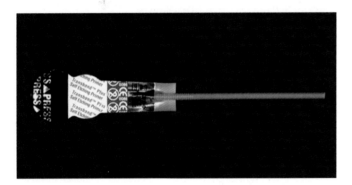

Fig. 18.15 Self-etching primer.

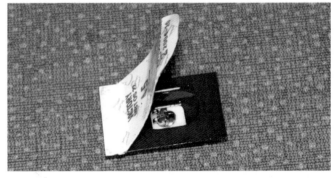

Fig. 18.16 Adhesive pre-coated bracket.

separate etch and prime technique, but these are still clinically acceptable.

Another recent innovation is the introduction of brackets with light-cure adhesive already applied to the base of the bracket, called Adhesive Precoated or APC brackets. The brackets are supplied in individual packages to prevent ambient light setting the adhesive. It is claimed that this approach gives a more consistent bond (Fig. 18.16).

Whatever material is used, any excess should be cleared from the perimeter of the bracket before the final set to reduce plaque retention around the bonded attachment.

18.3.4 Auxiliaries

Very small elastic bands, often described as elastomeric modules (Fig. 18.17), or wire ligatures (Fig. 18.18) are used to secure the archwire into the archwire slot (Fig. 18.19). Elastic modules are quicker to place and are usually more comfortable for the patient, but wire ligatures are still used selectively as they can be tightened to maximize contact between the wire and the bracket.

Intra-oral elastics for traction are commonly available in 2-, 3.5- and 4.5-ounce strengths and a variety of sizes, ranging from 1/8 to 3/4 inch (Fig. 18.20). For most purposes they should be changed every day. Class II and Class III elastic traction is discussed in Chapter 15. Latex-free varieties are now available.

Palatal or lingual arches can be used to reinforce anchorage, to achieve expansion (the quadhelix appliance), or molar de-rotation. They can be made in the laboratory from an impression of the teeth (Fig.18.21). Proprietary forms of most of the commonly used designs are also available, and these have the additional advantage that they are removable, thus facilitating adjustment (Fig. 18.22).

Springs are an integral part of the Tip Edge technique (see Section 18.6.2).

18.3.5 Archwires

Once an operator has chosen to use a particular type of bracket, the amount and type of force applied to an individual tooth can be controlled by varying the cross-sectional diameter and form of the archwire,

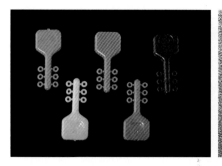

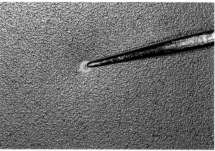

Fig. 18.17 Coloured elastomeric modules used to secure the archwire into the bracket slot.

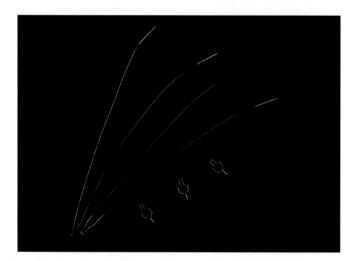

Fig. 18.18 Metal ligatures for securing the archwire into the bracket slot.

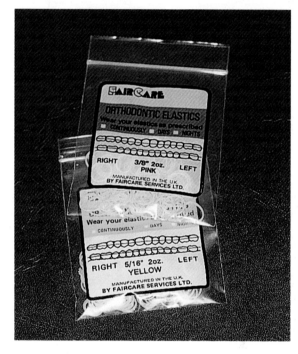

Fig. 18.20 Intra-oral elastics.

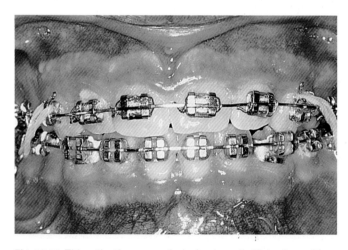

Fig. 18.19 This patient's upper archwire has been tied into place with wire ligatures in the upper arch and with elastomeric modules in the lower arch.

and/or the material of its construction (see also Box 18.2). In the initial stages of treatment a wire which is flexible with good resistance to permanent deformation is desirable, so that displaced teeth can be aligned without the application of excessive forces. In contrast, in the later stages of treatment rigid archwires are required to engage the archwire slot fully and to provide fine control over tooth position while resisting the unwanted effects of other forces, such as elastic traction.

The most popular wire is stainless steel (Fig. 18.23), because it is relatively inexpensive, easily formed and exhibits good stiffness. Because of these characteristics, stainless steel is particularly useful in the later stages of treatment.

Alternatively, other alloys which have a greater resistance to deformation and greater flexibility can be used. Of these, nickel titanium (Fig. 18.24) is the most popular. Archwires made of nickel titanium are capable of applying a light force without deformation, even when deflected several millimetres, but this alloy is more expensive than stainless steel. By virtue of their flexibility, nickel titanium wires provide less control against the unwanted side-effects of auxiliary forces. Modifications of nickel titanium include thermally active wires which are even more flexible when chilled. Other alloys which are less commonly used include titanium molybdenum alloy, known as TMA (Fig. 18.25).

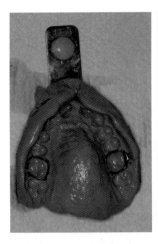
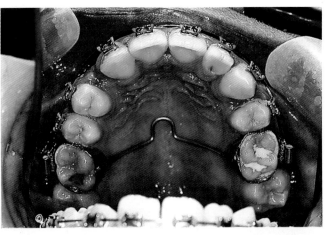

Fig. 18.21 A palatal arch, which is used to help provide additional anchorage in the upper arch by helping to resist forward movement of the maxillary molars. This arch has been constructed from an impression taken over the bands in situ. The bands are then removed and re-sited into the impression before disinfection and transfer to the laboratory for construction.

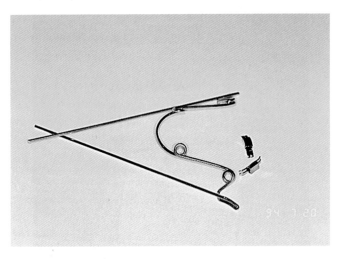

Fig. 18.22 A proprietary removable quadhelix. The distal aspect of the arms of the helix slot into the lingual sheaths (also shown) which are welded onto the palatal surface of bands on the upper molars.

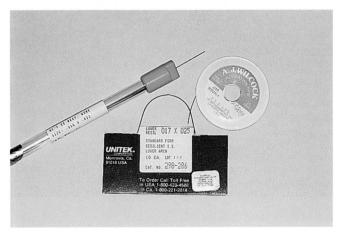

Fig. 18.23 The most popular archwire material is stainless steel which is available in straight lengths, as a coil on a spool, or pre-formed into archwires.

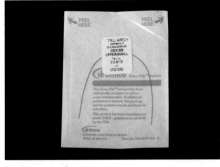
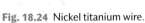
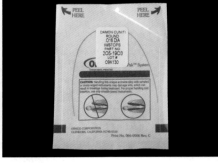
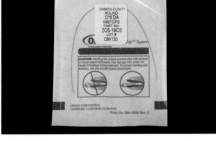

Fig. 18.24 Nickel titanium wire.

Archwires are described according to their dimensions. An archwire described as 0.016 inches (0.4 mm) is a round archwire, and that described as 0.016 × 0.022 inches (0.4 × 0.55 mm), is a rectangular archwire.

Archwires are available in straight lengths, as coils, or as preformed archwires (see Fig. 18.23). The latter variant is more costly to buy but saves chairside time. There are a wide variety of archform shapes; however, regardless of what design is chosen, some adjustment of the

Box 18.2 Physical properties of archwire materials

- Springback. This is the ability of a wire to return to its original shape after a force is applied. High values of springback mean that it is possible to tie in a displaced tooth without permanent distortion.

- Stiffness. The amount of force required to deflect or bend a wire. The greater the diameter of an archwire the greater the stiffness.

- Formability. This is the ease with which a wire can be bent to the desired shape, for example the placement of a coil in a spring, without fracture.

- Resilience. This is the stored energy available after deflection of an archwire without permanent deformation.

- Biocompatibility.

- Joinability. This is whether the material can be soldered or welded.

- Frictional characteristics. If tooth movement is to proceed quickly a wire with low surface friction is preferable.

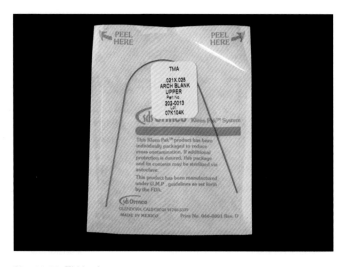

Fig. 18.25 TMA wire.

archwire to match the pre-treatment archform of the patient will be required (see Section 18.4).

The force exerted by a particular archwire material is given by the formula

$$F \propto \frac{dr^4}{l^3}$$

where d is the distance that the spring/wire is deflected, r is the radius of the wire, and l is the length of the wire.

Thus it can be appreciated that increasing the diameter of the archwire will significantly affect the force applied to the teeth, and increasing the length or span of wire between the brackets will inversely affect the applied force. As mentioned earlier, the distance between the brackets can be increased by reducing the width of the brackets, but the inter-bracket span can also be increased by the placement of loops in the archwire. Prior to the introduction of the newer more flexible alloys, multilooped stainless steel archwires were commonly used in the initial stages of treatment. Loops are still utilized in retraction archwires, but with the advent of the pre-adjusted appliance and sliding mechanics they are not used routinely.

18.4 Treatment planning for fixed appliances

By virtue of their coverage of the palate, removable appliances inherently provide more anchorage than fixed appliances. It is important to remember that, with a fixed appliance, movement of one tooth or a segment of teeth in one direction will result in an equal but opposite force acting on the remaining teeth included in the appliance. In addition, apical movement will place a greater strain on anchorage. For these reasons it is necessary to pay particular attention to anchorage when planning treatment involving fixed appliances and, if necessary, this can be reinforced extra-orally, for example, with headgear or intra-orally for example, with a palatal or lingual arch or temporary skeletal anchorage (see Chapter 15).

The importance of keeping the teeth within the zone of soft tissue balance has been discussed in Chapter 7. Therefore care is required to ensure that the archform, particularly of the lower arch, present at the beginning of treatment is largely preserved. It is wise to check the dimensions of any archwire against a model of the lower arch, taken before the start of treatment (Fig. 18.26), bearing in mind that the upper arch will of necessity be slightly broader. Of course, there are exceptions, as discussed in Chapter 7. However, these should be foreseen at the time of treatment planning and, if necessary, the implications discussed fully with the patient at that time.

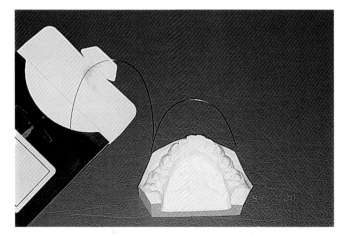

Fig. 18.26 The amount of adjustment required to a pre-formed lower archwire, as taken from the packet, to ensure that it conforms to the patient's pre-treatment archform and width.

18.5 Practical procedures

Accurate bracket placement is crucial to achieving success with fixed appliances. The 'correct' position of the bracket on the facial surface will depend upon the bracket system used. Most pre-adjusted systems require the bracket to be placed in the middle of the tooth along the long axis of the clinical crown. This can be quite difficult to judge, particularly if the tooth is worn. Bracket placement is particularly important with the pre-adjusted technique, as the values for tip and torque are calculated for the midpoint of the facial surface of the tooth. Incorrect bracket positioning will lead to incorrect tooth position and ultimately affect the functional and aesthetic result; therefore errors in bracket placement should be corrected as early as possible in the treatment. Alternatively, adjustments can be made to each archwire to compensate, but over the course of a treatment this can be time-consuming.

As mentioned in Section 18.3.5, when a fixed appliance is first placed a flexible archwire is advisable to avoid applying excessive forces to displaced teeth, which can be painful for the patient and result in bond failure. Usually, a round, pre-formed nickel titanium archwire is used to achieve initial alignment.

It is important to move on from these initial aligning archwires as soon as alignment is achieved, as by virtue of their flexibility they do not afford much control of tooth position. However, it is equally important to ensure that full bracket engagement has been achieved before proceeding to a more rigid archwire. Correction of inter-arch relationships and space closure is usually best carried out using rectangular wires for apical control. The exact archwire sequence will depend upon the dimensions of the archwire slot and operator preference.

Mesiodistal tooth movement can be achieved by one of the following:

(1) Moving teeth with the archwire: this is achieved by incorporating loops into the archwire which, when activated, move a section of the archwire and the attached teeth as shown in Fig. 18.27.

(2) Sliding teeth along the archwire either using elastic traction or (either opening or closing) coil springs (Fig. 18.28). This approach requires greater force to overcome friction between the bracket and the wire, and therefore places a greater strain on anchorage. This type of movement is known as 'sliding mechanics' and is applicable to pre-adjusted appliances where a straight archwire is used.

Fig. 18.29 shows the steps involved in the treatment of a maximum anchorage Class II division 2 malocclusion with fixed appliances.

Adjustments to the appliance need to be made on a regular basis, usually every 6–10 weeks. Once space closure is complete and incisor position corrected, some operators will place a more flexible full-sized archwire, often in conjunction with vertical elastic traction, to help 'sock-in' the buccal occlusion.

Following the attainment of the goals of treatment it is important to retain the finished result. This is covered in detail in Chapter 16.

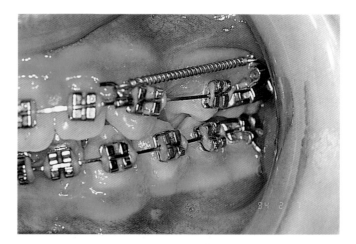

Fig. 18.28 Sliding teeth along the archwire using a nickel–titanium coil spring.

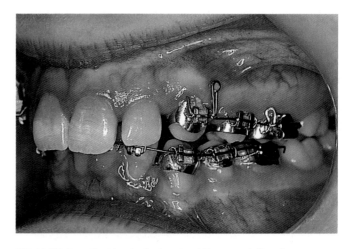

Fig. 18.27 A sectional archwire to retract the upper left canine.

18.6 Fixed appliance systems

18.6.1 Pre-adjusted appliances

Because of their advantages these systems are now universally accepted. The need for first-, second-, and third-order bends in the archwire during treatment is considerably reduced because the brackets are manufactured with the slot positioned to the bracket base in such a way that these movements are built in. Therefore plain preformed archwires can be used so that the teeth are moved progressively from the very start of treatment to their ideal position. Hence they are also known as the straight wire appliance.

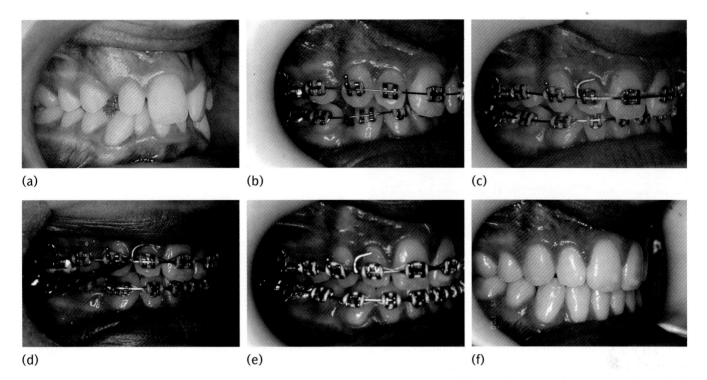

(a)   (b)   (c)

(d)   (e)   (f)

Fig. 18.29 The right buccal view of a 13-year-old with a Class II/2 malocclusion treated by extraction of all four first premolars. (a) Pre-treatment; (b) flexible nickel–titanium archwires were used to achieve alignment; (c) showing rectangular stainless steel working archwires and elastic chain being used to close spaces between the upper incisors; (d) following overbite reduction Class II traction is used in conjunction with space closure to correct incisor and buccal segment relationships; (e) the final stage of treatment is to detail the occlusion; (f) finished result.

As individual tooth positions are built into the bracket, it is necessary to produce a bracket for each tooth, but the time saved in wire bending and the superior results achieved more than compensate for the increased cost of purchasing a greater inventory of brackets. However, a pre-adjusted bracket system will not eliminate the need for wire bending as only average values are built into the appliance, and often additional individual bends need to be placed in the archwire.

Not surprisingly, there are many different opinions as to the correct position of each tooth, and many manufacturers keen to join a lucrative market. The result is an almost bewildering array of pre-adjusted systems, all with slightly differing degrees of torque and tip. Of these perhaps the best known are the Andrews' prescription, developed by Andrews, the father of the straight wire appliance (see Chapter 2, Section 2.4); the Roth system and the MBT prescription (see Table 18.1).

In practice treatment using pre-adjusting systems comprises six steps:

- Alignment
- Overbite reduction
- Overjet correction
- Space closure
- Finishing – this usually comprises placing small bends in the archwires to fine detail tooth position and occlusion
- Retention (Chapter 16)

Table 18.1 MBT prescription for tip and torque (at mid-point of facial surface)

	Torque (°)	Tip (°)
Maxilla		
Central incisor	17	4
Lateral incisor	10	8
Canine	−7	8
First premolar	−7	0
Second premolar	−7	0
First molar	−14	0
Second molar	−14	0
Mandible		
Central incisor	−6	0
Lateral incisor	−6	0
Canine	−6	3
First premolar	−12	2
Second premolar	−17	2
First molar	−20	0
Second molar	−10	0

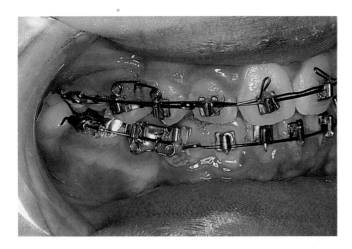

Fig. 18.30 The Begg appliance.

18.6.3 Self-ligating systems

In pre-adjusted systems, a proportion of active tooth movement is achieved by sliding teeth along the archwire, so-called sliding mechanics. Friction between the bracket and the archwire limits this movement and strains anchorage. Use of elastomeric modules or metal ligatures to tie the archwire into the bracket contributes to friction, therefore considerable research expertise has been directed towards self-ligating systems. The number of different types of self-ligating appliances is increasing all the time, but the most well-known include Damon (Fig. 18.32), Innovation and Smartclip. Self-ligating appliances are sub-divided into active or passive bracket designs depending upon whether or not closure of the clip or gate results in an active seating of the archwire in the bracket slot. Although initially manufacturers claimed reduced treatment times due to reduced friction, there is increasing evidence that overall treatment length is similar compared with conventional bracket designs.

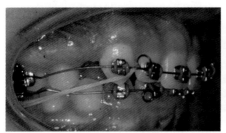 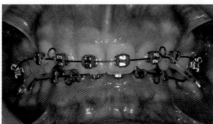 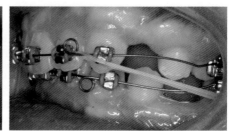

Fig. 18.31 A Tip Edge case in first stage of treatment.

18.6.2 The Tip Edge appliance

The Tip Edge appliance was developed from the Begg appliance with the aim of combining the advantages of both the straight wire and the Begg systems.

Named after its originator, the Begg appliance (Fig. 18.30) was based on the use of round wire which fitted fairly loosely into a channel at the top of the bracket. Light forces were used and tipping movements, with apical and rotational movement achieved by means of auxiliary springs or by loops placed in the archwire. However, the main drawback to the Begg system was that it was difficult to position the teeth precisely at the end of treatment.

The Tip Edge bracket (Fig. 18.31), allows tipping of the tooth in the initial stages of treatment when round archwires are employed, as in the Begg technique, but when full-sized rectangular archwires are used in the latter stages, the built-in pre-adjustments help to give a better degree of control of final tooth positioning.

18.6.4 Future developments

Not surprisingly there is increasing demand from patients, particularly adult patients, for more aesthetic appliances. This has translated into developments in three different approaches. Ceramic brackets (see Section 20.5.1); lingual appliances (see Section 20.5.3); and clear plastic aligners (see Section 20.5.2).

Future developments in the field of fixed appliances include:

- Customized brackets manufactured specifically for an individual patient. This is said to translate into a better finish at the end of treatment and a reduction in the need for adjustment to the archwires during treatment. In other words the bracket system is more complex, but 'simpler' wires can be used.
- Customized finishing wires used with 'standard' pre-adjusted brackets. The stainless steel finishing archwires are manufactured specifically for an individual patient. This is achieved using a cone-beam radiograph so that the final tooth position in all three planes of space can be planned.

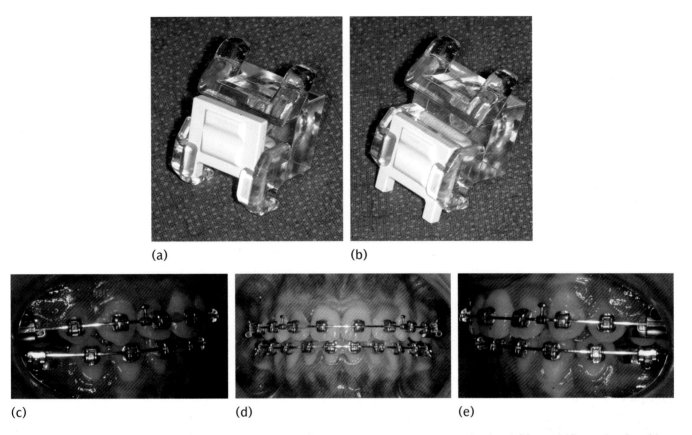

Fig. 18.32 The Damon self-ligating bracket system. (a) A model of a Damon bracket with the archwire slot closed; (b) a model Damon bracket with the archwire slot open; (c–e) a patient being treated with a Damon appliance (this is a newer modification of the Damon bracket).

18.7 Demineralization and fixed appliances

Placement of a fixed attachment upon a tooth surface leads to plaque accumulation. In addition, if a diet rich in sugar is consumed, this results in demineralization of the enamel surrounding the bracket and occasionally frank cavitation. The incidence of demineralization (Fig. 18.33) with fixed appliances has been variously reported as between 15 and 85 per cent. As any decalcification is undesirable, considerable interest has focused on ways of reducing this problem. The main approaches that have been used are as follows:

(1) Careful patient selection. It is unwise to embark upon treatment in a patient with a high rate of caries.

(2) Fluoride mouth rinses for the duration of treatment. The problem with this approach is that the individuals most at risk of demineralization are those least likely to comply fully with a rinsing regime.

(3) Local fluoride release from fluoride-containing cements and bonding adhesives. Variable results have been reported for those composites which have been marketed for their fluoride-releasing potential. Glass ionomer cements have been shown to be effective at reducing the incidence of demineralization around bands, whilst achieving equal or better retention results than conventional cements. Although glass ionomer cements appear effective at reducing demineralization around bonded attachments, this is at the expense of poorer retention rates (see Section 18.3.3).

(4) Dietary advice. This important aspect of preventive advice should not be forgotten. Patients are often advised to avoid chewy sweets during treatment, but the importance of avoiding sugared beverages and fizzy drinks, particularly between meals, should not be overlooked.

Fig. 18.33 Picture showing severe decalcification following fixed appliance treatment (naturally this patient was not treated by the author!).

18.8 Starting with fixed appliances

Some orthodontic supply companies offer the practitioner a kit containing brackets, bands, and a few archwires in return for an impression and a fee. Of course, this is an expensive alternative and, in addition, bands selected remotely from the patient using an impression are unlikely to be a good fit. However, it is extremely unwise, and arguably unethical, to embark on treatment with fixed appliances without first gaining adequate expertise in their use. This is best achieved by a longitudinal course in the form of an apprenticeship with a skilled operator. It is mandatory that this is supplemented by a thorough appreciation of orthodontic diagnosis and treatment planning, which is the most difficult aspect of orthodontics.

Key points

- Fixed appliances are capable of producing tooth movement in all three planes of space
- Fixed appliances are more demanding of anchorage so this must be planned and monitored carefully
- Training is required as fixed appliances have the potential to cause problems in all three planes of space
- A co-operative patient with good dental health is a pre-requisite for success

Relevant Cochrane reviews:

Adhesives for bonded molar tubes during fixed brace treatment
Millet, D.T *et al.* (2011)
http://onlinelibrary.wiley.com/doi/10.1002/14651858.CD008236.pub2/abstract
From the two well-designed and low risk of bias trials included in this review it was shown that the failure of molar tubes bonded with either a chemically-cured or light-cured adhesive was considerably higher than that of molar bands cemented with glass ionomer cement

Adhesives for fixed orthodontic bands
Millet, D.T *et al.* (2008)
http://onlinelibrary.wiley.com/doi/10.1002/14651858.CD004485.pub3/abstract
Concluded there is insufficient high quality evidence with regard to the most effective adhesive for attaching orthodontic bands to molar teeth

Adhesives for fixed orthodontic brackets
Mandall, N.A. *et al.* (2009)
http://onlinelibrary.wiley.com/doi/10.1002/14651858.CD002282/abstract
The authors were unable to draw any conclusions from this review

Fluorides for the prevention of white spot lesions on teeth during fixed brace treatment
Benson, P.E. *et al.* (2008)
http://onlinelibrary.wiley.com/doi/10.1002/14651858.CD003809.pub2/abstract
There is some evidence that the use of topical fluoride or fluoride-containing bonding materials during orthodontic treatment reduces the occurrence and severity of white spot lesions, however there is little evidence as to which method or combination of methods to deliver the fluoride is the most effective. Based on current best practice in other areas of dentistry, for which there is evidence, we recommend that patients with fixed braces rinse daily with a 0.05% sodium fluoride mouthrinse

Initial arch wires for alignment of crooked teeth with fixed orthodontic braces
Wang, Y. *et al.* (2010)
http://onlinelibrary.wiley.com/doi/10.1002/14651858.CD007859.pub2/abstract
There is some evidence to suggest that there is no difference between the speed of tooth alignment or pain experienced by patients when using one initial aligning arch wire over another. However, in view of the general poor quality of the included trials, these results should be viewed with caution

Interspace/interdental brushes for oral hygiene in orthodontic patients with fixed appliances
Goh, H.H. *et al.* (2008)
http://onlinelibrary.wiley.com/doi/10.1002/14651858.CD005410.pub2/abstract
Authors concluded that the present practice of recommending the use of interdental/interspace brushes in addition to standard toothbrushes is not supported by clinical investigations

Principal sources and further reading

Archambault, A., Lacoursiere, R., Badawi, H., Mahor, P.W., and Flores-Mir, C. (2010). Torque expression in stainless steel orthodontic brackets. A systematic review. *Angle Orthodontist*, **80**, 201–10.

Fleming, P.S. and Johal, A. (2010). Self-ligating brackets in orthodontics. A systematic review. *Angle Orthodontist*, **80**, 575–84.

Kapila, S. and Sachdeva, R. (1989). Mechanical properties and clinical applications of orthodontic wires. *American Journal of Orthodontics and Dentofacial Orthopedics*, **96**, 100–9.

An excellent, and readable, account of archwire materials.

Kusy, R. P. (1997). A review of contemporary archwires: their properties and characteristics. *Angle Orthodontist*, **67**, 197–207.

McLaughlin, R. P., Bennett, J., and Trevesi, H. J. (2001). *Systemised Orthodontic Treatment Mechanics*. Mosby, Edinburgh.

A clearly written and beautifully illustrated book, which should be read by anyone using fixed appliances.

Millett, D. T. and Gordon, P. H. (1994). A 5-year clinical review of bond failure with a no-mix adhesive (Right-on). *European Journal of Orthodontics*, **16**, 203–11.

O'Higgins, E. A. *et al*. (1999). The influence of maxillary incisor inclination on arch length. *British Journal of Orthodontics*, **26**, 97–102.

A fascinating article – a 'must read' for those practitioners using fixed appliances.

Pandis, N., Polychronopoulou, A., and Eliades, T. (2010). Active or passive self-ligating brackets? A randomized controlled trial of comparative efficiency in resolving maxillary anterior crowding in adolescents. *American Journal of Orthodontics and Dentofacial Orthopedics*, **137**, 12e.

Authors found no difference between the active and passive bracket systems investigated.

Rogers, S., Chadwick, B., and Treasure, E. (2010). Fluoride-containing orthodontic adhesives and decalcification in patients with fixed appliances: A systematic review. *American Journal of Orthodontics and Dentofacial Orthopedics*, **138**, 390e.

Russell, J. (2005). Aesthetic orthodontic brackets. *Journal of Orthodontics*, **32**, 146–63.

An easy to read résumé of currently available aesthetic brackets and their limitations.

Wright, N., Modarai, F., and Cobourne, M. (2011). Do you do Damon? What is the current evidence base underlying the philosophy of this appliance system? *Journal of Orthodontics*, **38**, 222–30.

As the title suggests!

References for this chapter can also be found at www.oxfordtextbooks.co.uk/orc/mitchell4e/. Where possible, these are presented as active links which direct you to the electronic version of the work, to help facilitate onward study. If you are a subscriber to that work (either individually or through an institution), and depending on your level of access, you may be able to peruse an abstract or the full article if available.

19

Functional appliances

S. J. Littlewood

Chapter contents

Learning objectives for this chapter

- Understand the best time to start functional appliance treatment and factors that may influence this
- Recognize malocclusions that may be treated successfully with functional appliances
- Be familiar with the common types of functional appliances
- Understand the clinical management of functional appliances
- Understand how functional appliances work and how successful they are

19.1 Definition

Functional appliances utilize, eliminate, or guide the forces of muscle function, tooth eruption and growth to correct a malocclusion.

19.2 History

The term 'functional appliance' is used, because initially it was believed that the appliance caused a change in muscle function, leading to a change in growth response. Although we now believe that function probably has little to do with the treatment effect, the term has remained.

The initial idea for functional appliances was derived from the monobloc, developed by Pierre Robin. This appliance was designed to posture the mandible forward in babies born with severely retrognathic mandibles and compromised airways. Andresen in the 1920s used this principle of forward posturing of the mandible to treat malocclusions with his activator appliance, the first functional appliance.

19.3 Overview

There are many different types of functional appliances, but most work by the principle of posturing the mandible forwards in growing patients. They are most effective at changing the anteroposterior occlusion between the upper and lower arches, usually in patients with a mild to moderate Class II skeletal discrepancy. They are not as effective at correcting tooth irregularities and improving arch alignment, so are often followed with a phase of fixed appliance treatment. There are many areas of controversy surrounding functional appliances, in particular treatment timing and mode of action. These areas will be addressed later in this chapter.

A typical functional appliance case is shown on pp. 236–40 to give an overview of the appliance in clinical use.

19.4 Case study: functional appliance

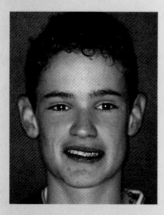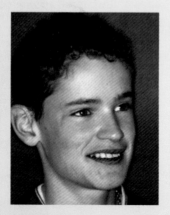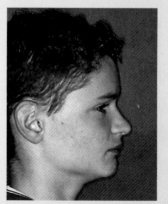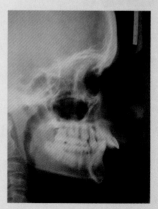

Fig. 19.1 (a) Extra-oral start records. Patient O.P. is 12 years old and complains of his prominent upper incisors. His clinical and radiographic records show he has a Class II division 1 incisor relationship on a Class II skeletal base. His principal problems are an increased overjet of 12 mm, due to proclined and spaced upper incisors and a retrognathic mandible.

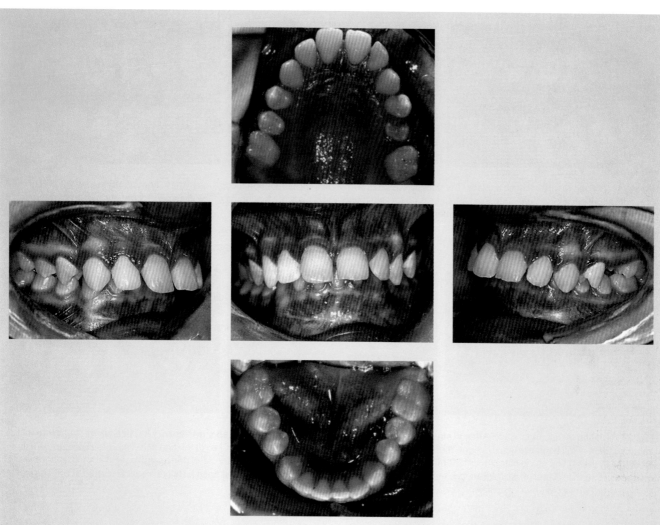

Fig. 19.1 (b) Intra-oral start records for O.P.

Aims of treatment

(1) Growth modification to improve skeletal pattern

(2) Camouflage any remaining skeletal discrepancy with fixed appliances

(3) Align the teeth and close the spaces

Treatment plan

(1) Growth modification with a functional appliance (twin-block)

(2) Towards end of functional appliance begin anterior alignment with fixed appliances

(3) Reassess case at end of functional appliance

(4) Upper and lower fixed appliances

(5) Retention

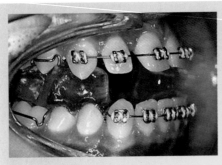
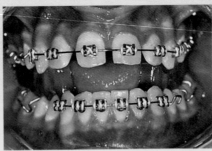
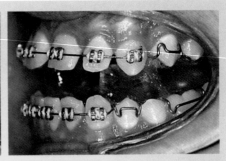

Fig. 19.1 (c) Functional appliance in place. The patient was fitted with a twin-block functional appliance. These photographs show the end of the functional appliance treatment, with fixed appliances on the labial segment. This is the beginning of the alignment of the teeth in preparation for transition to the fixed appliance phase of treatment.

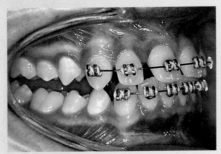
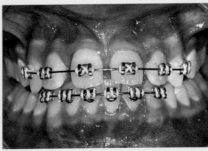
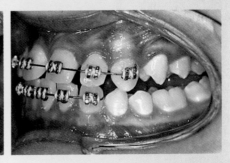

Fig. 19.1 (d) End of functional stage. After 10 months of the functional appliance the anteroposterior discrepancy has been corrected. Note that although there is still a small residual overjet, the buccal segments have been overcorrected to a Class III relationship. This is to allow for the risk of relapse in the second phase of treatment. At this stage full records are taken again to reassess the case, principally to see if any extractions are required before the second phase (extractions were not needed in this case). The posterior lateral open bites are a typical feature at this stage of a case treated with a twin-block appliance.

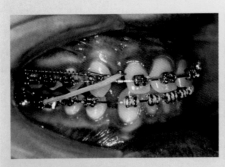
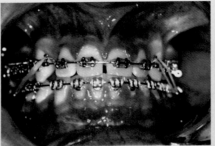
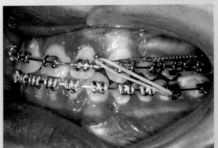

Fig. 19.1 (e) Fixed appliances in the second phase of treatment, with Class II elastics to maintain the changes achieved in the first phase of treatment. The fixed appliances were worn for 16 months.

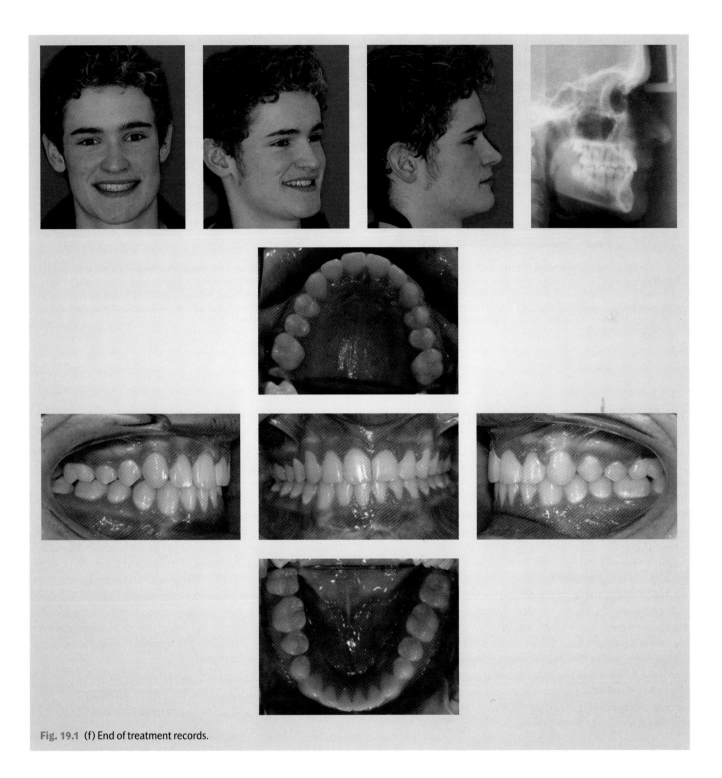

Fig. 19.1 (f) End of treatment records.

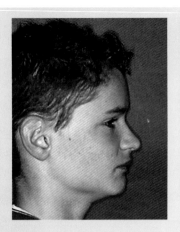
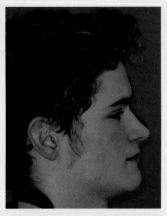
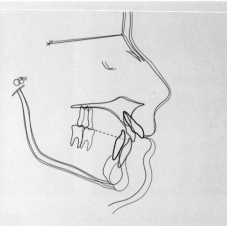

Fig. 19.1 (g) Effects of treatment. The treatment has been successful due to good patient compliance, an appropriate treatment plan, and favourable growth. The growth response to functional appliances is variable, and the growth shown here is better than average. As a result, in this case the skeletal discrepancy was corrected by the growth modification phase of the twin-block appliance. If growth had not been so favourable, then the residual skeletal discrepancy would have had to have been corrected either by orthodontic camouflage, or combined orthodontics and orthognathic surgery when the patient was older.

19.5 Timing of treatment

Functional appliances should be used when the patient is growing. As girls complete their growth slightly earlier than boys, functional appliances can be used a little later in boys. It has been suggested that treatment should, if possible, coincide with the pubertal growth spurt. There have been various attempts to predict this growth spurt, including taking multiple height measurements of the patient, as rapid changes in height coincide closely with the peak changes in the maxilla and mandible. However this does require multiple height measurements spread over a period of time. A more recent approach has been to use maturation changes seen on the cervical vertebrae visible on lateral skull radiographs. During the period of maximum mandibular, growth characteristic maturation changes are visible on cervical vertebrae C3 and C4. Further details about this are provided in the section on further reading at the end of this chapter. However, whichever technique is used it can be difficult to predict the pubertal growth spurt accurately. Fortunately studies have shown that favourable changes with functional appliances can occur outside this growth spurt. The key factor is that the patient is still actively growing.

19.5.1 Should treatment begin in the early mixed or late mixed dentition?

Whilst it is widely acknowledged that functional appliances must be used in growing patients, one area of controversy is whether to provide early treatment (in the early mixed dentition when the patient is under 10 years old) or wait until the late mixed dentition. Early treatment usually involves two phases of treatment: an initial phase with the functional appliance, followed by a pause while the adult dentition erupts, and then a second phase of fixed appliances. In contrast to this, if functional appliance treatment is started in the late mixed dentition, then by the end of the functional stage of treatment the adult dentition is usually erupted sufficiently to proceed straight onto the fixed appliances.

High quality studies comparing patients treated in the early mixed dentition with those treated in the late mixed dentition have now helped to answer this key question about the best time to start functional appliance treatment. This research has shown that both approaches successfully corrected the increased overjet, and there was no difference in the amount of skeletal change achieved or the quality of the final occlusal alignment. However, when patients had their functional appliance fitted earlier, their treatment lasted longer and they needed to attend more appointments. This means that early treatment is more expensive and more importantly, the treatment burden is greater for the patient.

19.5.2 Psychological factors and timing of functional appliance treatment

It has been suggested that one possible indication for early treatment with functional appliances is for psychological reasons. It has been shown that early treatment with functional appliances does produce a transient improvement in a patient's self-esteem and can reduce negative social experiences caused by their malocclusion.

19.5.3 Summary of timing of functional appliance treatment

Generally it is therefore better to start the functional appliance treatment in the late mixed dentition, provided there is still growth remaining.

This means that the patient is ready to progress onto the fixed appliance stage, which typically follows the functional appliance. If the functional appliance is started too early then there will be delay while waiting for the remaining deciduous teeth to exfoliate. The exception to this is when the younger patient is being teased about their teeth. In these situations the child can be given the choice of early treatment, hence addressing the cause of the teasing. However, both the child and the parent need to be aware that by starting the functional appliance earlier the patient will need to attend more appointments, and the total orthodontic treatment time will be longer.

19.6 Types of malocclusion treated with functional appliances

Although functional appliances have been used to treat a whole variety of malocclusions, they are usually used for the treatment of Class II malocclusions. They are typically used for treatment of Class II division 1, but with minor alterations can be used for the treatment of Class II division 2. Some functional appliances, such as a modified twin-block and FR3 Frankel appliance, have been described for the treatment of Class III malocclusions, but there is no evidence of any skeletal correction. These Class III malocclusions are often more simply treated by orthodontic camouflage using fixed appliances, so functionals are rarely used for the treatment of Class III malocclusions.

19.6.1 Treatment of Class II division 1 malocclusions

Functional appliances are most commonly used for the treatment of Class II division 1 malocclusions. If the arches are well aligned at the start of treatment, and the only problem is an anteroposterior discrepancy between the arches, then the functional appliance alone may be sufficient. In these cases it is wise to slightly over-correct the malocclusion to allow for some relapse, and ask the patient to wear the appliance at night until the end of their growth period.

Functional appliances are often used as a first phase of treatment, followed by a second phase of fixed appliances. The functional appliance corrects, or at least reduces, the skeletal discrepancy in a process known as growth modification or dentofacial orthopaedics. By correcting the anteroposterior problems with the functional appliance, the amount of anchorage required during the fixed appliance stage is reduced. However, since functional appliances also cause some tilting of the teeth, a significant part of the correction caused by a functional appliance is probably orthodontic camouflage.

Following the functional phase the patient is reassessed with regard to the need for possible extractions and fixed appliances to align the arches.

19.6.2 Treatment of Class II division 2 malocclusions

Class II division 2 malocclusions can also be treated using functional appliances. As mentioned in Chapter 10, this type of malocclusion can be difficult to treat, partly due to the increased overbite. The use of a functional appliance, before fixed appliances, may provide a more efficient alternative to treating these malocclusions with fixed appliances alone.

The approach to treatment is simple. The Class II division 2 incisor relationship is converted to a Class II division 1 relationship and then treated with a functional appliance. The retroclined upper incisors can be proclined forward using a pre-functional removable appliance, or a sectional fixed appliance on the upper labial segment. Alternatively some functional appliances can be modified to procline the upper incisors as part of the functional appliance phase of treatment. Figure 19.2 shows a Class II division 2 case treated with a modified twin-block appliance.

19.7 Types of functional appliance

There are many types of functional appliance, but most share the common feature of holding the mandible in a postured position. Functional appliances can be tissue-borne or tooth-borne, and may be removable or fixed. Some are also worn with headgear that may enhance the Class II correction. The use of headgear attached to a functional appliance attempts to restrict the anterior and vertical development of the maxilla. This can particularly helpful in cases where there is excess incisor show and a so-called 'gummy smile'. The disadvantage of using the additional headgear is that it is an extra burden for the patient, which may adversely affect overall compliance.

Five popular designs of functional appliances will be described here. There is no such thing as a standard functional appliance design, as every appliance should be individually tailored to the patient and their malocclusion.

19.7.1 Twin-block appliance

The twin-block appliance (Fig. 19.3) is the most popular functional appliance in the UK. The reason for its popularity is that it is well tolerated by patients as it is constructed in two parts. The upper and lower parts fit together using posterior bite blocks with interlocking bite-planes, which posture the mandible forwards. The blocks need to be at least 5 mm high, which prevents the patient from biting one block on top of the other. Instead the patient is encouraged to posture the mandible forwards, so that the lower block occludes in front of the upper block. The appliance can be worn full time, including during eating in some cases, which means that rapid correction is possible. It is also possible to modify the appliance to allow expansion of the upper arch during the functional appliance phase. A modification to allow correction of Class II division 2 malocclusions is shown in Fig. 19.2.

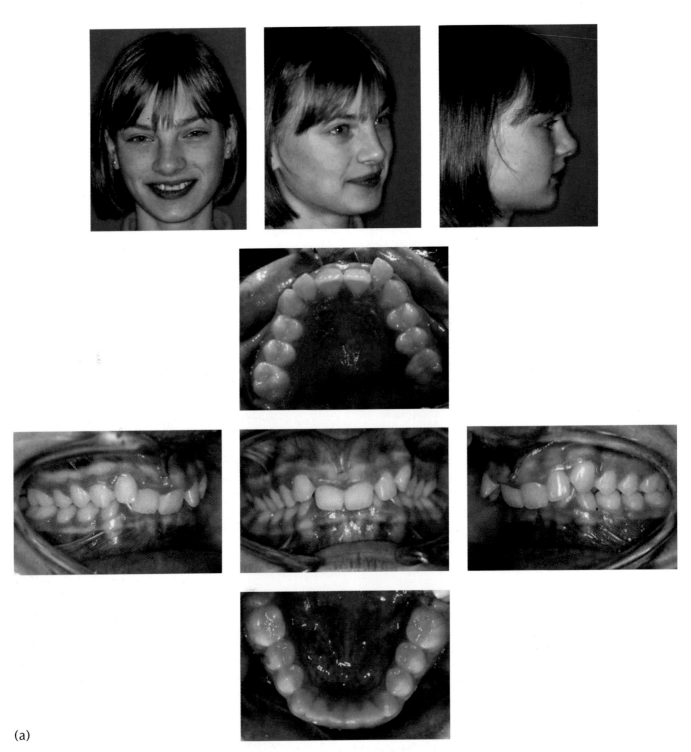

(a)

Fig. 19.2 Treatment of a Class II division 2 malocclusion with a twin-block. (a) Patient AD is 12 years old and complained of her crooked upper teeth. She presented with a Class II division 2 incisor relationship on a Class II skeletal base. Her principal problems were retroclined upper central incisors, an increased overbite and a retrognathic mandible. The treatment plan was to correct the anteroposterior discrepancy and procline the upper central incisors using a modified twin-block appliance. The functional appliance was then followed by a phase of fixed appliances and then retainers.

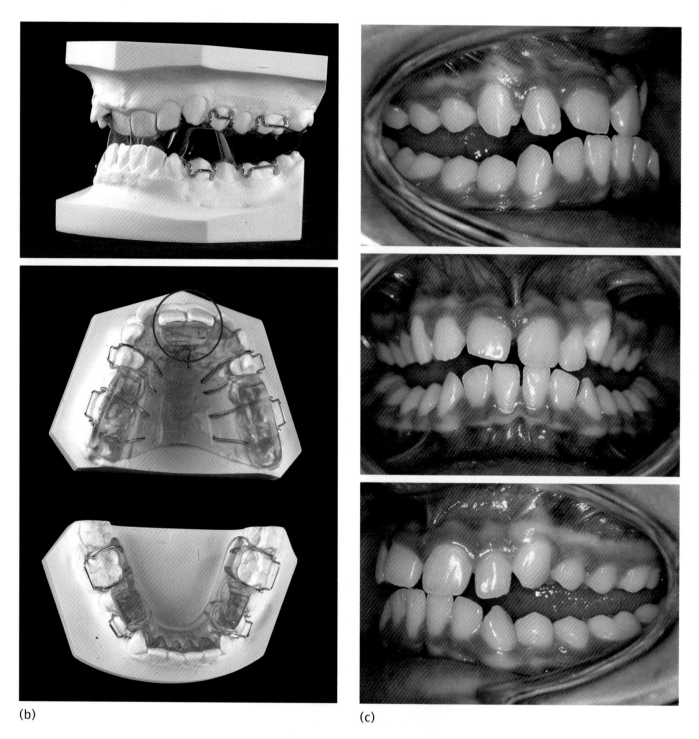

(b)

(c)

Fig. 19.2 (b) Twin-block appliance modified for treatment of a Class II division 2 malocclusion. Note the additional palatal double-cantilever spring (highlighted in red circle) in the upper arch, which is used to procline the central incisors. (c) End of functional stage. The anteroposterior discrepancy has been corrected and the retroclined upper central incisors proclined to normal inclinations. Note the posterior lateral open bites, which were closed in the second phase of fixed appliances.

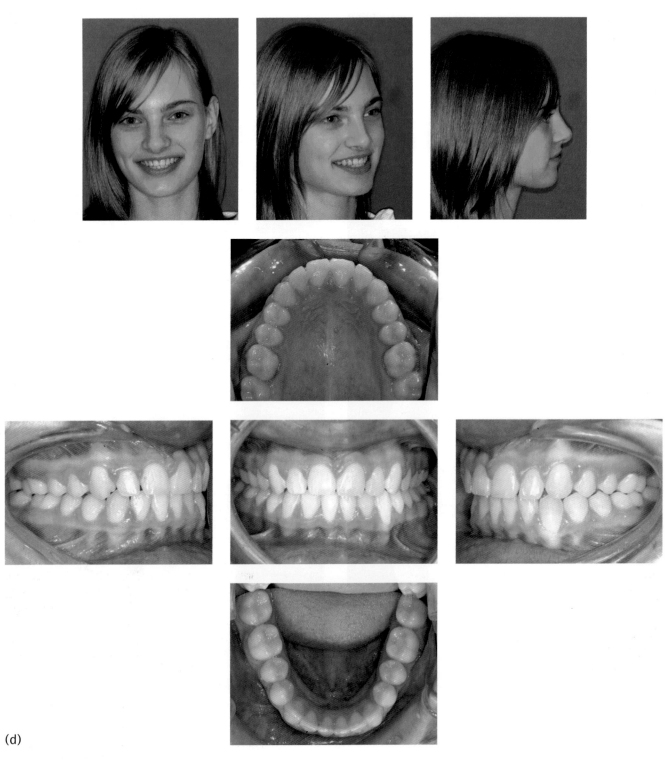

(d)

Fig. 19.2 (d) End of treatment.

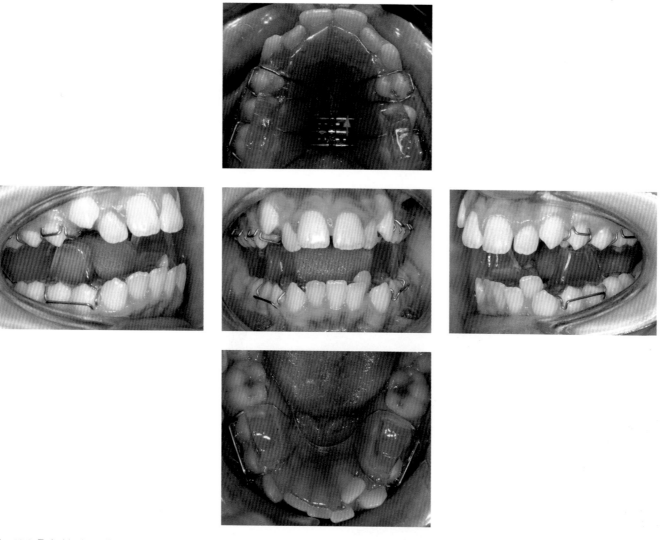

Fig. 19.3 Twin-block appliance. This twin-block also has an upper midline screw to permit expansion of the upper arch.

It is also easy to reactivate the twin-block appliance (Fig. 19.4). This means that during treatment if further advancement of the mandible is required, it is possible to modify the existing appliance rather than having to construct a new appliance.

One of the side-effects of the twin-block appliance is the residual posterior lateral open bites at the end of the functional phase (see Fig. 19.2). This is seen particularly in cases initially presenting with a deep overbite. The posterior teeth are prevented from erupting by the occlusal coverage of the bite blocks. Some clinicians will trim the acrylic away from the occlusal surfaces of the upper block to allow the lower molars to erupt. Any remaining lateral open bites are closed down in the fixed appliance phase of treatment.

19.7.2 Herbst appliance

The Herbst appliance (Figs 19.5 and 19.10) is a fixed functional appliance and is the most popular functional appliance in the US. There is a section attached to the upper buccal segment teeth and a section attached to the lower buccal segment teeth. These sections are joined by a rigid arm that postures the mandible forwards. As it is a fixed appliance, it removes some (but not all) compliance factors. It is as successful at reducing overjets as the twin-block appliance. It is however slightly better tolerated than the bulkier twin-block appliance, with patients finding it easier to eat and talk with it in place. The principle disadvantages are the increased breakages and higher cost of the Herbst appliance.

19.7.3 Medium opening activator (MOA)

This is a one-piece functional appliance, with minimal acrylic to improve patient comfort (Fig. 19.6). The lower acrylic extends lingual to the lower labial segment only, and the upper and lower parts are joined by two rigid acrylic posts, leaving a breathing hole anteriorly. As there is no molar capping on the lower posterior teeth, these teeth are free to erupt. The MOA is therefore useful when trying to reduce a deep overbite.

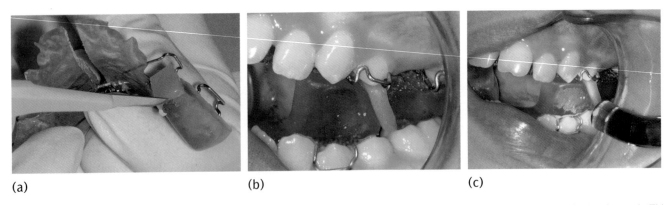

(a) (b) (c)

Fig. 19.4 Reactivation of the twin-block appliance. The twin-block can be reactivated during treatment to posture the mandible further forwards. This particular technique involves adding light-cured acrylic to the inclined bite-plane on the upper block. (a) Trimming the uncured acrylic to fit the left inclined bite-plane of the upper block. (b) The light-cured acrylic is placed on the upper block, forcing the lower block, and therefore the mandible, further anteriorly. (c) Light-curing the acrylic.

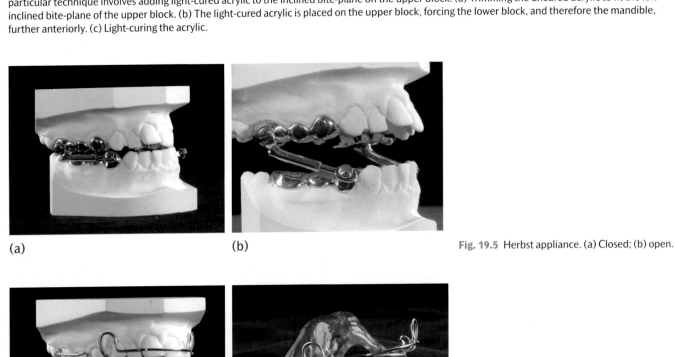

(a) (b)

Fig. 19.5 Herbst appliance. (a) Closed; (b) open.

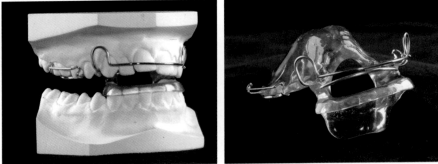

Fig. 19.6 Medium opening activator (MOA).

19.7.4 Bionator

The bionator (Fig. 19.7) was originally designed to modify tongue behaviour, using a heavy wire loop in the palate. We now know that the tongue is unlikely to be the cause of the increased overjet, but the lack of acrylic in the palate makes it easy to wear. A buccal extension of the labial bow holds the cheeks out of contact with the buccal segment teeth, allowing some arch expansion.

19.7.5 Frankel appliance

The Frankel appliance (Fig. 19.8) is the only completely tissue-borne appliance. It is named after the inventor, who originally called it the function regulator (or FR). There are different versions designed to treat different types of malocclusions. Like other functional appliances it postures the mandible forwards. It also has buccal shields to hold the cheeks away from the teeth and stretch the periosteum, allegedly to cause bone formation, although this has never been proved. It can be difficult to wear, is expensive to make and is troublesome to repair. As a result it is now used less frequently.

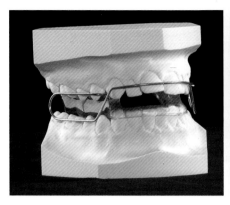
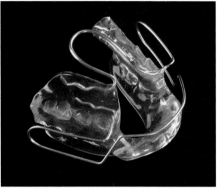

Fig. 19.7 Bionator.

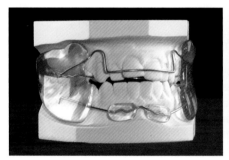
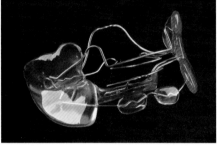

Fig. 19.8 Frankel appliance (FR1).

19.8 Clinical management of functional appliances

19.8.1 Preparing for the functional appliance

Well-extended upper and lower alginate impressions are required along with a recording of the postured bite. The bite recording should prescribe to the laboratory the exact position of the postured mandible in all three dimensions – anteroposteriorly, vertically and transversely. Figure 19.9 shows a wax bite recording for a functional appliance patient.

The degree of protrusion will depend on the size of the overjet and the comfort of the patient. For patients with a large overjet, protruding the patient's mandible more than 75 per cent of their maximum protrusion can make the appliance difficult to tolerate. It is relatively easy to reactivate some functional appliances during treatment if further protrusion is required (Fig. 19.4).

Research would suggest that it makes no difference to the final result whether we activate the appliance to the maximum advancement initially, or in increments of a few millimetres at a time during treatment. The decision of whether to protrude the patient to the maximum amount initially, or advance incrementally during treatment, should be based on patient comfort. For some patients incremental advancement of the mandible during treatment may make it easier to tolerate.

19.8.2 Fitting the functional appliance

The patient should be made aware that although the functional appliance will not be painful, it can be difficult to get used to

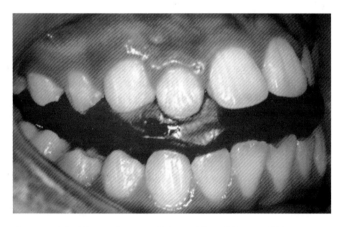

Fig. 19.9 Wax bite used to record the position of the mandible anteroposteriorly, vertically and transversely.

initially. Good motivation is important in all aspects of orthodontics, but this is particularly true with functional appliances. They can be demanding appliances to wear at first, but children will adapt to them very quickly provided they are worn sufficiently. The number of hours the appliance needs to be worn each day depends on the type of appliance. Functional appliances such as the twin-block and Herbst that can be worn full time often allow the patient to adapt more quickly.

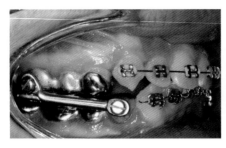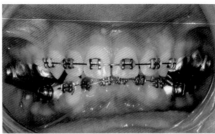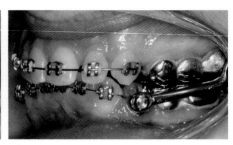

Fig. 19.10 Herbst appliance with sectional labial fixed appliances. Most functional appliances are followed by a stage of fixed appliances. The transition to fixed appliances can be complex. Some functionals, for example the Herbst appliance shown here, allows alignment of the upper and lower labial segments using fixed appliances, during the functional stage of treatment.

19.8.3 Reviewing the functional appliance

It is advisable to see the patient 2–3 weeks after fitting. At every review appointment motivation of the patient is vital, as well as checking the fit of the appliance and treatment progress. Once the clinician is confident that the patient is wearing the appliance as instructed the review appointments can be made at 6–10-week intervals.

If there is no progress this could be due to a number of factors:

- Poor compliance
- Lack of growth or an unfavourable growth rotation
- Problems with the design or fit of the appliance

Poor compliance is the most common potential problem with these appliances. Compliance tends to be better with the younger patients and those wearing fixed functionals, such as the Herbst appliance.

19.8.4 End of functional appliance treatment

At the end of the functional appliance treatment it is sensible to slightly over-correct the overjet reduction to edge-to-edge, due to the risk of relapse. Most functional appliances are followed by fixed appliances and this transition to fixed appliances is a complex area, best handled by a specialist (see Fig. 19.10). If the arches were initially well-aligned, and a second phase of fixed appliances is not required, then the patient is asked to wear the functional appliance at night for a period until growth is complete.

19.9 How functional appliances work

The mode of action of functional appliances is one of the most controversial areas in orthodontics. There seems to be little doubt that in patients who are growing, with good compliance, a favourable improvement in the occlusion can be achieved in most cases. When the mandible is postured, pressures are created by stretching of the muscles and soft tissues. These pressures are then transmitted to the dental arches and skeletal structures. However, it is not clear what proportion of the treatment effects are due to dental changes and what proportion are due to skeletal changes.

Early animal experiments seemed to suggest that substantial changes in the skeletal structure, including condylar growth, remodelling of the glenoid fossa, mandibular growth and maxillary restraint, could be achieved with functional appliances. However, these results should be interpreted with caution. Animals have different facial morphologies to humans and rarely have facial skeletal discrepancies and malocclusions. In addition, the functional appliances used in the animal experiments are fixed and posture the mandible in more extreme positions than would be realistic for human usage.

Clinical studies are more likely to give us an understanding of how these appliances work. Traditionally many of these studies have been retrospective. There are many inherent weaknesses in these retrospective trials, including lack of control of variables and a tendency to overestimate treatment effects due to loss of data from unsuccessful or failed treatments. The results of randomized controlled trials have helped to shed more light on what actually happens with functional appliance treatment.

It would appear that changes caused by functional appliances are principally due to dento-alveolar changes. This means there is distal movement of the upper dentition and mesial movement of the lower dentition, with tipping of the upper incisors palatally and the lower incisors labially. There are some minor skeletal changes, with some degree of maxillary restraint as well as mandibular growth. These changes, although clinically welcome, are too small (1–2 mm) to predictably replace the need for orthognathic surgery in severe skeletal discrepancies. The results of trials have also shown a large variability of response between individuals, with some patients showing more extensive skeletal changes (Fig. 19.1). This may explain why some cases seem to progress extremely well with obvious facial changes, while others show limited facial improvement. In some cases, even with minimal skeletal change, the patient's facial appearance can be improved. This is because the patient's incisor relationship has been corrected, often allowing the patient to comfortably obtain competent lips at rest.

Functional appliances have often been prescribed to cause 'growth modification'. There is some question as to whether this term is still relevant following the results of the randomized controlled clinical trials. The results of these studies suggest that on average growth changes achieved are smaller than was once initially hoped. This does not mean that total correction is impossible, but total correction of a severe deformity with growth modification alone rarely occurs. It is more likely that functional appliances improve the malocclusion, in many cases perhaps to a point where orthodontic camouflage rather than orthognathic surgery can be used to complete the treatment.

One area of difficulty for the clinician is whether to attempt growth modification for a child with a severe mandibular deficiency. The severity of the mandibular discrepancy is not a good indicator of the chance of a successful outcome. However, if the child, parents and clinician understand that the chance of major improvement is only about 20–30 per cent then the treatment can be undertaken. If the growth modification fails, or is insufficient to fully correct the problem, then camouflage or orthognathic surgery when the patient is older may need to be considered.

19.10 How successful are functional appliances?

This chapter has shown that functional appliances can be effective at reducing increased overjets and helping to treat Class II malocclusions in growing patients, but how successful are functional appliances?

The average failure rate for functional appliances is about 20 per cent. This needs to be explained to the patient and parents at the start of the treatment. The commonest reason for failure is lack of compliance, with the patient failing to wear the functional appliance as prescribed. It is therefore vital that treatment with functional appliances is focused on improving the compliance rate by motivating the patient, and making the appliance as comfortable as possible.

Key points about functional appliances

- Functional appliances posture the mandible and are used in growing patients
- They are usually used for correction of mild to moderate Class II skeletal problems
- In most cases they are followed by a second phase of fixed appliances
- They can be used alone to treat Class II division 1 malocclusions if the arches are well aligned
- They are used in the late mixed dentition, provided the patient is still growing
- They can be used earlier for psychological reasons if the patient is being teased, but this means more appointments and increased overall treatment time
- They produce predominantly dento-alveolar effects, with small skeletal changes
- Individual patient response to functional appliances is variable
- They can be difficult to wear initially and require encouragement and motivation from the clinician
- They are successful in approximately 80% of cases – the 20% failure rate is usually due to problems of patient compliance

---

Principal sources and further reading

Harrison, J. E., O'Brien, K. D., and Worthington, H. V. (2007). *The Cochrane Database of Systematic Reviews 2007*.

This systematic review discusses the evidence behind treatment of patients with increased overjets, and includes summaries of the best quality studies using functional appliances.

O'Brien, K.D. *et al.* (2009). Early treatment for Class II division 1 malocclusion with the Twin-Block appliance: a multi-center, randomized, controlled trial. *American Journal of Orthodontics and Dentofacial Orthopedics*, **135**, 573–9.

Dolce, C., McGorray, S.P., Brazeau, L. *et al.* (2007). Timing of Class II treatment: skeletal changes comparing 1-phase and 2-phase treatment. *American Journal of Orthodontics and Dentofacial Orthopedics*, **132**, 481–9.

O'Brien, K. D. *et al.* (2003). Effectiveness of treatment for Class II malocclusion with the Herbst or Twin-Block appliances: a randomised controlled trial. *American Journal of Orthodontics and Dentofacial Orthopedics*, **124**, 128–37.

Tulloch, J. F. C., Proffit, W. R., and Phillips, C. (2004). Outcomes in a 2-phase randomized clinical trial of early class II treatment. *American Journal of Orthodontics and Dentofacial Orthopedics*, **125**, 657–67.

The four papers above describe randomized controlled clinical trials involving functional appliances and are well worth reading.

Franchi, L., Bacetti, T., and McNamara, J. A. (2000). Mandibular growth as related to cervical vertebral maturation and body height. *American Journal of Orthodontics and Dentofacial Orthopedics*, **118**, 335–40.

This paper describes how to determine the peak stage of growth of the mandible by looking at the development and maturation of the cervical vertebrae visible on lateral skull radiographs

References for this chapter can also be found at www.oxfordtextbooks.co.uk/orc/mitchell4e/. Where possible, these are presented as active links which direct you to the electronic version of the work, to help facilitate onward study. If you are a subscriber to that work (either individually or through an institution), and depending on your level of access, you may be able to peruse an abstract or the full article if available.

20
Adult orthodontics
S. J. Littlewood

Chapter contents

20.1 Introduction

The demand for adult orthodontics is increasing. There are really two distinct groups of adults that request orthodontic treatment. The first group is looking for comprehensive treatment, having, for whatever reason, missed out on orthodontics as a child (Fig. 20.1). With dental awareness growing, an increasing demand for improved dental aesthetics and better social acceptance of orthodontic appliances, more adults are willing to wear appliances. The second group of adults requires orthodontic treatment to facilitate restorative and/or periodontal care. Tooth movement undertaken to facilitate other dental procedures is known as adjunctive orthodontic treatment.

20.2 Specific problems in adult orthodontic treatment

In many ways the approach to treatment in adult patients follows the same process as that for children. There are however some problems that are specific to adult patients:

- Lack of growth
- Periodontal disease
- Missing or heavily restored teeth
- Physiological factors affecting tooth movement
- Adult motivation and attitude towards treatment

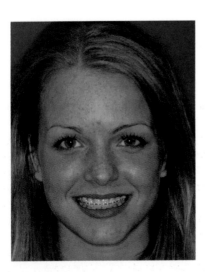

Fig. 20.1 Adult wearing ceramic brackets.

20.2.1 Lack of growth

Although growth continues at a very slow rate throughout adulthood, the majority of growth changes have occurred by the end of puberty. This means that there is no scope for growth modification, so skeletal discrepancies can only be treated with either orthodontic camouflage, or combined orthodontics and orthognathic surgery.

It can also be more difficult to reduce overbites without the benefit of growth. Where possible, overbite reduction should be achieved by intrusion of the incisors, rather than the more common method of extruding the molars (provided this does not compromise the smile aesthetics). This is because extrusion of posterior teeth is more prone to relapse in adults.

20.2.2 Periodontal disease

Adult patients are more likely to be suffering, or have suffered, from periodontal disease. A reduced periodontium is not a contraindication to orthodontic treatment, but it is vital that any active periodontal disease is treated and stabilized before orthodontic treatment can begin. This is discussed in more detail in Section 20.3.

20.2.3 Missing or heavily restored teeth

Tooth loss may lead to drifting and/or tilting of adjacent teeth and over-eruption of opposing teeth into the space. In addition, atrophy of the alveolar bone can occur, leading to a narrowing or 'necking' in the site of the missing tooth or teeth (Fig. 20.2). This can make tooth movement into these areas more difficult.

Heavily restored teeth are more common in adults and may complicate the orthodontic treatment. The choice of extractions may be

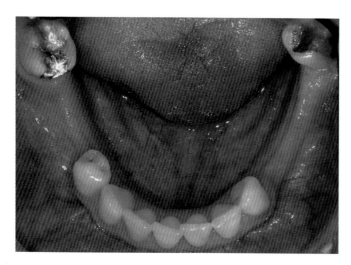

Fig. 20.2 Atrophy of alveolus after tooth loss.

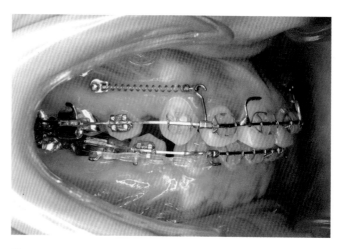

Fig. 20.3 Miniscrew used for anchorage (courtesy of Professor Hyo-Sang Park). The overjet is being reduced by traction applied to a miniscrew on each side. By avoiding traction to the molar teeth this limits the unwanted forward movement of the posterior teeth.

determined by the prognosis of the restored teeth, and bonding to certain restorative materials is more difficult than bonding directly to enamel. Specialist techniques and materials are needed when bonding fixed appliances to gold, amalgam and porcelain, and the patient needs to be warned that the restoration may be damaged when removing the fixed appliance. For this reason, if possible, it is best to leave any definitive restorations until after the orthodontic treatment.

20.2.4 Physiological factors affecting tooth movement

There is a reduced tissue blood supply and decreased cell turnover in adults, which can mean that initial tooth movement is slower in adults, and may be more painful. Lighter initial forces are therefore advisable.

20.2.5 Adult motivation and attitude towards treatment

Adults have the potential to be excellent, well-motivated patients. Physiological factors might suggest that adult treatment should take longer than it does in children; however, this is not always the case. It has been suggested that the increased co-operation may compensate for slower initial tooth movement.

Adults tend to be more conscious of the appearance of the appliance, so there has been a drive towards more aesthetic orthodontic appliances (see Section 20.5). Although distal movement of the upper molars with headgear is technically feasible, adults are more reluctant to wear extra-oral appliances. Alternative sources of anchorage are therefore more commonly used in adult patients, such as implant-based anchorage (Fig. 20.3).

20.3 Orthodontics and periodontal disease

Periodontal disease is more common in adults, and is therefore an important factor that must be considered in all adult orthodontic patients. It is wise to undertake a full periodontal examination in all adult patients to exclude the presence of active periodontal disease. Periodontal attachment loss is not a contraindication to orthodontic treatment, but active periodontal disease must be treated and stabilized before treatment begins. The presence of plaque is the most important factor in the initiation, progression and recurrence of periodontal disease. Teeth with reduced periodontal support can be safely moved provided there is adequate plaque control.

20.3.1 Malalignment problems caused by periodontal disease

Loss of periodontal support can lead to pathological tooth migration of a single tooth or a group of teeth. The commonest presentation of periodontal attachment loss is labial migration and spacing of the incisors (Fig. 20.4). The teeth lie in an area of balance between the tongue lingually and the lips and cheeks buccally. The forces from the tongue are higher than those exerted by the lips and cheeks, but a normal healthy periodontium resists these proclining forces from the tongue. If however periodontal attachment is lost as a result of disease, then the teeth will be proclined forwards. In addition, if posterior teeth are lost then this lack of posterior support produces more pressures on the labial segment, leading to further proclination of the incisors.

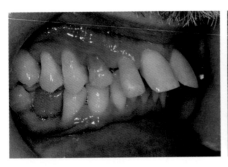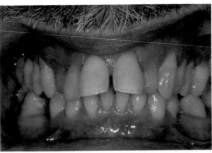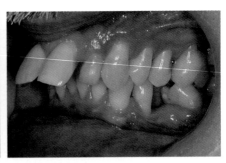

Fig. 20.4 Proclination and spacing of incisors secondary to the loss of periodontal attachment. This patient initially presented with a Class II division 1 incisor relationship with an overjet of 6 mm. However, due to periodontal disease and the subsequent loss of periodontal attachment around the upper labial segment, these upper incisors have flared forward, and become spaced.

20.4 Orthodontic treatment as an adjunct to restorative work

With an increasing number of patients keeping their teeth for longer, there is a greater need for interdisciplinary treatment of patients with complex dental problems. Where collaboration is needed between the orthodontist and the restorative dentist, it is helpful to see the patients jointly to formulate a co-ordinated and appropriate treatment plan. Orthodontic treatment in these cases does not necessarily require comprehensive correction aiming for an ideal occlusion. The aims of adjunctive orthodontic treatment are to:

- Facilitate restorative work by appropriate positioning of teeth
- Improve the periodontal health by reducing areas that harbour plaque, and making it simpler for the patient to maintain good oral hygiene
- Position the teeth so that occlusal forces are transmitted along the long axis of the tooth, and tooth wear is more evenly distributed throughout the arch

The following are examples of problems that benefit from a joint approach between the orthodontist and the restorative dentist:

- *Uprighting of abutment teeth*: following tooth loss adjacent teeth may drift into the space. Uprighting these abutment teeth can facilitate the placement of replacement prosthetic teeth (Fig. 20.5).
- *Redistribution or closure of spaces*: following tooth loss it may be possible to close the remaining space, or move a proposed abutment tooth into the middle of an edentulous span, in order to aid construction of a more robust prosthesis. If implants are required then the roots may need to be repositioned to permit surgical placement.
- *Intrusion of over-erupted teeth*: one of the side effects of tooth loss is over-eruption of the opposing tooth. This can interfere with restora-

tion of the space, so the over-erupted tooth can be intruded using orthodontics.

- *Extrusion of fractured teeth*: sometimes it is necessary to extrude a fractured tooth, to bring the fracture line supragingivally to allow placement of a crown or restoration. There is a limit to this, as excess extrusion will reduce the amount of tooth supported by bone, reducing the crown-to-root ratio.

20.4.1 Orthodontic management of patients with periodontal disease

Once the periodontal disease has been fully stabilized, and the patient is able to maintain a good standard of oral hygiene, treatment can begin (Fig. 20.5). Lighter forces are required, due to the reduced periodontal support, and ideally bonds rather than bands should be used on the molars to aid oral hygiene. Removal of excess adhesive will also help to reduce plaque retention. Due to the reduced alveolar bone support the centre of resistance of the tooth moves apically. This means there is a greater tendency for teeth to tip excessively, so this must be carefully controlled with appropriate treatment mechanics.

Retention at the end of treatment needs to be carefully considered. Even when the teeth are aligned and the periodontium is healthy, the problem of reduced periodontal support remains. With reduced periodontal attachment there will always be a tendency for the forces of the tongue to procline the incisors. These cases require permanent retention, often in the form of bonded retainers, and the patient must be taught how to maintain excellent oral hygiene around these retainers (see Chapter 16).

Fig. 20.5 Adjunctive orthodontic treatment. (a) Patient PM is 50 years old and was referred from her general dental practitioner with combined restorative and orthodontic problems. She had initially presented with moderate chronic periodontitis, with extensive bone loss (see DPT radiograph). This had led to migration of the teeth, particularly the upper right lateral incisor and upper right canine, which had both drifted and extruded. Following treatment and stabilization of the periodontal disease, restoration of the upper central incisor space was complicated by the position of these two teeth. The treatment plan was adjunctive fixed appliance treatment to re-position these teeth, align the upper arch and allow provision of an upper removable prosthesis. (b) Following 8 months of upper fixed appliance treatment, the upper arch was aligned and appropriate space made for the prosthesis. No attempt was made at comprehensive orthodontic correction, with no treatment in the lower arch and no reduction in overjet. (c) A removable partial denture was made. A well-fitting aesthetic prosthesis was made possible by the adjunctive orthodontic treatment.

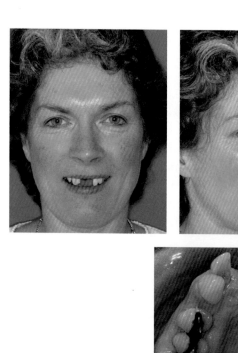
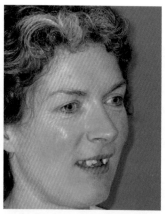
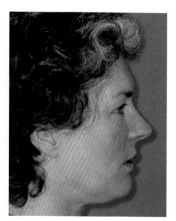
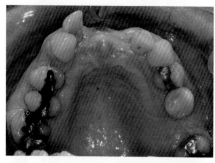
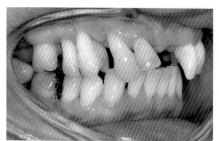
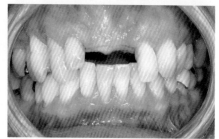
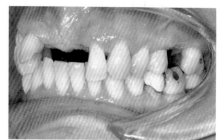
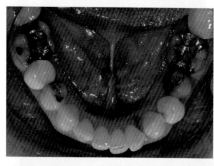
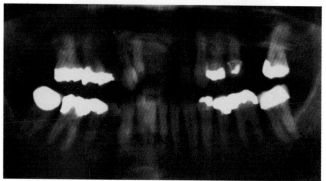

(a)

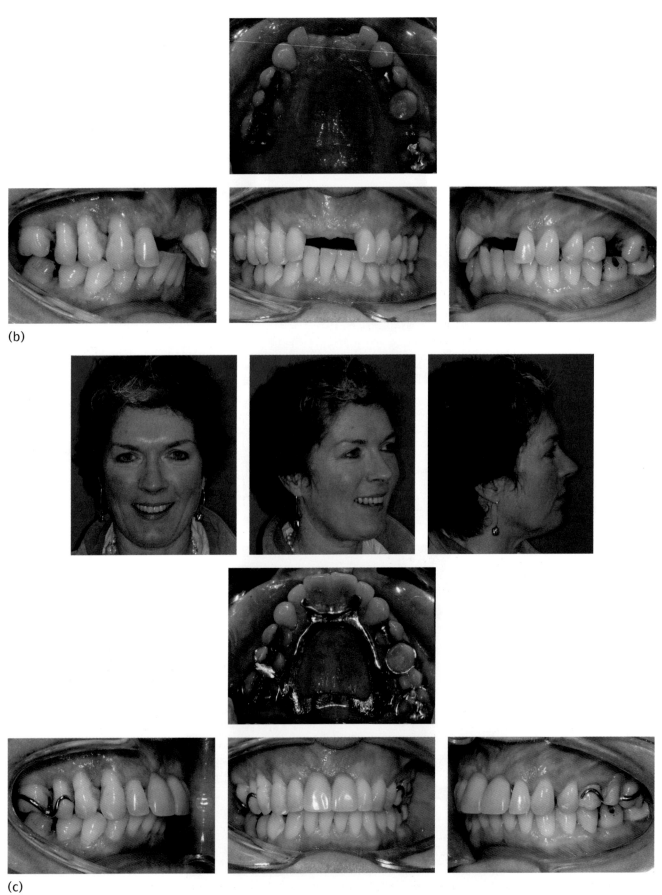

(b)

(c)

Fig. 20.5 (*continued*)

20.5 Aesthetic orthodontic appliances

Although aesthetic orthodontic appliances are not restricted to adult patients, the drive for less visible appliances has come from adults. This demand has led to the development of a number of orthodontic appliances with improved aesthetics (see Box 20.1).

20.5.1 Aesthetic orthodontic brackets and wires

Aesthetic orthodontic brackets (Fig. 20.1) are made of clear or tooth-coloured material. Although not invisible, they can significantly reduce the appearance of fixed appliances. They can either be made of ceramic materials or polycarbonate (plastic) brackets. Original plastic brackets showed problems with staining and a lack of stiffness, which led to deformation of the bracket when trying to apply torque. Although improvements to plastic brackets have been made, by the addition of metal slots or the addition of ceramic particles, they still have a problem with loss of torque and this lack of control means that at the present time ceramic brackets are preferred.

All ceramic brackets are composed of aluminium oxide in either a polycrystalline or monocrystalline form, depending on their method of fabrication. Despite their undoubted aesthetic advantages, ceramic brackets do have some potential disadvantages:

> ### Box 20.1 Different approaches to reduce the negative aesthetic impact of orthodontic treatment
>
> - Aesthetic orthodontic brackets and wires
> - Clear orthodontic aligners
> - Lingual orthodontics

- *Bonding and bond strength.* Ceramic brackets cannot bond chemically with composite resin, because the aluminium oxide is inert. In an attempt to address this, early ceramic brackets were coated with a silane-bonding agent, but this produced bonds that were too strong, resulting in enamel fractures at debond. Most current ceramic brackets therefore bond by mechanical retention using a variety of ingenious designs.

- *Frictional resistance.* Ceramic brackets offer more friction to sliding of the archwire, than standard metal brackets, which may increase the treatment time.

- *Bracket breakage.* Bracket breakage, particularly of the tie-wings, is more common with ceramic brackets, but improvements in the bracket morphology as well as refining of the manufacturing process have helped to reduce the number of breakages.

- *Iatrogenic enamel damage.* Ceramic brackets are harder than enamel, so if these brackets are in occlusal contact with the opposing teeth there is a significant risk of enamel wear. Consequently these brackets should be avoided in the lower arch if there is a possibility of occlusal contact. Most patients will accept metal brackets on the lower arch, as they will be barely visible in many patients (Fig. 20.6).

- *Debonding.* Removing metal brackets at the end of treatment is not usually a problem, as they are relatively pliable and the base can be easily distorted. Ceramic brackets are more rigid and the sudden force used to debond brackets can shatter the bracket, or on occasion, may cause enamel fractures. It is recommended that excess adhesive flash is removed from around the bracket before debonding. It is also vital to follow the bracket manufacturer's instructions, as different brands of brackets are designed to be removed in different ways.

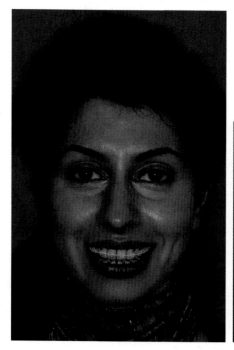
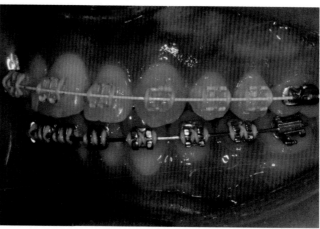

Fig. 20.6 Patient wearing upper ceramic brackets and lower metal brackets. Note the aesthetic wire in the upper arch.

Attempts to make orthodontic wires more aesthetic have proved more challenging. Two broad approaches have been attempted to produce aesthetic orthodontic wires:

- Coated metallic wires (Fig. 20.7)
- Non-metallic aesthetic wires

Both stainless steel and nickel titanium wires are available coated with white epoxy or Teflon. Unfortunately in both cases the coating can become discoloured and wear off during clinical use. An alternative that has been tried is rhodium coating, which reduces the reflectivity of the wire, giving it a matt white or frosted appearance, which although not tooth coloured is more aesthetic than the normal metallic wire appearance.

Attempts to make non-metallic aesthetic wires have so far been unsuccessful, as the wires have proved to be unreliable, with their mechanical properties failing to match their improved aesthetic appearance.

One of the commonest complaints from patients wearing aesthetic brackets with conventional ligation is that the elastomeric modules or 'o' ring that holds the wire in the place have a good appearance initially (Fig 20.8), but discolour with time, usually due to food colouring in the diet. Self-ligating aesthetic brackets have recently been developed to overcome this problem, as they require no elastomeric modules (see Fig 20.9).

20.5.2 Clear orthodontic aligners: the Invisalign® concept

The use of clear plastic appliances was first described using plastic retainer materials. Mildly irregular cases were treated by producing a series of patient casts with the teeth cut off and progressively repositioned until the teeth were in the correct position. A series of clear plastic tooth positioners, or aligners, were fabricated over these casts. The patient would then wear this series of clear plastic appliances to move the teeth. This technique was demanding and labour intensive, until the process was computerized by Align Technology in the late 1990s and the Invisalign® concept was created (Fig. 20.10). There are now several companies offering variations of this clear aligner treatment.

Accurate impressions (usually using poly-vinyl siloxane) are taken to allow the construction of precision casts which can be scanned to produce a virtual 3-D model. This 3-D model can then be manipulated by the orthodontist and the malocclusion 'virtually' corrected using proprietary software. It is important that the clinician has a good understanding of orthodontic principles before undertaking this type of treatment, recognizing the limitations of the technique and communicating this clearly to the patient as part of the consent process.

A series of clear plastic aligners are produced that gradually correct the malocclusion towards the clinician's goals. Each aligner is worn for 2 weeks, and is only removed for eating, drinking, brushing and flossing. Each aligner will move the teeth approximately 0.25 mm.

The potential advantages of Invisalign® are:

- Excellent aesthetics
- Ease of use and comfort for patient
- Ease of care and oral hygiene

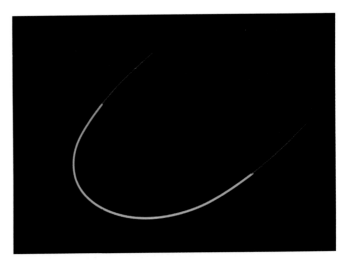

Fig. 20.7 Coated metallic aesthetic archwire.

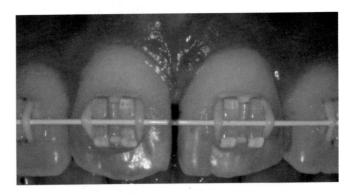

Fig. 20.8 Tooth-coloured modules on brackets using conventional ligation. The photograph shows the appearance when they are first placed. However, with time the elastomeric modules often discolour, compromising the aesthetic appearance of the appliance.

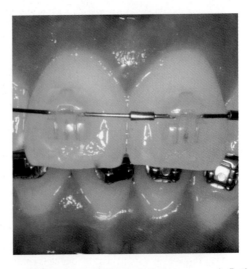

Fig. 20.9 Self-ligating aesthetic brackets in the upper arch. Both the bracket and the sliding clip mechanism are made from polycrystalline ceramic material. This removes the need for the wire to be held in place by elastomeric modules, which can discolour.

Potential disadvantages are:

- Limited control over root movement
- Limited intermaxillary correction (limited anteroposterior changes) without the use of elastics between the aligners
- Cost

The limited control over root position means that movements such as root paralleling, correction of severe rotations, tooth uprighting and tooth extrusion, are more difficult. This makes space closure more challenging, so in general Invisalign® is better at treating simple to moderate non-extraction alignments, rather than corrections requiring extractions.

The technology is constantly developing to try and improve the control over tooth movements. This includes the addition of customized composite attachments to the teeth, designed to offer more control over tooth movements, power ridges built into the plastic anteriorly to improve torque control, and customized attachments for intermaxillary elastics.

At the present time, Invisalign® is most effective at treating milder malocclusions presenting with malalignment, but it may be used successfully in combination with other techniques to treat more complex cases. The other treatment techniques may include restorative work, such as veneers, and even a short phase of fixed appliances. In more complex cases clear aligner treatment may not replace the use of fixed appliances, but it may reduce the amount of time the patient needs to wear less aesthetic labial fixed appliances.

20.5.3 Lingual orthodontics

Lingual appliances (Fig. 20.11) in many ways offer the ultimate in aesthetic appliances, as the whole system is bonded to the lingual aspect of the teeth. After much attention in the early 1980s their popularity

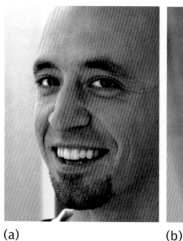
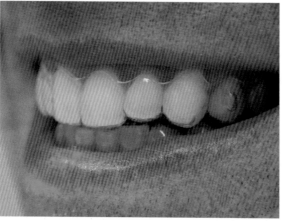

(a)　　　　　　　　　　(b)

Fig. 20.10 Invisalign® (courtesy of Align Technology, Inc.). (a) Facial view of a patient wearing an aligner. (b) Close-up of aligner in place.

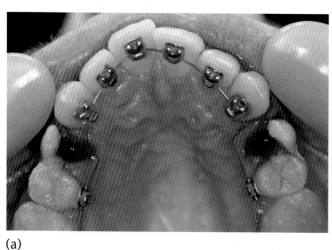
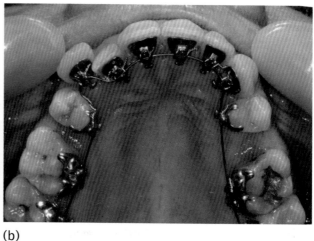

(a)　　　　　　　　　　(b)

Fig. 20.11 Lingual orthodontics (photographs courtesy of Dr Rob Slater). (a) Ormco STb lingual brackets. This patient has a non-customized lingual appliance in place. Note the temporary pontics that have been placed in the first premolar areas immediately following extractions. This is because not only does the patient want to hide the orthodontic appliance, but also the extraction spaces. These pontics will be gradually trimmed as the spaces are closed. Note the mushroom-shaped archwire. This is because the canine and first premolars have markedly different buccal–palatal widths. In order for the labial surfaces to be properly aligned, the archwire has to be offset between the canine and the first premolar. (b) Customized Incognito® lingual appliance. This patient has a lingual appliance with customized brackets and wires.

fell, partly due to the introduction of ceramic brackets, but also due to a number of problems with the appliance. Recent technological improvements and an increased demand for 'invisible' appliances have led to a recent increase in interest in lingual orthodontics.

Lingual orthodontics offers a number of advantages:

- Aesthetics
- No risk to the labial enamel through decalcification
- Position of the teeth can be seen more accurately as it is not obscured by the appliance
- Some lingual brackets create a bite-plane effect on the upper incisors and canines, making these types of brackets useful for treating deep overbites

Lingual orthodontics also has some potential disadvantages:

- Speech alteration
- Discomfort to the patient's tongue
- Masticatory difficulties
- More technically demanding for the operator, which increases the chair-time and therefore the cost of this approach
- Operator proficiency in indirect bonding is required and rebonding failed brackets can be difficult

- More difficult to clean
- Initial alignment can be more challenging in more crowded cases due to reduced interbracket span
- Increased bracket loss

The majority of tongue discomfort is related to the mandibular arch, so patients may choose to have a lingual appliance in the upper arch, where aesthetics is more crucial and a labial appliance in the lower.

Lingual orthodontics can range from simple alignment of the upper labial segment (the so-called 'social six') using round wires, to comprehensive treatment using appliances made using state-of-the-art computer-assisted design/manufacture (CAD/CAM) technology (Fig. 20.11b). CAD/CAM has allowed the production of fully customized appliances, with individualized production of brackets and wires. One of the challenges of aligning teeth from the lingual aspect is the unique morphology of the lingual aspect of teeth, and the range of bucco-lingual thickness of teeth. Customization of appliances overcomes these problems, improving the fit of the appliances, increasing the finishing control, as well as reducing speech problems and tongue irritation. Also if the customized brackets debond during treatment they can be rebonded directly, as the bracket base-to-tooth fit is so good that incorrect positioning is unlikely.

It remains to be seen if these new developments will continue to lead to more widespread use of lingual orthodontics.

20.6 Obstructive sleep apnoea and mandibular advancement splints

20.6.1 Introduction to Obstructive Sleep Apnoea (OSA)

Removable mandibular advancement splints can be successfully used in the treatment of adults suffering from obstructive sleep apnoea (OSA), a sleep-related breathing disorder. These splints are similar to orthodontic functional appliances that are used for the treatment of Class II problems in children, because they posture the mandible forwards. As a result, orthodontists have undertaken a lot of the research in this area.

OSA is characterized by repeated collapse of the upper airway during sleep, with cessation of breathing. The aetiology is complex, but involves anatomical and pathophysiological factors that produce obstruction of the airflow in the upper airway, often in the pharyngeal region. The compromised airflow often leads to snoring noise, or in more severe cases occlusion of the airway. The collapse of the upper airway can lead to periodic cessation of breathing (apnoea) or reduced airflow (hypopneoa). This can lead to cardiovascular and respiratory complications, as well as affecting the quality of life of both the patient and their families. The symptoms of OSA are summarized in Box 20.2 below. These symptoms can be worsened by certain aggravating factors:

- Alcohol consumption before bedtime
- Obesity
- Supine sleeping position

- Co-existing respiratory disease
- Medication that suppresses the central nervous system, which may lead to further relaxation of the pharyngeal musculature

20.6.2 Diagnosis of OSA

Accurate diagnosis of OSA requires a comprehensive history, examination, use of screening questionnaires and specialist sleep tests.

Box 20.2 Symptoms of OSA

Nocturnal symptoms

- Anti-social snoring
- Choking/gasping and witnessed apnoeas
- Restlessness
- Nocturia

Daytime symptoms

- Excessive daytime sleepiness
- Depression
- Headaches

The history must include a dental, medical and sleep history, and if appropriate a history from the partner can be useful to describe the sleep disturbances. Screening questionnaires, such as the validated Epworth Sleepiness Scale which provides a subjective measurement of the degree of daytime sleepiness, may be used to determine whether formal sleep tests are indicated.

In addition to a normal extra-oral and intra-oral examination, a specialist ear, nose and throat examination may be indicated to identify any clear physical obstructions that may be compromising the airway. The patient's body mass index (providing a measurement of possible obesity) and the neck circumference are both measured, as both are known to affect the patency of the upper airway.

If the history, examination and screening questionnaires are suggestive of OSA, then the diagnosis can be confirmed using sleep tests. This can be done with an overnight sleep study, known as polysomnography, but more recently multi-channel monitoring systems have been used for the patient to wear at home while they are asleep, and the data from these can help confirm the diagnosis of OSA.

20.6.3 Treatment of OSA including the use of mandibular advancement splints

Treatment of obstructive sleep apnoea may be surgical or non-surgical. Unless a clear anatomical problem can be identified the surgical approaches often only provide a temporary improvement, and the side-effects of the surgery are potentially severe.

Non-surgical approaches include the following:

(1) Removal of aggravating factors

(2) Continuous positive airway pressure (CPAP)

(3) Mandibular advancement splints

The first stage of treatment for all patients suffering from OSA is to identify and if possible remove the aggravating factors discussed earlier. This can often reduce the severity of OSA.

CPAP is a continuous stream of filtered air delivered via a nasal mask and is considered the gold standard for the treatment of obstructive sleep apnoea. To be effective the CPAP needs to be worn at least 4-6 hours per night, seven days a week. However, some patients find it difficult to wear the mask and long-term compliance can be a problem.

Mandibular advancement splints are used for the treatment of simple snoring, mild to moderate obstructive sleep apnoea, and for patients with severe OSA who cannot tolerate CPAP. By advancing the mandible they increase the pharyngeal airway, pulling the tongue anteriorly and increasing the muscle tone of the palatal muscles and reducing airway collapsibility.

There are various designs of mandibular advancement appliances, but customized appliances constructed from accurate impressions have been shown to be more successful than semi-customized versions that the patient adapts to their dentition. The appliances can be one-piece, or two-piece with interconnection of the maxillary and mandibular portions. Both types of appliances protrude the mandible. Figure 20.12 shows a one-piece example. The key to success is a comfortable, retentive appliance, which protrudes the mandible, with minimal vertical opening. Excessive vertical opening tends to rotate the mandible backwards and downwards, which may compromise the airway.

Patients need to be made aware that the splints can reduce the symptoms of OSA, but they are not a cure, so long-term wear is usually required. They also need to be aware of the possible side-effects (see Box 20.3). The sleep physician may suggest a repeat sleep test with the splint in place to ensure that it has addressed the OSA, particularly in more severe cases.

20.6.4 Conclusion about removable appliances and OSA

Mandibular advancement splints can play a vital role in the treatment of OSA. Due to the multi-factorial nature of OSA, these patients must be treated as part of a team, involving not only the dentist, but also sleep physicians and ENT surgeons. With a careful diagnosis and liaison with the other team members, mandibular advancement splints clearly have an important role in the treatment of some patients with OSA.

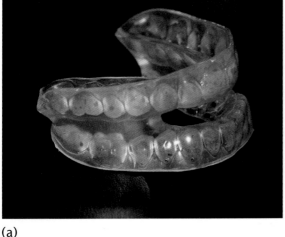 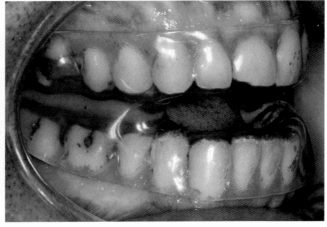

(a) (b)

Fig. 20.12 (a, b). A one-piece mandibular advancement splint, protruding the mandible forwards, with limited vertical opening.

Box 20.3 Possible side effects of mandibular advancement splints

Short term

- Discomfort of teeth, muscles of mastication, temporomandibular joints
- Excess salivation
- Dry mouth

- Occlusion is incorrect on wakening, before gradually returning to normal

Long-term

- Possible minor dento-alveolar changes, with long-term changes in the occlusion

---

Key points about adult orthodontics

- The demand for adult orthodontics is increasing.
- Certain problems are particularly relevant in adult orthodontics: lack of growth, periodontal disease, missing or heavily restored teeth, different physiological response in tooth movement, different attitudes to treatment.
- Adult patients are more likely to present with periodontal disease. Orthodontic treatment is possible in patients with periodontal disease, provided this is treated, stabilized and maintained throughout treatment. Treatment mechanics and retention must be adapted to allow for the reduced periodontal support.
- Adjunctive orthodontic treatment is tooth movement to facilitate other dental procedures and is more common in adults.
- There is an increased demand for aesthetic orthodontic appliances in adults. This can include aesthetic labial fixed appliances, clear aligners and lingual appliances.

Principal sources and further reading

Boyd, R. L., Leggot, P. J., Quinn, R. S., Eakle, W. S., and Chambers, D. (1989). Periodontal implications of orthodontic treatment in adults with reduced or normal periodontal tissues versus those of adolescents. *American Journal of Orthodontics and Dentofacial Orthopedics*, **96**, 191–9.

The periodontal implications of orthodontic treatments in adults are discussed.

Bressler, J. M., Hamamoto, S., King, G. J., and Bollen, A. (2011) Invisalign Therapy – a systematic review of lower quality evidence, Chapter 11 in *Evidence-based Orthodontics*, Wiley-Blackwell.

This chapter provides an overview of the current evidence available for the use of clear aligner treatment.

Cousley, R. R. J. (2011). Orthodontic bone anchorage, Chapter 30 in *Orthodontics: Principles and Practice*, Wiley-Blackwell.

This provides a clear overview on the topic of bone anchorage devices.

Creekmore, T. (1989). Lingual orthodontics – its renaissance. *American Journal of Orthodontics and Dentofacial Orthopedics*, **96**, 120–37.

This article highlights some of the initial problems with lingual appliances and how they were overcome.

Joffe, L. (2003). Invisalign®: early experiences. *Journal of Orthodontics*, **30**, 348–52.

An easy-to-read overview of the Invisalign® concept.

Johal, A. and Battagel, J. M. (2001). Current principles in the management of obstructive sleep apnoea with mandibular advancement appliances. *British Dental Journal*, **190**, 532–6.

This paper provides a good overview of the use of mandibular advancement splints in the treatment of OSA, emphasizing a multi-disciplinary approach to treatment.

Nattrass, C. and Sandy, J. R. (1995). Adult orthodontics – a review. *British Journal of Orthodontics*, **22**, 331–7.

This review covers a range of issues involved in adult orthodontics.

Ong, M. A., Wang, H-L., and Smith, F. N. (1998). Interrelationship between periodontics and adult orthodontics. *Journal of Clinical Periodontology*, **25**, 271–7.

As the title suggests, this review describes the interface between periodontal and orthodontic treatment.

Russell, J. R. (2005). Aesthetic orthodontic brackets. *Journal of Orthodontics*, **32**, 146–63.

A summary of the advantages and disadvantages of contemporary aesthetic brackets.

Shah, H. V., Boyd, S. A., Sandy, J. R., and Ireland, A. J. (2011). Aesthetic labial appliances – an update. *Orthodontic Update*, **4**, 70–7

Singh, P. and Cox, S. (2011) Lingual orthodontics: an overview. *Dental Update*, **38**, 390–5.

Wiechmann, D., Rummel, V., Thalheim, A., Simon, J-S., and Wiechmann, L. (2003). Customized brackets and archwires for lingual orthodontic treatment. *American Journal of Orthodontics and Dentofacial Orthopedics*, **124**, 593–9.

This paper describes how computer-aided design and manufacturing technology is used to produce custom-made brackets to overcome some of the problems of lingual orthodontics.

 References for this chapter can also be found at www.oxfordtextbooks.co.uk/orc/mitchell4e/. Where possible, these are presented as active links which direct you to the electronic version of the work, to help facilitate onward study. If you are a subscriber to that work (either individually or through an institution), and depending on your level of access, you may be able to peruse an abstract or the full article if available.

21

Orthodontics and orthognathic surgery

S. J. Littlewood

Chapter contents

Learning objectives for this chapter

- Understand the indications for combined treatment using orthodontics and orthognathic surgery
- Understand the process of diagnosis and treatment planning for patients with dentofacial deformity and the importance of the patient's soft tissues in this process
- Be familiar with the sequence of treatment of extractions, pre-surgical treatment, surgery and post-surgical orthodontics
- Be familiar with the common surgical approaches used to correct dentofacial deformity, and the risks involved in surgery
- Recognize that the development of new 3-D technology will change combined orthodontic and orthognathic surgery in the future

21.1 Introduction

Orthognathic surgery is surgery aimed at correcting dentofacial deformity. A dentofacial deformity is a deviation from normal facial proportions and dental relationships that is severe enough to be handicapping to a patient. The patient can be handicapped in two possible ways: jaw function, or aesthetics. It is estimated that 2–3 per cent of the population has a dentofacial deformity.

Jaw function problems may include eating difficulties or speech problems. The malocclusion is rarely so extreme that eating is not possible at all, but it may be difficult and embarrassing for the patient to try and eat certain types of food, particularly in public (Fig. 21.1). Speech difficulties may also be related to an underlying dentofacial deformity. However, the most common reason for patients seeking combined orthodontic and surgical treatment is dental and/or facial aesthetic problems, which can lead to psychological and social problems.

For correction of a dentofacial deformity, a combined orthodontic and surgical approach is required. Successful treatment requires close interdisciplinary work involving a number of specialists. Joint planning sessions and combined clinics are helpful to ensure that the whole team provides a co-ordinated approach to treatment. The patient should also be provided with appropriate information leaflets and DVDs to help them fully understand the implications of treatment as part of the overall consent process (Fig. 21.2).

21.2 Indications for treatment

Combined orthodontics and orthognathic surgery is indicated for patients who have a severe skeletal or very severe dento-alveolar problem that is too extreme to correct with orthodontics alone. The presence of a skeletal discrepancy does not automatically mean that a patient requires surgical intervention. When faced with a skeletal discrepancy the clinician has three choices:

- Growth modification
- Orthodontic camouflage
- Combined orthodontics and orthognathic surgery

Growth modification is only possible in growing patients and usually means treatment with headgear or functional appliances (see Chapter 19). On average, growth modification can only alter skeletal relationships by a limited amount and is often unpredictable. There is inevitably some correction by displacement of the teeth, so when using growth modification at least part of the correction is due to dental compensation for the skeletal discrepancy.

Once growth is complete, the only non-surgical option is orthodontic camouflage. This means moving the teeth into the correct dental relationships, but accepting the skeletal discrepancy. Major tooth movements may help to produce a good dental occlusion, but there is a danger of compromising facial aesthetics (Fig. 21.3). In these cases, a combined surgical approach may be required.

Clinical examples of cases when orthognathic surgery is commonly used include:

- Severe Class II skeletal malocclusions
- Severe Class III skeletal malocclusions
- Severe vertical disproportions leading to anterior open bite or a severely increased overbite
- Skeletal asymmetries

Combined orthodontic and surgical treatment is only started once growth has slowed to adult levels. This is important, because if the patient experiences significant facial growth after treatment has finished, this could compromise the result.

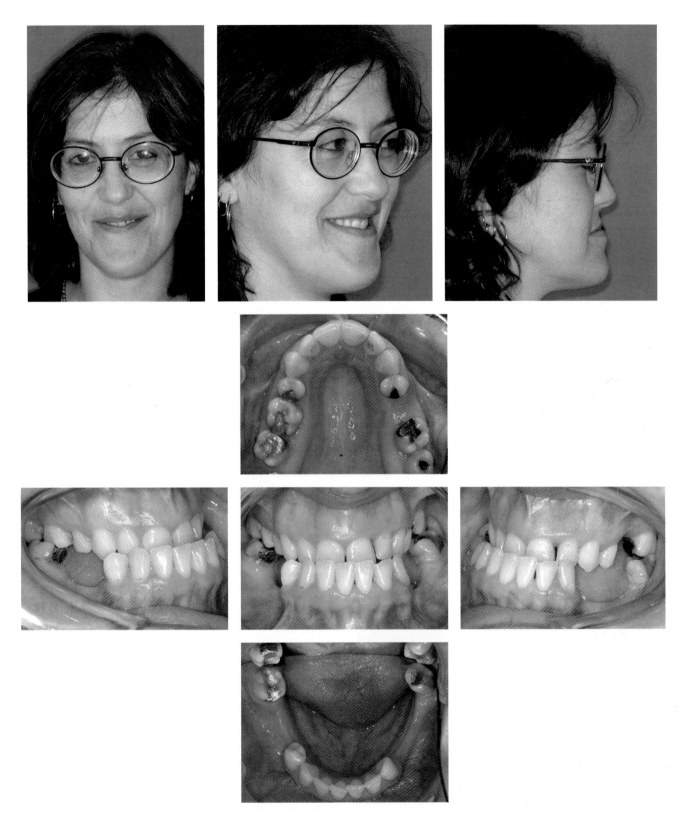

Fig. 21.1 Initial presentation of patient with severe Class III skeletal pattern. Patient I.E is 35 years old and presented complaining of the poor appearance of her bite, her prominent chin and difficulty eating in public. She had a marked Class III skeletal relationship with a reverse overjet. This patient's computer planning is shown in Fig. 21.8, her pre-surgical photographs in Fig. 21.12, and her end of treatment photographs in Fig. 21.16.

21.3 Objectives of combined orthodontics and orthognathic surgery

The objectives of treatment are the same as for orthodontic treatment:

- Acceptable dental and facial aesthetics
- Good function
- Optimal oral health
- Stability

21.4 The importance of the soft tissues

The appearance of the face is affected by the underlying facial skeleton, so any skeletal disproportions will affect the facial soft tissues. As a result, for many years diagnosis and treatment planning was focused on the hard tissues of the face (the dentition and the bony skeleton), with treatment aiming to achieve a perfect occlusion and ideal skeletal proportions. However, we are now aware that the soft tissue is the key area to focus on for two reasons:

- It is the soft tissues we see, so it is the soft tissue proportions that determine the aesthetic result. The soft tissue proportions are related to, but not necessarily identical, to the underlying skeletal pattern
- The soft tissues determine the limit of orthodontic and orthognathic treatment. It is not possible to create the same ideal dental and

skeletal result in every case, as the outcome is strongly influenced by the surrounding soft tissues. It is the soft tissues that determine the limit of treatment and how well a patient can adapt to the new position of the teeth and jaws. This includes the pressures exerted by the lips, cheeks, tongue and facial musculature, as well as soft tissues around the teeth – the periodontal ligament.

As a result the diagnosis should start with an analysis of the soft tissues, followed by analysis of the underlying bones and teeth. In terms of planning a process called 'reverse engineering' is used. This means the clinician decides what has to be done to the hard tissues (dentition and facial skeleton) to achieve the appropriate soft tissue outcomes.

21.5 Diagnosis and treatment plan

Diagnosis and treatment planning for combined orthodontic and orthognathic surgical patients should follow the same logical sequence used for routine orthodontic treatment planning (see Chapter 7). By taking an appropriate history, clinical examination and collection of appropriate diagnostic records, the necessary database of information

can be collected. This database can then be used to make a problem list (see Chapter 7, Fig. 7.1). This chapter will focus on the areas of direct relevance to orthognathic surgical patients.

21.5.1 History

The purpose of the history is to determine the patient's concerns, motivation for treatment, expectations of treatment, psychological status and medical and dental history.

Patient's concerns

The patient should be allowed to describe whether their concerns are aesthetic, functional or both. Functional problems could be masticatory and/or speech problems. While masticatory problems can often be markedly improved, care should be taken when promising resolution of speech problems, which are often firmly established by adulthood. Full correction of the speech problems may not be possible with the orthodontics and orthognathic surgery, and it is wise to seek the expert advice of a speech therapist.

In addition to aesthetic and functional problems, the patient may present complaining of pain. This pain could be due to a traumatic overbite or temporomandibular joint dysfunction. Traumatic overbites can be successfully addressed during combined treatment, but there is no guarantee that surgery to correct a dentofacial deformity will correct temporomandibular joint dysfunction.

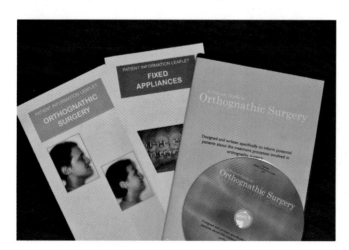

Fig. 21.2 Patient information leaflets and DVD. Information leaflets and DVDs about orthognathic surgery are often provided for patients considering this complex combined orthodontic and orthognathic surgery treatment. They play a key part in the informed consent process.

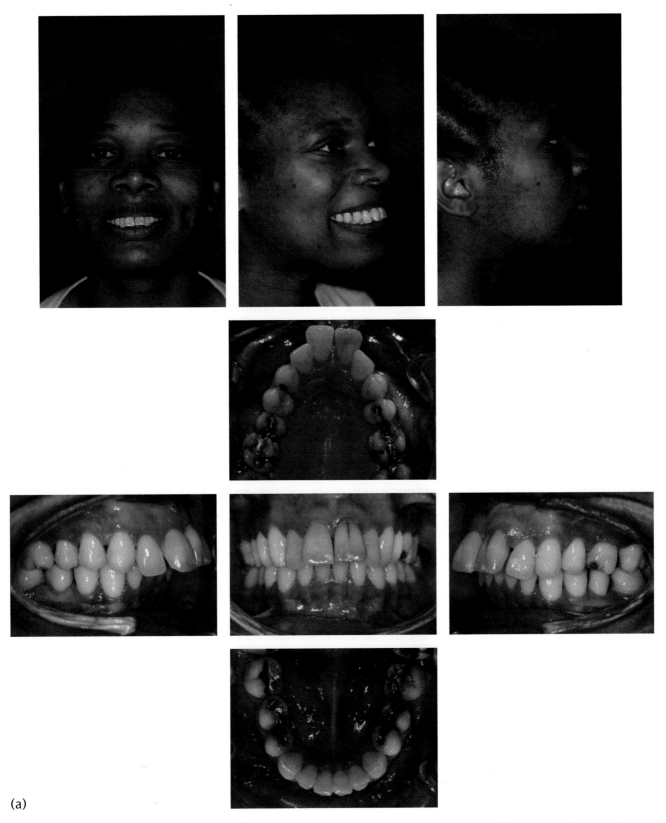

(a)

Fig. 21.3 Patient with Class II skeletal discrepancy. (a) Before treatment. This patient complained of her prominent upper teeth. She had a 14 mm overjet and a retrognathic mandible. It may have been possible to correct her dental malocclusion with orthodontics alone, but excessive retraction of the upper labial segment would have resulted in an unfavourable facial profile.

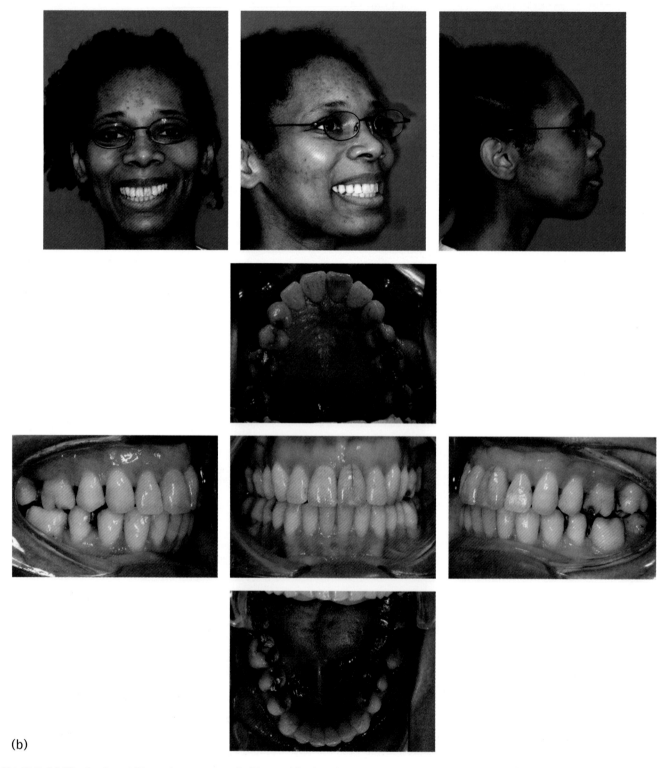

(b)

Fig. 21.3 (b) After treatment. The patient was treated with a combination of extractions, fixed appliances and mandibular advancement surgery.

Patient's motivation, expectations and psychological status

It is important to assess why the patient is seeking treatment at this time and what they expect the effect of the treatment will be. A small number of patients may have unrealistic expectations that combined treatment will not only improve their facial and dental appearance, but also have remarkable effects on their relationships and career prospects. The involvement of a clinical psychologist during the assessment and treatment planning of these cases is often helpful. A clinical psychologist should ideally be part of the interdisciplinary team.

The psychologist can help to assess a patient's expectations and determine their ability to cope with the treatment. They can also identify patients who may have underlying psychological or psychiatric problems that need to be addressed before beginning any treatment. There is one particular group of patients to be aware of who suffer from a condition known as body dysmorphic disorder. These patients present with a non-existent or very minor facial deformity and they have an obsession with this imagined or greatly exaggerated defect in their appearance. A close liaison with a clinical psychologist or psychiatrist is required in the management of this group of patients.

Patients with dentofacial deformities may present expressing concerns about their facial appearance, but some may have no concerns about their teeth. These patients may be surprised that prolonged fixed appliances are required as part of the treatment. In very rare circumstances it is possible to achieve a reasonable result with surgery alone. However, in most cases surgery without orthodontic involvement produces a compromised result. If the patient is not prepared to wear fixed appliances, then it is usually better not to proceed.

Medical and dental history

Patients who will be undergoing combined treatment must be fully dentally fit. They must also have a medical history that is compatible with a general anaesthetic. Conditions such as diabetes, hypothyroidism, adrenal insufficiency, bleeding disorders, cardiac and respiratory disorders and many other medical conditions, may complicate or prevent treatment. If there is any doubt about this, then an early consultation with an anaesthetist and their general medical practitioner is advised, before embarking on treatment.

21.5.2 Clinical examination

A systematic approach to the clinical examination will be required to assess the facial and dental aesthetics, the malocclusion and identify any pathology.

When assessing the facial appearance it is the proportions of the face that are important. The aim of combined orthodontic and orthognathic treatment is not necessarily to try and make the patient beautiful – it is about moving them towards more normal facial proportions (see section on further reading for more details on this). When assessing facial proportions it is important to take into account the patient's racial background, gender and age. This will help the clinician to decide whether the clinical features are within normal limits.

The extra-oral assessment is really a facial soft tissue assessment. The information from the extra-oral examination can then be combined with the information obtained from the radiographs. The radiographs will explain the hard tissue (dental and skeletal) contribution to the facial appearance.

Full face assessment

The symmetry and vertical proportions of the face are assessed from the frontal view. No face is completely symmetrical, but marked deviations should be noted (Fig. 21.4).

The 'ideal' face can be vertically divided by horizontal lines at the hairline, nasal base and the chin. The lower third can be further divided so that the meeting point of the lips is one-third of the way from the base of the nose to the chin (Fig. 21.5).

Profile assessment

For assessment of the patient's profile the patient should be assessed in the natural head position: the position the head is held when the patient is relaxed and looking into the distance. The middle and lower thirds are assessed in relation to the forehead area. In normal profile, the base of the nose lies approximately vertically below the most anterior portion of the forehead. The shape and size of the nose and paranasal areas should also be assessed. All things being equal the bigger the

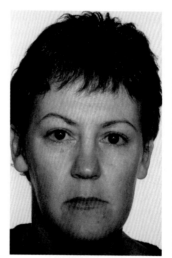
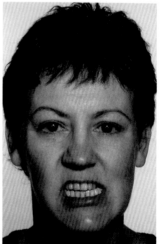
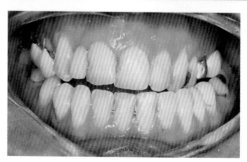

Fig. 21.4 Facial asymmetry. This patient shows a mandibular asymmetry to the left. Note the large centreline discrepancy between the arches. This is partly because the upper centreline is to the right by 2 mm (for dental reasons), but mostly because the lower centreline is to the left by 5 mm due to the underlying mandibular skeletal asymmetry.

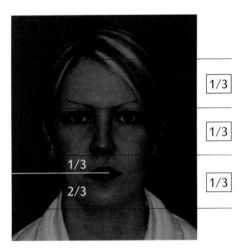

Fig. 21.5 Vertical proportions. In normal proportions the face can be divided into three equal thirds, with the lower third further divided so that the commisures of the lips are one-third of the way from the base of the nose to the chin.

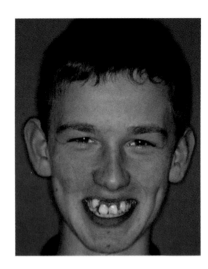

Fig. 21.6 'Gummy smile'. This 'gummy smile' is due to vertical maxillary excess.

nose, the more lip and chin prominence is needed to achieve facial balance. The nasolabial angle should also be noted, as it can be affected by excessive retraction or proclination of the upper incisors.

It is worth noting at this point that a full assessment of the patient's nose should form part of the assessment. It is possible the patient may benefit from a rhinoplasty as part of the overall treatment plan. It is also important to recognize that surgery to the maxilla may affect the shape of the nose, and this needs to be assessed and discussed with the patient as part of the consent process.

The chin projection is affected by the position of the mandible, the prominence of the bony chin point and the amount of soft tissue coverage. When a patient has a retrognathic mandible it is possible to get an idea of the effect of surgery by asking the patient to posture their mandible forwards the desired amount. The likely effects of other surgical movements are more difficult to assess clinically, and usually involve manipulation of the patient's photographic and radiographic records. Surgical planning and predictions are discussed in more detail in Section 21.6.

Smile aesthetics

One of the most important features to assess is the position of the dentition in relation to the lips and face, both transversely and vertically. Transversely, it is important to check whether the centrelines of the upper and lower dentitions are coincident with each other, and whether they are coincident with the centre of the face. It should be noted whether any centreline problem is of dental or skeletal origin.

Vertically the amount of upper incisor show should be assessed. At rest this should be 1 mm for males and 3 mm for females. On full smiling the full height of the upper incisors should be visible. Any occlusal cant of the dentition should also be noted.

If there is excess gingivae showing the patient may refer to this as a 'gummy smile'. When a 'gummy' smile is noted it is important that the aetiology is understood, as this will dictate the type of treatment required. 'Gummy' smiles do not always require surgical treatment.

Possible aetiological causes of a 'gummy' smile include true vertical maxillary excess (Fig. 21.6), a short upper lip, a localized dento-alveolar problem, short crowns (due to incisal wear), gingival overgrowth or hyperactive lip musculature.

Temporomandibular joints

The presence of any signs or symptoms of temporomandibular joint dysfunction should be noted. Ideally any symptoms should be treated conservatively prior to treatment. Often placing fixed appliances will at least temporarily relieve some of the symptoms. This may be due to the tenderness of the teeth reducing parafunctional habits such as clenching and grinding. However, it is unwise to promise any marked long-term improvement in the temporomandibular dysfunction, as a direct result of the combined orthodontics and orthognathic surgery (see also Section 1.7).

Intra-oral assessment

A full assessment of the dentition and occlusion needs to be undertaken. Any dental disease needs to be identified, treated and stabilized before combined orthodontics and orthognathic surgery can begin.

The relationship of one arch to the other is less important in orthognathic cases, as this part of the problem is often addressed by the surgery. However, each arch should be individually assessed for alignment and symmetry. The amount of crowding in each arch should be assessed, as well as the inclination of the teeth. The inclination of the incisors is important, because in most patients with a skeletal discrepancy the teeth have been tilted. This is due to the action of the lips and tongue attempting to achieve an anterior oral seal. This process is called 'dento-alveolar compensation' for the underlying skeletal pattern. In a Class II skeletal problem, the lower incisors are often proclined by the tongue. Conversely in a Class III skeletal pattern the lower incisors are often retroclined by the lower lip, with the upper incisors proclined by the tongue (Fig. 21.7). It is important to recognize any dento-alveolar compensation, as one of the aims of pre-surgical orthodontic treatment is to undo this compensation – a process known as 'decompensation'.

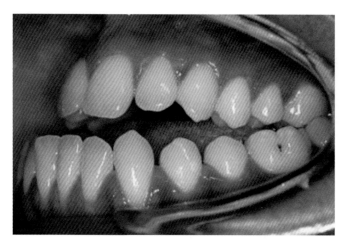

Fig. 21.7 Class III malocclusion showing dento-alveolar compensation. In this case the lower lip has retroclined the lower incisors and the upper incisors have been proclined by the tongue.

21.5.3 Radiographic examination

This usually includes those radiographs taken as part of the routine orthodontic assessment of a patient with a skeletal discrepancy: a panoramic dental view (DPT), a lateral cephalometric radiograph, and if indicated a view of the upper incisors. Additional views may be needed, depending on the case. For example, a posteroanterior skull radiograph may be taken to assess asymmetry.

21.5.4 Cephalometric assessment

In addition to a routine cephalometric analysis (Chapter 6), many surgeons and orthodontists will carry out more specialized analyses to determine the underlying aetiology of the particular problem. Many such analyses exist, and for further details the reader is referred to the section on further reading at the end of the chapter. The purpose of the analysis is to provide detailed information about the relationships between the different parts of the dentofacial complex:

- cranium and cranial base
- nasomaxillary complex
- mandible
- maxillary dentition
- mandibular dentition

The detection of any imbalances and disproportions in these dentofacial relationships is based on comparing the data for the individual with so-called normal data. As with the assessment of soft tissue proportions, the normal data for the hard tissues must be relevant to the patient being treated, in terms of age, gender and racial background.

21.6 Planning

Using the information gathered from the history, examination and diagnostic records, it should be possible to create a problem list, followed by the aims of treatment. This is discussed in greater detail in Chapter 7, Sections 7.3 and 7.4. Once the aims of the treatment are identified, the various specialists involved in the case should consider, as a team, the advantages and disadvantages of different approaches to treatment.

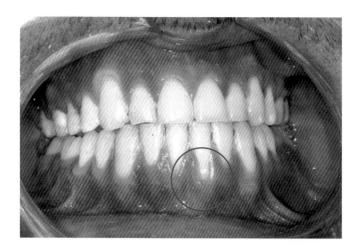

Fig. 21.8 Periodontal problems associated with proclination of the lower incisors during decompensation in a Class III skeletal case.

One of the orthodontist's responsibilities in the planning process is to consider reversing any dento-alveolar decompensation. It may not always be possible, or desirable, to fully decompensate incisors. For example, a narrow mandibular symphysis and/or thin labial periodontal tissues may make full decompensation impossible without compromising the periodontal support around the teeth. Figure 21.8 shows lower incisors that were decompensated to their ideal angulations, but this resulted in perforation of the labial plate, producing gingival recession. This is an example of a treatment aimed at producing an ideal occlusal result that has produced a compromised result, because it was beyond the limitations of the soft tissues (see Section 21.4).

One of the principle aims of combined orthodontics and orthognathic surgery is to obtain ideal facial aesthetics. This means appropriate soft tissue positioning in all three dimensions. The treatment actually moves the hard tissues: the orthodontist positions the teeth and the surgeon positions the facial skeleton. The challenge is to move the hard tissues to produce the best possible position of the soft tissues. Accurately predicting the soft tissue changes in response to hard tissue treatment changes is not an exact art, as the hard and soft tissues do not move in a 1:1 ratio.

Planning can be undertaken with a combination of cephalometric tracings, digital photographs and dental casts. Computer prediction software can predict the likely responses of the soft tissues, so when

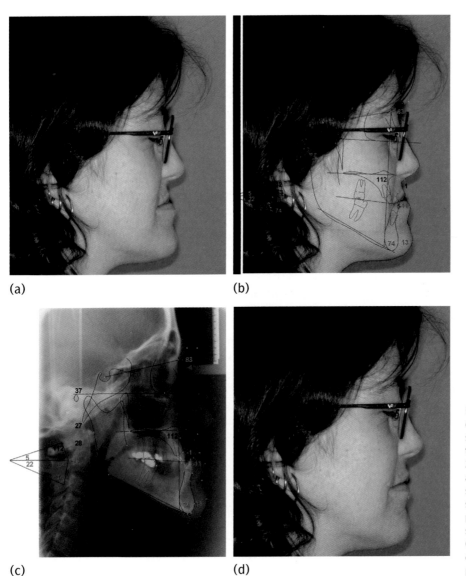

(a)

(b)

(c)

(d)

Fig. 21.9 Computer predictions. This figure demonstrates the use of Dolphin Imaging® software to predict the facial appearance of the proposed plan for the patient shown in Fig. 21.1. The proposed plan is a Le Fort I maxillary advancement of 5 mm and mandibular saggital split setback of 3 mm. The actual result of surgery is shown in Fig. 21.16. (a) Lateral facial photograph before treatment. (b) Analysis superimposed on lateral facial photograph. (c) Analysis superimposed on lateral cephalometric radiograph. (d) Computer prediction of proposed plan.

the proposed orthodontic and surgical movements are undertaken virtually on the computer, the likely soft tissue profile can be produced. Specialist planning software can be used to link the patient's digital photograph with their cephalometric tracing, so that the patient's image can be automatically 'morphed' in response to the planned surgical and orthodontic movements (Fig. 21.9). These predictions are only as good as the data that they are based on, but they give the clinicians an idea of the feasibility and likely success of different treatment plans. The computerized prediction can be shown to the patient to give them a better understanding of the likely possible outcome, but it must be made clear that this is simply a prediction and not a guarantee of the final outcome.

21.7 Common surgical procedures

Only a brief overview of some of the more popular surgical techniques is included here. Additional information is available in the literature cited in the section on further reading.

As aesthetics are of major importance, where possible an intra-oral approach should be used to avoid unsightly scars. Segmental procedures have an increased morbidity, as damage to the teeth or disruption of the blood supply to a segment is more likely.

21.7.1 Maxillary procedures

Le Fort I

This is the most widely used maxillary technique (Fig. 21.10). The standard approach is a horseshoe incision of the buccal mucosa and underlying bone, which results in the maxilla being pedicled on the palatal soft tissues and blood supply. The maxilla can then be moved upwards (after removal of the intervening bone), downwards (with interpositional bone graft), or forwards. Movement of the maxilla backwards is not feasible in practice.

Le Fort II

This is employed to achieve mid-face advancement. The surgery is more extensive than for a Le Fort I and therefore carries more risks.

Le Fort III

This usually necessitates the raising of a bicoronal flap for access and is commonly used in the management of craniofacial anomalies.

Surgical Assisted Rapid Palatal Expansion (SARPE)

Stable correction of the transverse dimension is notoriously difficult. SARPE is an attempt to address the transverse problem, without resorting to segmental surgery of the maxilla and its inherent risks. It involves the use of corticotomies, and the use of a rapid palatal expander that is used to rapidly widen the upper arch. The advantage of the technique is that it enlarges the maxilla transversely, expanding the upper arch considerably more than can be achieved with orthodontic appliances alone. The disadvantage is that an additional surgical intervention is required.

21.7.2 Mandibular procedures

Ramus procedures

The most commonly used ramus techniques are the following.

- Sagittal split osteotomy (Fig. 21.11). This procedure can be used to advance or push back the mandible or to correct mild asymmetry. The bony cut extends obliquely from above the lingula, across the retromolar region, and vertically down the buccal plate to the lower border. The main complication is damage to the inferior alveolar nerve.

- Vertical subsigmoid osteotomy. This is used for mandibular prognathism and involves a bone cut from the sigmoid notch to the lower border. This can be performed intra-orally using special instruments or extra-orally using standard instruments at the expense of a scar.

- Body osteotomy. This operation is useful if there is a natural gap in the lower arch anterior to the mental foramen in a patient with mandibular prognathism. It is rarely used.

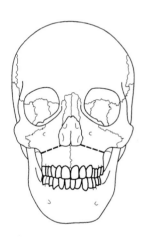
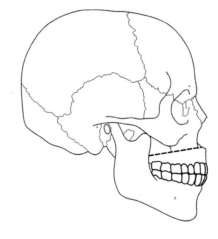

Fig. 21.10 Diagram showing the position of the surgical incisions (broken lines) for a Le Fort I procedure.

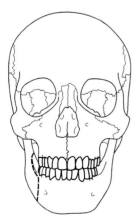
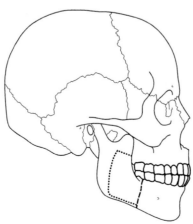

Fig. 21.11 Diagram to show the position of the surgical incisions (broken and dotted lines) for a sagittal split osteotomy.

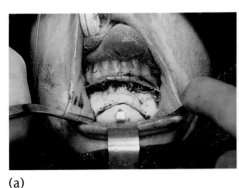

(a)

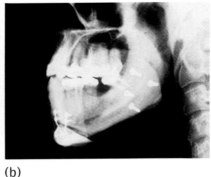

(b)

Fig. 21.12 (a) A genioplasty being carried out. (b) Lateral cephalometric radiograph of a patient who had a genioplasty carried out in addition to a sagittal split ramus procedure (note the plates securing the genioplasty).

Genioplasty

The tip of the chin can be moved in almost any direction, limited by sliding bony contact and the muscle pedicle (Fig. 21.12). This technique may be used to supplement mandibular ramus surgery where there is a localized abnormality of the chin area in addition to the general mandibular position. It can also be usefully employed as an isolated operation, where it is used as a masking procedure, thus avoiding more complex treatment (for example, mild mandibular asymmetry).

21.7.3 Bimaxillary surgery

Many patients require surgery to both jaws to correct the underlying skeletal discrepancy (see clinical case illustrated in Figs 21.1, 21.9, 21.13 and 21.16).

21.7.4 Distraction osteogenesis

This is a technique that involves osteomomy cuts followed by a slow mechanical separation of the bone fragments with an expandable device. It is a technique that was originally developed for lengthening limbs.

It offers exciting potential for larger movements than can be achieved with traditional orthognathic surgery, and has been found to be useful in the treatment of patients with severe jaw deficiencies, particularly those associated with craniofacial syndromes.

After the bone cuts, there is a latent period of 4–5 days before the bones are separated gradually by the mechanical device. The mechanical device is turned each day and the tension leads to the production of new bone, while allowing time for the soft tissues to adapt. The technique avoids the problems of harvesting and maintaining a viable bone graft and in addition the adaptation of the soft tissues allows movements to be larger than with traditional approaches.

Initially external fixators were used, but there are now an increasing number of intra-oral devices available, which reduce the risk of extra-oral scarring. The potential problems of the devices – discomfort, difficulty achieving the correct vector of force and the need for good patient compliance – have meant that this technique has not been seen as a replacement for conventional osteotomies in routine cases. However, cases that were previously thought to be beyond the scope of orthognathic treatment (principally due to soft tissue restrictions) can now be treated.

21.8 Sequence of treatment

21.8.1 Extractions

Extractions may be required to relieve crowding, level arches and allow correction of the inclination of the incisors (decompensation). In addition, the surgeon may wish to extract unerupted third molars before the start of treatment, in case they interfere with the future osteotomy site. This is particularly true for mandibular ramus surgery.

21.8.2 Pre-surgical orthodontics

There are four aims of pre-surgical orthodontics:

- Alignment and levelling
- Co-ordination (ensuring arches will be compatible with each other after surgery)
- Decompensation
- Creation of space for osteotomy cuts if segmental surgery is required

The pre-surgical orthodontics is undertaken with fixed appliances to allow the correct anterior–posterior and vertical positioning of the incisors. This allows the surgical movements to take place. The fixed appliances also act as a method of intra-operative intermaxillary fixation and a means of attaching the intermaxillary elastics used post-operatively.

Although levelling of the arches is typically undertaken before surgery, there are two exceptions to this:

- In cases of anterior open bite, attempts to level the arch before surgery will lead to extrusion of the upper incisors, which is unstable. In these cases the anterior and posterior segments are aligned in separate segments. Space is made between these segments and the arch is levelled by aligning the segments surgically.

- In Class II cases presenting with deep overbite and a reduced face height, the lower arch is not levelled before surgery. When the mandible is advanced the lower incisor position ensures the lower face height is increased. This approach is called a '3 point landing' because

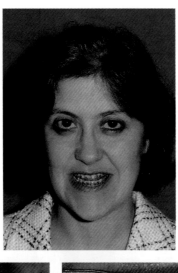
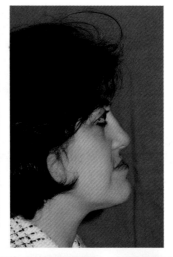

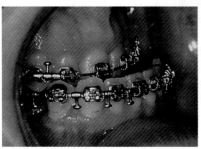
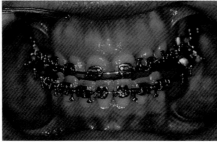
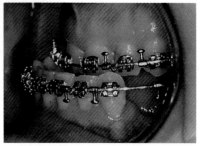

Fig. 21.13 End of pre-surgical orthodontics. Patient IE (from Fig. 21.1) has now been decompensated for surgery. Note the upright lower incisors and the associated worsening of the facial aesthetics due to the protruding lower lip. The patient was warned about this temporary worsening of the profile before surgery.

immediately post-surgery the only tooth contact is between the incisors and the posterior molars. The arch is levelled post-surgery by extruding the premolar teeth.

Decompensation is undertaken to correct the angulations of the incisors. There is a tendency for the decompensation during presurgical orthodontics to make the patient look worse, as the full extent of the skeletal discrepancy becomes clear (Fig. 21.13). The patient should be warned about this before treatment begins and reassured that this is just temporary until the surgery is completed.

Traditionally the majority of orthodontic treatment is undertaken before surgery, producing aligned, levelled, co-ordinated and decompensated arches. The advantage of this approach is that it offers a more predictable surgical phase and more accurate planning immediately pre-surgery. An alternative view is that minimal orthodontics should be undertaken before surgery, as the soft tissue environment may be more conducive to some orthodontic movements once the skeletal pattern is corrected.

21.8.3 Preparing for surgery

Pre-surgical orthodontics takes about 12–18 months, depending on the complexity of the case. At the end of this stage a new set of records are taken – impressions, photos, radiographs – to check the pre-surgical movements have been achieved and to modify or confirm the surgical

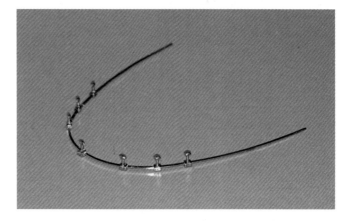

Fig. 21.14 Crimpable hooks added to the archwire. These can be used for intermaxillary fixation during surgery and for attachment of intermaxillary elastics post-operatively.

plan. Rigid stainless steel archwires are placed. Intermaxillary fixation is required during surgery, so hooks are usually added to the archwire (Fig. 21.14) or brackets. Alternatively the orthodontist can use brackets that incorporate a hook on every tooth from the start.

Study models are produced which can be used for model surgery to mimic the surgical plan. Model surgery is undertaken to verify that the planned surgical moves are appropriate, and to allow construction of intermaxillary wafers. These acrylic wafers are used during surgery to help the surgeon position the jaws correctly. A face-bow recording is required to mount the models on a semi-adjustable articulator, for single jaw maxillary procedures and bimaxillary procedures (Fig. 21.15). If the condyles are to be separated from the dentition by mandibular surgery alone, then the semi-adjustable articulator (and therefore face-bow recording) is not required.

21.8.4 Surgery

This is an in-patient procedure usually involving a stay of 1–3 days in hospital, depending on the complexity of the surgery. In the past, patients were placed in intermaxillary wires to fix the bony segments in place during healing. This meant the patient's upper and lower arches were tied together for 6 weeks. This is now rarely required due to the introduction of small bone plates that are used to fix the bony segments semi-rigidly in the maxilla and the use of plates and/or screws in the mandible. This has significantly reduced the morbidity post-operatively, with a reduced risk to the airway, early mobilization of the jaws, earlier return to a good palatable diet and easier oral hygiene. As a result the procedure is much better tolerated by patients and also has resulted in better final bone stability.

A brief description of the common surgical procedures has been given in Section 21.7. The surgery carries a number of risks, the exact nature of these risks depending on the procedure undertaken. These risks should be explained by the surgeon before any treatment is started as part of the informed consent process (see Box 21.1).

21.8.5 Post-surgical orthodontics

Immediately post-surgery the patient is usually wearing intermaxillary traction to guide the arches into the desired position. The aims of post-surgical orthodontics are:

- Complete any movements not undertaken pre-surgery (e.g. correction of posterior crossbite and levelling by extrusion of premolars)

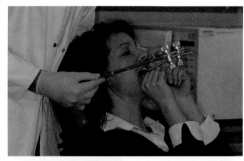

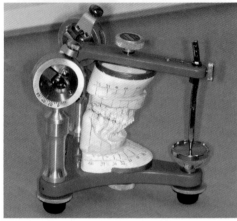

Fig. 21.15 Model surgery. A face-bow recording is taken and the models mounted on a semi-adjustable articulator.

- Root paralleling at any segmental osteotomy sites
- Detailing and settling

Within a few weeks, lighter round stainless steel wires are often used in conjunction with the intermaxillary elastics to aid settling. Final detailing can then be undertaken to produce a well-interdigitated occlusion (Fig. 21.16). Post-surgical orthodontics typically takes 3–9 months.

Box 21.1 Possible risks of orthognathic surgery

These depend on the type and extent of the surgery. The patient needs to be made aware of these surgical risks before treatment begins as part of the consent process. Based on the article by Ryan *et al.* (2011).

Expected surgical risk

- Swelling
- Bleeding
- Limited mouth opening
- Dietary changes and associated weight loss in the short term
- Time off work and recovery
- Changes in facial appearance
- Changes in nerve sensation

Possible surgical risks

- Permanent nerve damage to ID nerve
- Need for re-operation
- Infection
- Need to remove plates
- TMJ problems
- Relapse
- Problems swallowing
- Bleeding requiring further intervention
- Tooth avulsion or other damage to periodontal support
- Ophthalmic complications
- Reduction in auditory capacity

Risks of anaesthetic

- The risks associated with a general anaesthetic need to be discussed

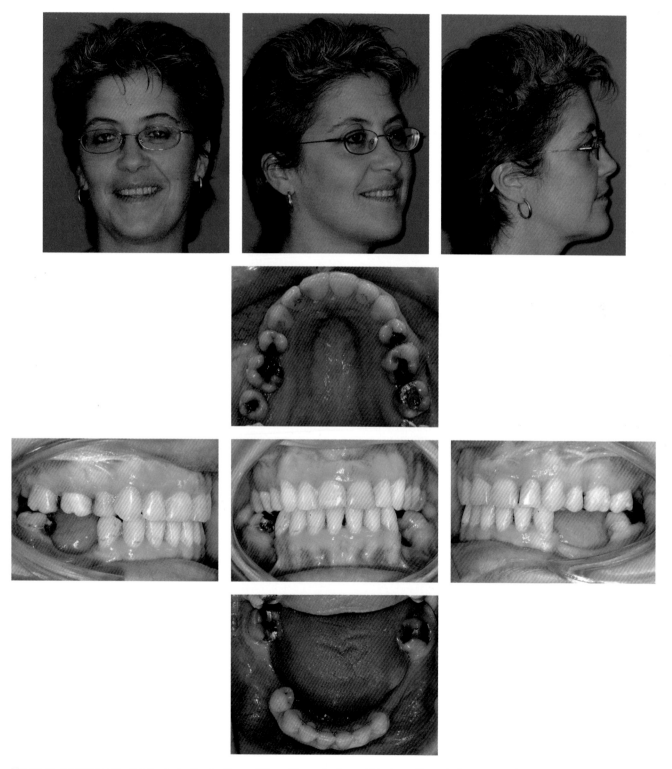

Fig. 21.16 End of treatment following orthodontics and bimaxillary osteotomy. This shows the end of treatment photographs for the patient shown in Figs 21.1, 21.9 and 21.13.

21.9 Retention and relapse

Orthodontic retainers are used to retain the teeth in the correct position at the end of treatment, along similar lines as for conventional fixed appliance therapy (see Chapter 16). However, in addition to the usual relapse factors, there are additional aetiological factors in combined orthodontic and orthognathic surgery.

21.9.1 Surgical factors

- Poor planning.
- The size of the movement required. Movement of the maxilla by more than 5–6 mm in any direction is more susceptible to relapse, as is movement of the mandible by more than 8 mm.
- Direction of movement required (see Box 21.2).
- Distraction of the condylar heads out of the glenoid fossa during surgery.
- Inadequate fixation.

21.9.2 Orthodontic factors

- Poor planning.
- Movement of the teeth into zones of soft tissue pressure will lead to relapse when appliances are removed. Therefore treatment should be planned to ensure that the teeth will be in a zone of soft tissue balance post-operatively and that the lips will be competent.
- Extrusion of the teeth during alignment tends to relapse post-treatment, particularly in cases of anterior open bite.

21.9.3 Patient factors

- The nature of the problem; for example, anterior open bites associated with abnormal soft tissue behaviour, are notoriously difficult to treat successfully, and have a marked potential to relapse. Patients should be warned of this prior to treatment.

> **Box 21.2 Stability of orthognathic surgery**
>
> Most stable at the top, gradually moving down to the least stable at the bottom of the list). Based on the article by Proffit *et al.* (2007).
>
> Very stable
> - Maxillary impaction
> - Mandibular advancement
> - Genioplasty (any direction)
>
> Stable
> - Maxillary advancement
> - Correction of maxillary asymmetry
>
> Stable (with rigid fixation)
> - Maxillary impaction with mandibular advancement
> - Maxillary advancement with mandibular setback
> - Correction of mandibular asymmetry
>
> Problems with stability
> - Mandibular setback
> - Movement of maxilla downwards
> - Surgical expansion of maxilla

- In patients with cleft lip and palate, advancement of the maxilla is difficult and prone to relapse because of the scar tissue of the primary repair.
- Failure to comply with treatment; for example, patient does not wear intermaxillary elastic traction as instructed.

21.10 Future developments in orthognathic surgery: 3D surgical simulation

The conventional methods used to plan orthognathic surgery described in this chapter rely on lateral radiographic images, and occasionally posterioranterior radiographs in cases of asymmetry. Both these radiographs only provide a two-dimensional (2D) presentation of the dentition and facial skeleton. Model surgery allows some appreciation of the dentition and occlusion in three dimensions (3D), but not the maxilla and mandible.

The traditional approach provides only a limited understanding of the complex 3D structures of the dentofacial skeleton. It is only at the time of surgery that the surgeon has a better understanding of the contours, thickness and quality of bone, and is able to gain a more detailed appreciation of the position of key anatomical structures, such as the inferior dental nerve. Osteotomy cuts, alignment of the segments and fixation are effectively undertaken in a freehand manner, and are reliant on the skill and experience of the surgeon. The anatomy of the region is complex and the surgeon is often working in a field with restricted visibility.

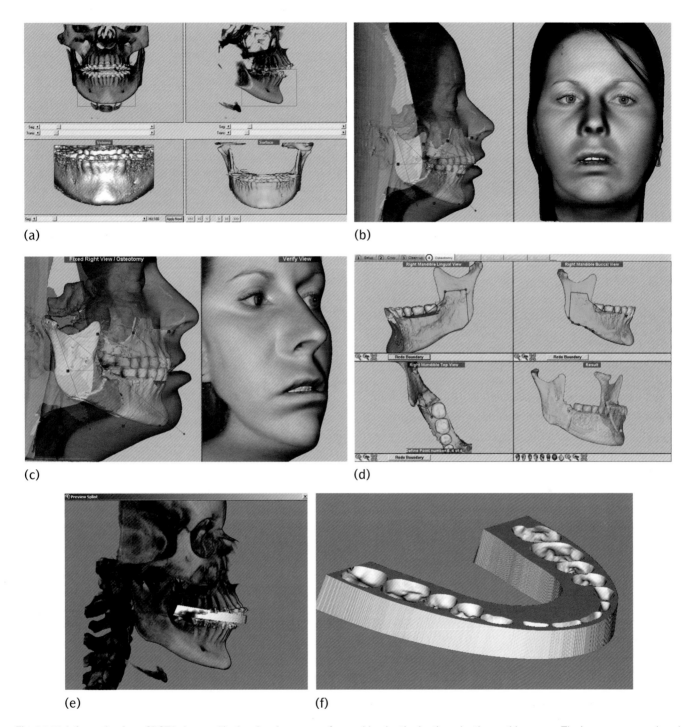

Fig. 21.17 Information from CBCT being used in the planning process for combined orthodontic and orthognathic surgery. The images were produced using Dolphin Imaging 3D software (kindly provided by Paul Thomas).

(a) Detailed 3D information of the anterior mandible captured from CBCT.
(b) Information from the CBCT has been combined with information from 3D facial camera system.
(c) 3D prediction of bimaxillary osteotomy.
(d) Virtual osteotomy cuts in the mandible. Note the inferior alveolar nerve clearly marked in green.
(e, f) Designing a surgical splint to be used during the operation.

21.10.1 Use of Cone Beam CT technology and implications for treatment in the future

Cone beam computed tomography (CBCT) now allows the acquisition of detailed 3D images of the face in high resolution. Using this 'virtual' 3D information, software is being developed that could revolutionize the way that orthognathic planning and surgery is undertaken. In dentistry we are familiar with the use of CAD/CAM (computer-aided design/computer-aided manufacture) for the manufacture of complex 3-dimensional restorations. Computer-aided surgery (CAS) is now being introduced that will allow surgical planning and simulation using the information captured from CBCT.

This technology offers a number of potential exciting possibilities:

- A more detailed appreciation of the anatomy of the patient in three dimensions (Fig. 21.17a).
- The data from CBCT can be combined with the data captured from 3D facial camera systems. This allows the clinicians to see the relationship of the soft tissues with the underlying hard tissues (Fig. 21.17b). Virtual surgery can then be undertaken on this 3D model and the effect on the overlying soft tissues assessed (Fig. 21.17c). The accuracy of these 3D predictions will improve as we gather more data on the 3D effects on soft tissues of combined orthodontics and orthognathic surgical treatment.
- Virtual surgery will allow the surgeon to calculate the most appropriate and safest osteotomy lines in advance of the operation (Fig. 21.17d).
- Once the team is happy with the final virtual surgery, this virtual set-up can be used to manufacture positioning splints (Fig. 21.17e) and construct customized fixation plates.
- The developments described so far have been based on the surgery being planned and executed virtually. However, the surgeon, not the computer, will perform the actual surgery, so the next challenge is to ensure the surgeon follows the virtual plan. Surgical navigation systems are being developed to help transfer the information from the virtual plan into the operating room. They will use tracking devices to follow surgical instruments and the patient's changing anatomy, and using a navigation screen will help to guide the surgeon in making the appropriate cuts and ensure correct positioning and fixation of the bone segments.

Future developments in 3D technology are likely to fundamentally change our approach to combined orthodontic and orthognathic treatment in the future, in terms of diagnosis, treatment planning and, eventually, in the execution of the surgery.

Key points about orthodontics and orthognathic surgery

- Orthognathic surgery is aimed at correcting dentofacial deformity
- It is indicated for patients that have a severe skeletal or very severe dento-alveolar problem that is beyond the scope of orthodontics alone
- Planning and treatment should be undertaken by an interdisciplinary team
- The typical sequence of treatment is extractions, a phase of pre-surgical orthodontics, the surgery and then a shorter phase of post-surgical orthodontics
- The aims of pre-surgical orthodontics are alignment and levelling, co-ordination of the arches, decompensation, and creation of space for osteotomy cuts if segmental surgery is used
- Fixed appliances are used to fulfil the pre-surgical aims, provide a method of intermaxillary fixation during surgery, and offer a means of attaching intermaxillary elastics post-operatively
- Post-surgical orthodontics aims to correct any movements not undertaken at surgery, root paralleling at any segmental osteotomy sites and detailing and settling
- Developments in 3D technology are likely to change the way combined orthodontic and orthognathic treatment is undertaken in the future

---

Principal sources and further reading

Cevidanes, L.H.C., Tucker, S., Styner, M., Kim, H., Chapuis, J., Reyes, M., Proffit, W., Turvey, T., and Jaskolkai, M. (2010). Three-dimensional surgical simulation. *American Journal Orthodontics and Dentofacial Orthopedics*, **138**, 361–71.
   This paper provides a detailed overview of contemporary 3D technology that is being developed for orthognathic surgery planning and simulation

Cunningham, S. J. and Feinmann, C. (1998). Psychological assessment of patients requiring orthognathic surgery and the relevance of body dysmorphic disorder. *British Journal of Orthodontics*, **25**, 293–8.
   An article alerting the clinician to the condition body dysmorphic disorder.

Edler, R.J. (2001). Background considerations to facial aesthetics. *Journal of Orthodontics*, **28**, 159–68.

This paper discusses how to improve facial aesthetics and the importance of moving towards average facial proportions

Hajeer, M. Y., Millett, D. T., Ayoub, A. F., and Siebert, J. P. (2004). Applications of 3D imaging in orthodontics: Part I. *Journal of Orthodontics*, **31**, 62–70.

An overview of the new 3D imaging systems is discussed.

Hunt, N. P. and Rudge, S. J. (1984). Facial profile and orthognathic surgery. *British Journal of Orthodontics*, **11**, 126–36.

A detailed account of assessment of a patient for orthognathic surgery.

Lee, R. T. (1994). The benefits of post-surgical orthodontic treatment. *British Journal of Orthodontics*, **21**, 265–74.

The potential advantages of undertaking minimal orthodontic treatment pre-surgically are discussed.

Proffit, W.R., Turvey, T.A., and Phillips, C. (2007). The hierarchy of stability and predictability in orthognathic surgery with rigid fixation: an update and extension. *Head & Face Medicine*, **3**, 21.

The stability of various types of orthognathic procedures is described.

Proffit, W. R., White, R. P., and Sarver, D. M. (2003). *Contemporary Treatment of Dentofacial Deformity*. Mosby, St Louis, MO.

This textbook is highly recommended for readers wanting more information on this subject. It is a comprehensive and well-written account of the treatment of dentofacial deformity.

Ryan, F., Shute, J., Cedro, M., Singh, J., Lee, E., Lee, S., Lloyd, T. W., Robinson, A., Gill, D., Hunt, N. P., and Cunningham, S. J. (2011). A new style of orthognathic clinic. *Journal of Orthodontics*, **38**, 124–33.

An innovative approach to the orthognathic clinic, aiming to provide key information to patients deciding on whether or not to proceed with treatment.

References for this chapter can also be found at www.oxfordtextbooks.co.uk/orc/mitchell4e/. Where possible, these are presented as active links which direct you to the electronic version of the work, to help facilitate onward study. If you are a subscriber to that work (either individually or through an institution), and depending on your level of access, you may be able to peruse an abstract or the full article if available.

22

Cleft lip and palate and other craniofacial anomalies

Chapter contents

Relevant sections in other chapters
4.2 Craniofacial embryology

Learning objectives for this chapter

- Gain an appreciation of the different presentations of cleft lip and/or palate and the problems they present for the patient and the clinician
- Gain an understanding of the basic principles of management of patients with a cleft

22.1 Prevalence

Cleft lip and palate is the most common craniofacial malformation, comprising 65 per cent of all anomalies affecting the head and neck. There are two distinct types of cleft anomaly; cleft lip with or without cleft palate, and isolated cleft palate, which result from failure of fusion at two different stages of dentofacial development (see Section 4.2).

22.1.1 Cleft lip and palate

The prevalence of cleft lip and palate varies geographically and between different racial groups. Amongst Caucasians, this anomaly occurs in approximately 1 in every 700 live births and the prevalence is increasing. A family history can be found in around 40 per cent of cases of cleft lip with or without cleft palate, and the risk of unaffected parents having another child with this anomaly is 1 in 20 (Box 22.1). Males are affected more frequently than females, and the left side is involved more commonly than the right. Interestingly, the severity of the cleft is usually more marked when it arises in the less common variant.

> **Box 22.1 Genetic risks of cleft lip and palate**
>
> - Parents with no cleft but with one affected child: risk for next child = 1 in 25 (4 per cent)
> - One parent with CLP: risk for first child = 1 in 50 (2 per cent)
> - One parent with CLP and first child with CLP: risk for next child = 1 in 10 (10 per cent)
> - Both parents affected: risk for first child = 3 in 5 (60 per cent)

22.1.2 Isolated cleft of the secondary palate

Isolated cleft occurs in around 1 in 2000 live births and affects females more often than males. Clefts of the secondary palate have a lesser genetic component, with a family history in around 20 per cent and a reduced risk of further affected offspring to normal parents (1 in 80).

Isolated cleft palate is also found as a feature in a number of syndromes including Down's, Treacher–Collins, Pierre–Robin, and Klippel–Fiel syndromes.

22.2 Aetiology

In normal development, fusion of the embryological processes that comprise the upper lip occurs around the sixth week of intra-uterine life. 'Flip-up' of the palatal shelves from a vertical to a horizontal position followed by fusion to form the secondary palate occurs around the eighth week. Before fusion can take place the embryological processes must grow until they come into contact. Then breakdown of the overlying epithelium is followed by invasion of mesenchyme. If this process is to take place successfully, a number of different factors need to interact at the right time. Evidence from population studies and experimental data suggests that both genetic and environmental factors play a part in the aetiology of clefts. Specific gene mutations have been shown to be linked to cleft lip and/or cleft palate. Environmental factors that have been implicated include anticonvulsant drugs, folic acid deficiency and maternal smoking.

It is postulated that isolated cleft palate is more common in females than males because transposition of the palatal shelves occurs later in the female foetus. Thus greater opportunity exists for an environmental insult to affect successful elevation, which is further hampered by widening of the face as a result of growth in the intervening period (see Chapter 4, Section 4.2.4).

22.3 Classification

A number of classifications exist but, given the wide variation in clinical presentation, in practice it is often preferable to describe the presenting deformity in words (Fig. 22.1).

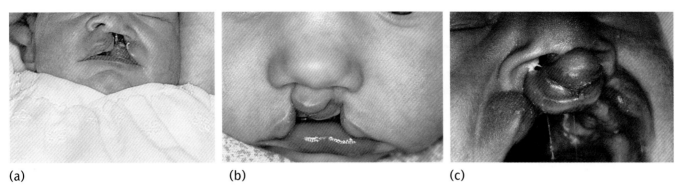

(a)   (b)   (c)

Fig. 22.1 (a) Baby with a complete unilateral cleft lip and palate on the left side; (b) baby with a bilateral incomplete cleft lip; (c) baby with a complete bilateral cleft lip and palate.

22.4 Problems in management

22.4.1 Congenital anomalies

The disturbances in dental and skeletal development caused by the clefting process itself depend upon the site and severity of the cleft.

Lip only

There is little effect in this type, although notching of the alveolus adjacent to the cleft lip may sometimes be seen.

Lip and alveolus

A unilateral cleft of the lip and alveolus is not usually associated with segmental displacement. However, in bilateral cases the premaxilla may be rotated forwards. The lateral incisor on the side of the cleft may exhibit some of the following dental anomalies:

- congenital absence
- an abnormality of tooth size and/or shape
- enamel defects
- or present as two conical teeth, one on each side of the cleft

Lip and palate

In unilateral clefts rotation and collapse of both segments inwards anteriorly is usually seen, although this is usually more marked on the side of the cleft (the lesser segment). In bilateral clefts both lateral segments are often collapsed behind a prominent premaxilla (Fig. 22.2).

Palate only

A widening of the arch posteriorly is usually seen.

It has been shown that individuals with a cleft have a more concave profile, and whilst a degree of this is due to a restriction of growth (see below), research indicates that cleft patients have a tendency towards a more retrognathic maxilla and mandible and also a reduced upper face height compared with the normal population.

22.4.2 Post-surgical distortions

Studies of individuals with unoperated clefts (usually in Third World countries) show that they do not experience a significant restriction of facial growth, although there is a lack of development in the region of the cleft itself, possibly because of tissue hypoplasia. In contrast, individuals who have undergone surgical repair of a cleft lip and palate exhibit marked restriction of mid-face growth anteroposteriorly and transversely (Fig. 22.3). This is attributed to the restraining effect of the scar tissue, which results from surgical intervention. It has been estimated that approximately 40 per cent of cleft patients exhibit marked maxillary retrusion. Limitation of vertical growth of the maxilla coupled with a tendency for an increased lower facial height results in an excessive freeway space, and frequently overclosure (Fig. 22.4).

22.4.3 Hearing and speech

Speech development is adversely affected by the presence of fistulae in the palate and by velopharyngeal insufficiency, where the soft palate is not able to make an adequate contact with the back of the pharynx to close off the nasal airway (Fig. 22.5).

A cleft involving the posterior part of the hard and soft palate will also involve the tensor palati muscles, which act on the Eustachian tube. This predisposes the patient to problems with middle-ear effusion (known colloquially as 'glue ear'). Obviously, hearing difficulties will also retard a child's speech development. Therefore management of the child with a cleft involving the posterior palate must include audiological assessments and myringotomy with or without grommets as indicated.

22.4.4 Other congenital abnormalities

Cleft lip with or without cleft palate, and isolated cleft palate are associated with other congenital abnormalities (Box 22.2). The actual figures vary between populations, but the prevalence is greater in babies with isolated cleft palate. The most common anomalies affect the heart and extremities.

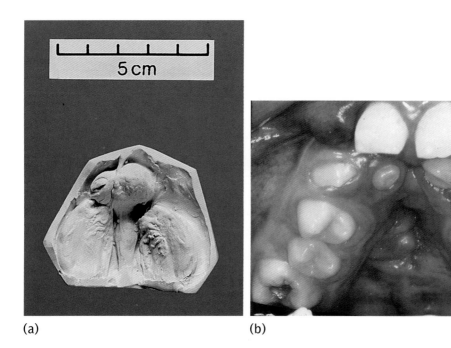

(a)   (b)

Fig. 22.2 (a) Upper model of a bilateral complete cleft lip and palate showing the inward collapse of the lateral segments behind the premaxillary segment; (b) upper arch of a patient in the late mixed dentition with a bilateral complete cleft lip and palate.

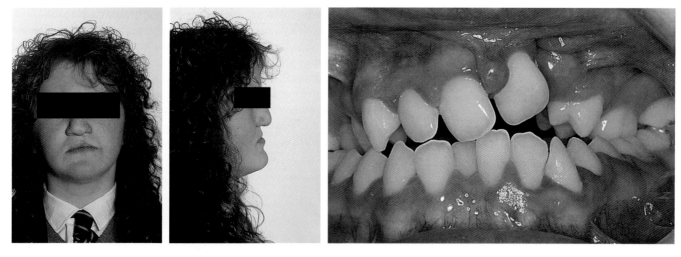

Fig. 22.3 Patient with a repaired unilateral cleft lip and palate of the left side showing mid-face retrusion.

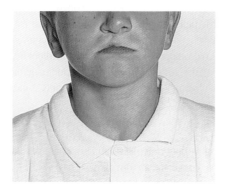

Fig. 22.4 Patient with a repaired cleft lip and palate of the right side who had a degree of overclosure, believed to be due to the restricting effect of the primary repair on vertical growth.

22.4.5 Dental anomalies

In addition to the affects on the teeth in the region of the cleft discussed above, the following anomalies are more prevalent in the remainder of the dentition:

- delayed eruption (delay increases with severity of cleft)
- hypodontia
- supernumerary teeth
- general reduction in tooth size
- abnormalities of tooth size and shape (Fig. 22.6)
- enamel defects

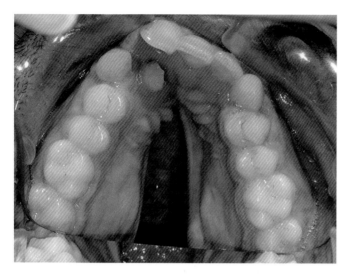

Box 22.2 In a study of nearly 4000 patients with isolated CP (Calzolari *et al*. 2004):

- 55% had cleft palate only
- 27% had a recognized syndrome
- 18% had other anomalies

Fig. 22.5 Patient with unrepaired cleft palate. As a result their speech was unintelligible.

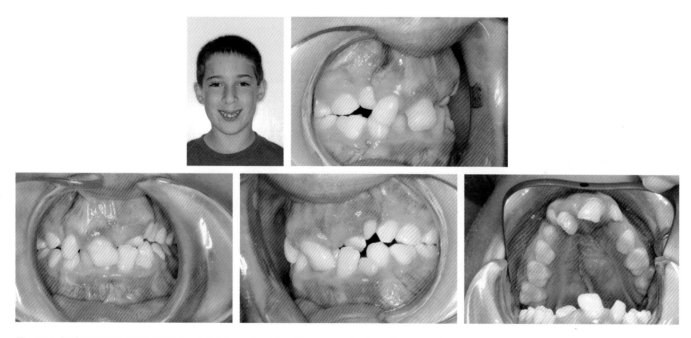

Fig. 22.6 Patient with a repaired bilateral cleft lip and palate with abnormally shaped upper incisors.

22.5 Co-ordination of care

In order to minimize the number of hospital visits and to ensure integrated interdisciplinary management, it is essential to employ a team approach with joint clinics. In order to build up expertise within the team and for meaningful audit, care should be centralized within a region. The core members usually include the following:

- cleft surgeon
- orthodontist
- psychologist
- speech and language therapist
- health visitor/ specialized nurse
- ear, nose, and throat (ENT) surgeon

22.6 Management

It is now accepted practice that patients with a cleft lip and/or palate should be managed to a standardized protocol. The rationale for this is two-fold. Firstly, a standard regime reduces the temptation for additional 'touch-up' surgical procedures, the benefits of which are limited. A standardized protocol also permits useful audit of the outcome of all aspects of cleft care and thereby leads to the refinement and improvement of the management of subsequent generations of cleft children (see Section 22.7).

22.6.1 At birth

With improved foetal ultrasound screening, an increasing proportion of clefts are detected prenatally. This has the advantage that the parents can be counselled and prepared for the arrival of a child with a cleft. Otherwise, the birth of a child with a cleft anomaly will come as a shock and a disappointment for the parents. It is common for them to experience feelings of guilt and they will need time to grieve for the emotional loss of the 'normal' child that they anticipated. It is important to provide support for the mother at this time to ensure that bonding develops normally and that help with feeding is available straightaway for those infants with a cleft. This is now usually provided by a trained cleft health visitor. Because an affected child will have difficulty in sucking, a bottle and teat which help direct the flow of milk into the mouth is helpful, for example a soft bottle which can be squeezed (Fig. 22.7). An early explanation from a member(s) of the cleft team of probable future management and the possibilities of modern treatment is appreciated by parents. Further support can be obtained from CLAPA (the Cleft Lip and Palate Association www.clapa.com), which is a voluntary group largely comprising parents of, and individuals with a cleft (Fig. 22.8).

Some centres still advocate the use of acrylic plates designed to help with feeding or to move the displaced cleft segments actively towards a more normal relationship to aid subsequent surgical apposition. This approach, which is known as pre-surgical orthopaedics, is becoming less fashionable because of a lack of evidence of its efficacy, the additional burden of care for the parents and the good results achieved by a number of cleft teams (for example in Oslo) who do not employ pre-surgical plates.

22.6.2 Lip repair

There is a wide variation in the timing of primary lip repair, depending upon the preference and protocol of the surgeon and cleft team involved. Neonatal repair is still being evaluated. In the UK, primary lip repair is, on average, carried out around 3 months of age. A number of different surgical techniques have been described (for example Millard, Delaire, and straight line). The best techniques aim to dissect out and re-oppose the muscles of the lip and alar base in their correct anatomical position. However, there is some controversy as to whether tissue movement should be achieved by subperiosteal dissection or supraperiosteal dissection and skin-lengthening cuts. The degree to which the alar cartilage is dissected is also contentious, as is the use of a vomer flap.

Most centres repair bilateral cleft lips at the same procedure, but some still carry out two separate operations. Primary bone grafting of the alveolus at the time of lip repair has fallen into disrepute owing to the adverse effects upon subsequent growth.

22.6.3 Palate repair

The goal of hard palate closure is to separate the oral and nasal cavities, with minimal effects upon normal growth and development. In order to achieve the latter, surgery should avoid wide undermining of the palatal soft tissues. Two-layered closure is currently often employed with vomer flaps used to close the nasal layer and mucoperiosteal flaps with minimal bone exposure used for the oral layer.

The goal of soft palate surgery should be re-apposition of the muscle sling to facilitate normal velopharyngeal function and closure for intelligible speech.

In some European centres closure of the hard palate is delayed until 5 years of age or older in an effort to reduce the unwanted effects of early surgery upon growth. There is some evidence to suggest that transverse

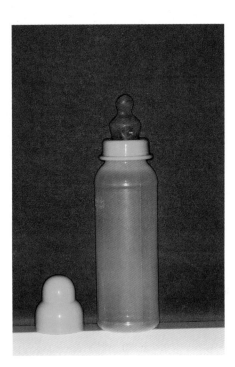

Fig. 22.7 A soft squeezable bottle and special teat for feeding cleft babies.

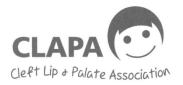

Fig. 22.8 The Cleft Lip and Palate Association logo.

growth of the maxilla is improved. However, the adverse effect upon speech development has been well documented. In the UK, hard and soft palate repair is undertaken, on average, between 6 to 9 months of age with the philosophy that any unwanted effects upon growth caused by repair at this stage (which can be compensated for to a degree by orthodontics and surgery) are preferable to fostering the development of poor articulatory habits, which can be extremely difficult to eradicate after the age of 5 years.

22.6.4 Primary dentition

The first formal speech assessment is usually carried out around 18 months of age, however, monitoring of a patient's speech should continue throughout childhood. This is usually done at certain predefined ages, but will depend upon the needs and circumstances of the child.

An assessment with an ENT surgeon should also be arranged, if this specialty has not been involved at the time of primary repair.

It is important to minimize surgical interference with the cleft child's life and 'minor' touch-ups should be avoided. Lip revision, prior to the start of schooling, should be performed only if clearly indicated. Closure of any residual palatal fistulae may be considered to help speech development. In a proportion of cases the repaired cleft palate does not completely seal off the nasopharynx during speech and nasal escape of air may occur, resulting in a nasal intonation to the child's speech. This is called velophargngeal incompetence (VPI). If from evidence from investigations such as speech assessment, videofluroscopy, and nasoendoscopy, VPI is diagnosed, a pharyngoplasty may help. This operation involves moving mucosal or musculomucosal pharyngeal flaps to augment the shape and function of the soft palate. If indicated, this should be carried out around 4 to 5 years of age.

Orthodontic treatment in the primary dentition is not warranted. However, during this stage it is important to develop good dental care habits, instituting fluoride supplements in non-fluoridated areas.

22.6.5 Mixed dentition

During this stage the restraining effect of surgery upon growth becomes more apparent, initially transversely in the upper arch and then anteroposteriorly as growth in the latter dimension predominates. With the eruption of the permanent incisors, defects in tooth number, formation, and position can be assessed. Often the upper incisors erupt into lingual occlusion and commonly are also displaced or rotated (Fig. 22.9).

In order to avoid straining patient co-operation, it is better if orthodontic intervention is concentrated into two phases. The first stage is usually carried out during the mixed dentition with the specific aim of preparing the patient for alveolar or secondary bone grafting. Subsequent management is discussed in Section 22.6.6.

Alveolar (secondary) bone grafting

This technique has significantly improved the orthodontic care of patients with an alveolar cleft involving the alveolus as it involves repairing the defect with cancellous bone (Box 22.3).

For optimal results this procedure should be timed before the eruption of the permanent canines, at around 9–10 years, particularly as eruption of a tooth through the graft helps to stabilize it. However, in some patients earlier bone grafting is indicated to provide bone for an unerupted viable lateral incisor to erupt.

Before bone grafting is carried out, any transverse collapse of the segments should be corrected to allow complete exposure of the alveolar defect and to improve access for the surgeon. This is most commonly carried out by using a fixed expansion appliance called the quadhelix (see Chapter 13, Section 13.4.4). This appliance has the advantage that the arms can be extended anteriorly, if indicated, to procline the upper incisors, but in cases with more severe displacement and/or rotation of the incisors a simple fixed appliance can be used concurrently (Fig. 22.11). However, care is required to ensure that the roots of the teeth adjacent to the cleft are not moved out of their bony support, and it may be necessary to defer their complete alignment to the post-grafting stage. A palatal arch may be fitted to retain the expansion achieved whilst bone grafting is carried out (Fig. 22.12).

In patients with a bilateral complete cleft lip and palate the premaxillary segment is often mobile. In these cases, in order to ensure that the graft takes and bony healing occurs, it is necessary to stabilize the premaxilla during the healing period after bone grafting. This can be accomplished by placement of a relatively rigid buccal archwire prior to bone grafting, which is left *in situ* for at least 3 months after the operation.

If space closure on the side of the cleft is planned, consideration should be given to the need to extract the deciduous molars on that side prior to grafting in order to facilitate forward movement of the

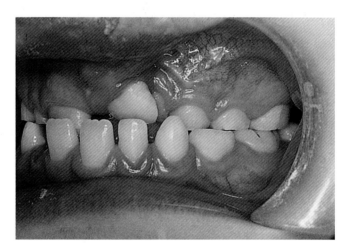

Fig. 22.9 A repaired unilateral cleft lip and palate in the mixed dentition.

Box 22.3 Benefits of alveolar bone grafting

- provision of bone through which the permanent canine (or lateral incisor) can erupt into the arch (Fig. 22.10);
- the possibility of providing the patient with an intact arch;
- improved alar base support;
- aids closure of residual oronasal fistulae;
- stabilization of a mobile premaxilla in a bilateral cleft.

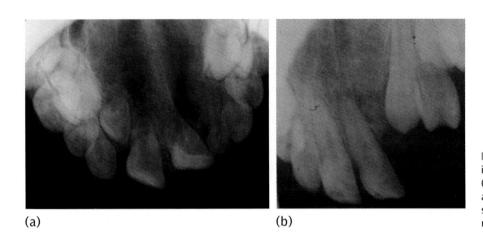

(a) (b)

Fig. 22.10 Radiographs of the patient shown in Fig. 22.13, who had an alveolar bone graft: (a) prior to bone grafting showing cleft of left alveolus; (b) 1 month after bone grafting. The supernumerary tooth lying in the cleft was removed at the time of surgery.

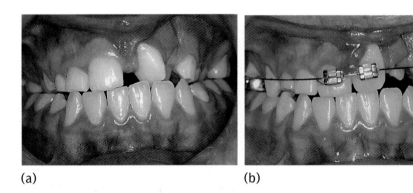

(a) (b)

Fig. 22.11 Patient with a repaired unilateral cleft of the lip and palate of the left side: (a) pre-treatment; (b) following expansion and alignment of the rotated upper left central incisor.

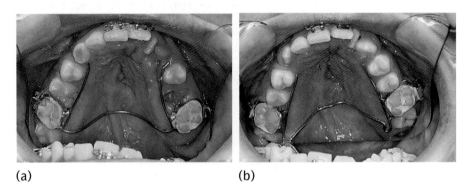

(a) (b)

Fig. 22.12 The same patient as in Fig. 22.11: (a) palatal arch and sectional archwire to retain position of the upper central incisors, prior to bone grafting; (b) after bone grafting, showing the upper left canine erupting.

first permanent molar. However, any extractions should be carried out at least 3 weeks prior to bone grafting in order to allow healing of the keratinized mucosa for the surgeon to raise flaps.

Cancellous bone is currently used for bone grafting because it assumes the characteristics of the adjacent bone; however, this may change in the future as bone morphogenesis proteins become cheaper and more readily available. Cancellous bone can be harvested from a number of sites, but the iliac crest is currently the most popular site. Keratinized flaps should be raised and utilized for closure, as mucosal flaps may interfere with subsequent tooth eruption. Unerupted supernumerary teeth are commonly found in the cleft itself, and these can

be removed at the time of operation. There is no substantive evidence to support the contention that simultaneous bone grafting of bilateral alveolar clefts jeopardizes the integrity of the premaxilla.

The complications of this technique include the following:

- granuloma formation in the region of the graft – this often resolves with increased oral hygiene, but surgical removal may be required
- failure of the graft to take – this usually only occurs to a partial degree
- root resorption – relatively rare
- around 10–15 per cent of canines on the grafted side subsequently require exposure

22.6.6 Permanent dentition

Once the permanent dentition has been established, but before further orthodontic treatment is planned the patient should be assessed as to the likely need for orthognathic surgery to correct mid-face retrusion (see Chapter 21). The degree of maxillary retrognathia, the magnitude and effect of any future growth, and the patient's wishes should all be taken into consideration, however, it has been shown that around 25 per cent of cleft lip and palate patients treated to a standardized protocol require orthognathic surgery. This is because scar tissue from the original primary repair restricts growth of the maxilla. If surgical correction is indicated, this should be deferred until the growth rate has slowed to adult levels (and be preceded by pre-surgical orthodontic alignment) (Box 22.4).

If orthodontics alone is indicated, this can be commenced once the permanent dentition is established. Usually fixed appliances are necessary (Fig. 22.13). If space closure in the region of the cleft is not feasible, treatment planning should be carried out in collaboration with a restorative opinion regarding how the resultant space will be restored in the longer term e.g. implant, bridgework.

At the end of orthodontic treatment, retention will be required. If the maxillary arch has been expanded, this will be particularly prone to relapse, and retention of the arch width with either a removable retainer

> **Box 22.4 Orthognathic surgery in cleft patients**
> - Surgical advancement of the maxilla may affect velophrayngeal function therefore a speech assessment should be carried out before planning surgery
> - Scar tissue may restrict the amount of forward movement of the maxilla that is possible
> - Reduced blood supply to the maxilla due to scarring
> - Maxillary distraction may overcome these problems (Section 21.7.4)

worn at night long-term or a partial denture (if indicated for prosthetic reasons) is advisable. For further details on retention and the different types of retainer see Chapter 16 and Section 16.6 in particular.

22.6.7 Completion of growth

A final surgical revision of the nose (rhinoplasty) may be carried out at this stage. However, if orthognathic surgery is planned this should be carried out first, as movement of the underlying facial bones will affect the contour of the nose.

22.7 Audit of cleft palate care

Audit of cleft palate management is difficult because of the different disciplines involved in providing care and the range of clinical presentations. As in all branches of medicine, concentration of expertise and experience at a centre of excellence produces superior results to those obtained by a lone practitioner carrying out small numbers of a particular procedure each year. Therefore, it has been suggested that each team should 'treat' a minimum of 50 cleft patients per year to provide sufficient numbers for meaningful audit and to develop adequate expertise. In order to try to evaluate the effects of treatment, careful records taken before and after any intervention

(surgical or orthodontic) must be a priority. If the results of one surgical team carrying out a particular treatment protocol are to be compared with another treatment regimen carried out at a different centre, some standardization of these records is required. These should include study models and photographs of the cleft prior to primary closure, so that the size and morphology of the original cleft can be taken into consideration. The recommended minimum data set for each cleft sub-group for the United Kingdom is given on the website of the Craniofacial Society of Great Britain and Ireland (http://www.craniofacialsociety.org.uk/info/audit.html).

22.8 Other craniofacial anomalies

22.8.1 Hemifacial microsomia

This is the second most common craniofacial anomaly, with a prevalence of 1 in 5000 births. It is a congenital defect characterized by a lack of both hard and soft tissue on the affected side of the face, usually in the area of the mandibular ramus and external ear (i.e. in the region of the first and second branchial arches, hence its older name of first arch syndrome). This anomaly usually affects one side of the face (Fig. 22.14), but does present bilaterally in around 30 per cent of cases. A wide spectrum of ear and cranial nerve deformities are found. Goldenhar syndrome or oculo-auriculovertebral dysplasia (the latter name neatly explains the affected sites, but is more difficult to remember) is a variant of hemifacial microsomia.

Management usually involves a combination of surgery and orthodontic treatment. However, milder cases can sometimes be

managed with orthodontic appliances alone. Orthodontic treatment usually involves the use of a specialized type of functional appliance known as a hybrid appliance, so called because components are selected according to the needs of the individual malocclusion, for example encouraging eruption of the buccal segment teeth on the affected side.

The degree and type of surgery depends upon the severity of the defect:

- Early reconstruction (5 to 8 years of age) – is usually reserved for severe cases with no functioning TMJ.
- In the growing child – distraction osteogenesis (see Section 21.7.4) where a functioning TMJ exists.
- Late teens – to enhance the contour of the skeleton and soft tissues – conventional orthognathic and reconstructive techniques.

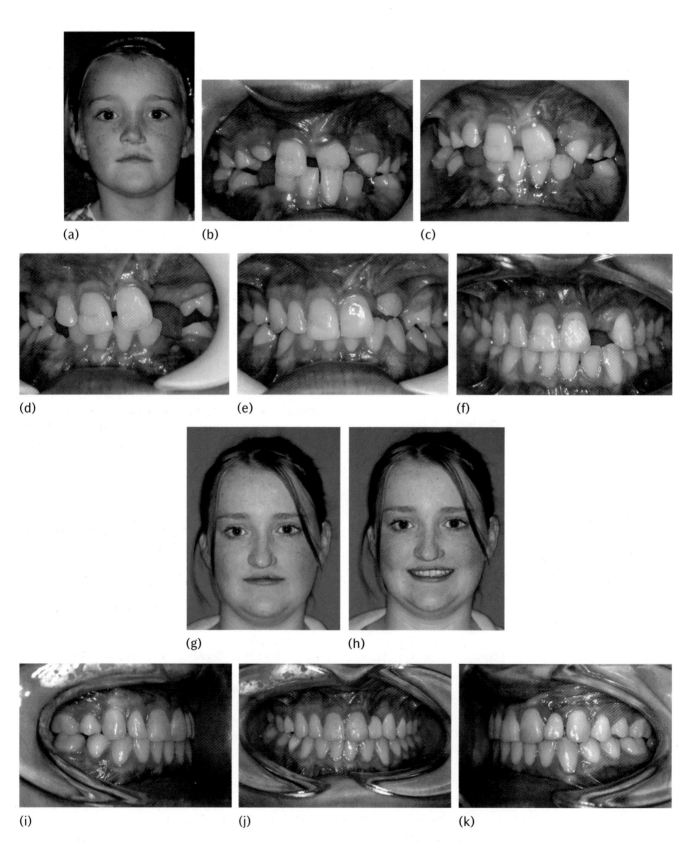

Fig. 22.13 Patient with a repaired unilateral left cleft lip and palate (see also Fig. 22.10 which shows radiographs of same patient pre- and post-bone graft). (a, b) Aged 9 years, pre-treatment; (c) following correction of anterior crossbite and prior to alveolar bone graft of left alveolus; (d) post-alveolar bone graft; (e) at age 12 years after eruption of upper left canine; (f) following comprehensive fixed appliance treatment to localize space for prosthetic replacement of absent upper left lateral incisor; (g–k) following bridgework to replace absent upper left lateral incisor.

22.8.2 Treacher–Collins syndrome

This syndrome is also known as mandibulofacial dysostosis. It is inherited in an autosomal dominant manner and consists of the following features, which present bilaterally:

- downward sloping (anti-mongoloid slant) palpebral fissures and colobomas (notched iris with a displaced pupil);
- hypoplastic malar bones;
- mandibular retrognathia;
- deformed ears, including middle and inner ear which can result in deafness;
- hypoplastic air sinuses;
- cleft palate in one-third of cases;
- most have completely normal intellectual function.

The specifics of management depend upon the features of the case, but usually staged craniofacial surgery is required.

22.8.3 Pierre–Robin sequence

This anomaly consists of retrognathia of the mandible, cleft palate, and glossoptosis (the tongue position restricts the pharynx), which together

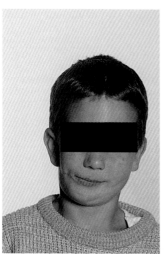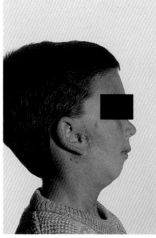

Fig. 22.14 Patient with hemifacial microsomia.

cause airway problems in the infant. Previously it was thought that due to raised intra-uterine pressure the head of the foetus was compressed against the chest, thus restricting normal development of the mandible, however, recent research would suggest a metabolic aetiological factor. The first priority at birth is to maintain the airway; in a proportion of cases it is necessary to use a nasopharyngeal airway for the first few days, but once the child is older, or in less severe cases, prone nursing will suffice. Rarely, tracheostomy for medium-term airway protection is required. Subsequent management is as for cleft palate (see above). For affected patients with a compromised airway or poor aesthetics, early distraction osteogenesis can be considered, or alternatively, orthognathic surgery towards the end of growth (see Chapter 21). In milder cases conventional orthodontic mechanotherapy for Class II skeletal patterns can be planned.

22.8.4 Craniosynostoses

In craniosynostosis and craniofacial synostoses, premature fusion of one or more of the sutures of the bones of the cranial base or vault occurs. The effects depend upon the site and extent of the premature fusion, but all have a marked effect upon growth. In some cases restriction of skull vault growth can lead to an increase in intracranial pressure which, if untreated, can lead to brain damage. If raised intracranial pressure is detected, release of the affected suture(s) before 6 months of age is indicated. This may be the only intervention needed in isolated craniosynostoses. Combined craniofacial synostoses (e.g. Crouzon syndrome, Apert syndrome) require subsequent staged orthodontic and surgical intervention. This may become the prime indication for telemetric distraction osteogenesis.

Relevant Cochrane reviews:

Feeding interventions for growth and development in infants with cleft lip, cleft palate or cleft lip and palate
Glenny, A. *et al.* (2008)
http://onlinelibrary.wiley.com/o/cochrane/clsysrev/articles/CD003315/frame.html
Secondary bone grafting for alveolar cleft in children with cleft lip or cleft lip and palate
Guo, J. *et al.* (2011)
http://onlinelibrary.wiley.com/doi/10.1002/14651858.CD008050.pub2/full

---

Key points

- Cleft care is complex and requires a co-ordinated multidisciplinary team approach
- Each team should manage sufficient cases to build up expertise and provide numbers for meaningful audit
- Management should be to a pre-determined protocol
- To facilitate audit and inter-centre comparisons, records should be collected to a standardized national protocol
- Interventions should be restricted to the minimum to reduce the burden on the cleft patient and their family

Principal sources and further reading

Bergland, O., Semb, G., and Abyholm, F. E. (1986). Elimination of the residual alveolar cleft by secondary bone grafting and subsequent orthodontic treatment. *Cleft Lip and Palate Journal*, **23**, 175–205.

This paper is now a classic. It describes the pioneering work by the Oslo cleft team on alveolar bone grafting.

Calzolari, E. Bianchi, F., Rubini, M. Ritvanen, A., and Neville, A.J. (2004). EUROCAT working group. Epidemiology of cleft palate in Europe: implications for genetic research. *Cleft Palate – Craniofacial Journal*, 41, 244–9.

The source of the figures for the study of nearly 4000 patients with isolated cleft palate referred to in Box 22.2.

Clinical Standards Advisory Group (1998). *Cleft Lip and/or Palate*. Stationery Office, London.

The results of a national audit of cleft care in the UK that led to a transformation in the way cleft care is delivered.

Cousley, R. R. J. (1993). A comparison of two classification systems for hemifacial microsomia. *British Journal of Oral and Maxillofacial Surgery*, **31**, 78–82.

Daskalogiannakis, J., Ross, R. B., and Tompson, B. D. (2001). The mandibular catch-up controversy in Pierre Robin sequence. *American Journal of Orthodontics and Dentofacial Orthopedics*, **120**, 280–5.

Eppley, B. L. and Sadove, A. M. (2000). Management of alveolar cleft bone grafting – State of the Art. *Cleft Palate – Craniofacial Journal*, **37**, 229–33.

An interesting read for those clinicians involved in alveolar bone grafting.

Jones, M. C. (2002). Prenatal diagnosis of cleft lip and palate: detection rates, accuracy of ultrasonography, associated anomalies and strategies for counseling. *Cleft Palate – Craniofacial Journal*, **39**, 169–73.

LaRossa, D. (2000). The state of the art in cleft palate surgery. *Cleft Palate and Craniofacial Journal*, **37**, 225–8.

Mossey, P., Little, J., Munger, R.G., Dixon, M.J., and Shaw, W.C. (2009). Cleft Lip and Palate. *The Lancet*, **374**, 1773–85.

An excellent review article which focuses on the aetiology of clefts.

Ranta, R. (1986). A review of tooth formation in children in cleft lip/palate. *American Journal of Orthodontics and Dentofacial Orthopedics*, **90**, 11–18.

Steinberg, M. D. *et al.* (1999). State of the art in oral and maxillofacial surgery: treatment of maxillary hypoplasia and anterior palatal and alveolar clefts. *Cleft Palate – Craniofacial Journal*, **36**, 283–91.

Uzel A., Alparslan, N. (2010). Long-term Effects of Presurgical Infant Orthopedics in Patients with Cleft Lip and Palate: A Systematic Review. *Cleft Palate-Craniofacial Journal*. **48**, 587–95.

This review found no long-term benefits from the use of pre-surgical orthopedic plates prior to primary surgery.

Wyatt, R., Sell, D., Russell, J, Harding, A., Harland, K., and Albery, E. (1996). Cleft palate speech dissected: a review of current knowledge and analysis. *British Journal of Plastic Surgery*, **49**, 143–9.

An excellent article – recommended reading for any professional treating cleft children.

23

Orthodontic first aid

Chapter contents

Whenever a patient presents with an orthodontic problem it is important to carry out:

- A medical history
- A full history of the 'problem'

- If the patient is the patient of another operator then a history of the treatment should also be taken
- A thorough examination
- When in doubt seek expert advice

Table 23.1 Fixed appliance

Patient's presenting complaint	Possible causes	Management	Learning points
Wire sticking out distally from molar tube/band	Ends of wire not trimmed	(1) NT round wires: cut leaving 1–2 mm, remove wire, flame ends and turn-in (2) SS round wires: cut leaving 1–2 mm to turn-in (3) rectangular wires: cut flush with distal aspect of tube	Always check with patient that ends are not sticking out before they leave chair
	Archwire has moved round	(1) Round wires: re-position archwire and turn ends in (2) Rectangular wires: re-position archwire and crimp hook or piece of tubing; or bond composite blob onto wire in convenient position	This is a particular problem with reduced friction bracket systems. Use a 'stop' (see management column) to prevent wire sliding round when using these systems
	In initial stages as teeth align excess wire has moved distally through tubes	NT round wires: cut leaving 1–2 mm, remove wire, flame ends and turn-in	
Wire sticking out mesial to molar	Ligature wire end turned out	Turn end in	
	Ligature wire has broken	Replace	
Bracket has detached wrom tooth	Bracket is in traumatic occlusion with opposing tooth	Consider these options: (1) Use a band instead of a bonded attachment (2) Place GI cement blob to either occlusal surface of molar teeth or palatally to upper incisors (depending upon overbite) (3) Fit a removable bite-plane appliance (4) Place an intrusion bend in wire in opposing arch (5) Leave off bond until further overbite reduction has been achieved	
	Archwire over-activated to engage bracket	Replace bracket and then place more flexible archwire to align tooth	
	Patient has knocked bracket off	Replace bracket in 'ideal position' on tooth. May need to drop down a wire size to fully engage bracket	Educate patient: (1) Reasons for avoiding hard foods (2) To avoid pen chewing
Band loose	Band is too big for tooth	Select correct sized band for 'snug' fit and cement in place	
	Patient is eating sticky foods/ sweets	Remove any remaining cement and re-cement band	Educate patient about reasons for avoiding sticky foods
		When one band of a quad/TPA becomes loose it is necessary to remove the quad/ TPA and re-cement both bands	
Teeth feel loose	A slight increase in mobility is normal during tooth movement	Check mobility of affected tooth/teeth. Reassure patient	Warn patient in advance that this is likely to happen

Table 23.1 (*continued*)

Patient's presenting complaint	Possible causes	Management	Learning points
	Tooth in traumatic occlusion with opposing arch	Check occlusion. Consider these options: (1) Fit a removable bite-plane appliance (2) Place an intrusion bend in wire in opposing arch (3) Take steps to reduce overbite	
	Root resorption	(1) Take radiographs to check how many teeth are affected and to what extent (2) Discuss with patient (3) If limited – rest for 3 months before re-commencing active tooth movement (4) If marked ? discontinue treatment	
Tooth/teeth are painful	Some discomfort is normal after fitting and adjustment of FA	Reassure patient. Advise proprietary painkillers	Warn patient in advance that this is likely to happen especially for first few days after fitting/adjustment
	Tooth/teeth in traumatic occlusion	Check occlusion. Consider following: (1) Fit a removable bite-plane appliance (2) Place an intrusion bend in wire in opposing arch (3) Take steps to reduce overbite	
	Periapical pathology	(1) Take careful history (2) Check vitality (3) Check response to percussion (4) Take periapical X-ray If diagnosis confirmed, remove attachment from tooth and refer patient to their dentist for further management. If practicable, defer further active tooth movement until radiographic signs of apical healing	
	Periodontal problem	(1) Take careful history (2) Probe affected tooth/teeth (3) Take periapical radiograph If diagnosis confirmed, remove attachment from tooth/teeth and refer patient to their dentist for further management	
Nance bulb or quad digging into palate		(1) Reassess need to continue with nance/quad (2) If need to continue, remove and adjust so that no longer digging into palate	Use gentle forces to minimize strain on anchorage (excessive forces can result in forward movement of molars to which nance is attached)
Sheath soldered to band on molar for attachment of palatal arch or quad has detached	Often occurs due to patient factors (e.g. eating hard/chewy foods)	Remove palatal arch/quad and band. Re-solder new sheath and replace band and palatal arch/quad	Advise patient to avoid hard/sticky foods or 'fiddling' with arch/quad
Patient hit in/around mouth		(1) Take periapical radiograph of affected tooth/teeth, if root fracture, splint affected tooth/teeth with heavy archwire (2) If brackets knocked off replace if moisture control possible (if not defer for 1 week) (3) If archwire distorted, remove archwire and place light flexible archwire (4) If teeth displaced, attempt re-positioning and place light flexible archwire (5) Monitor vitality (6) Warn of risks of delayed concussion	

Table 23.2 Removable appliance

Patient's presenting complaint	Possible causes	Management	Learning points
Mouth watering	Inevitable when appliance first fitted. If persists usually reflects insufficient wear	Reassure patient and advise that will resolve as mouth adapts to strange plastic object	Warn patient at time of fitting
Problems with speech	Inevitable when appliance first fitted. If persists usually reflects insufficient wear	Reassure patient and advise that will resolve once mouth adapts to strange plastic object	Warn patient at time of fitting
Appliance loose	Appliance unretentive due to poor design	Consider adding additional clasps and/or a labial bow. If not feasible then re-make appliance with improved design	
	Clasps not retentive. NB If patient habitually clicks appliance in and out the clasps flex and become less retentive	Adjust clasps	It is advisable to warn patients when fitting appliance not to click appliance in and out
Clasp fractured	Can occur if patient habitually clicks appliance in and out	Replace clasp (if working model not available will need new impression) Will need to fit repair as often some adjustment is required at chair-side	
Acrylic fractured (including bite-plane, buccal capping)		Check whether fractured portion needs to be replaced or not. If not, smooth fractured edge. If repair required, take new impression if working model not available. Will need to fit repair as often some adjustment is required at chair-side	
Redness on roof of mouth	Candida	(1) OHI and dietary advice (2) If marked infection or does not respond to (1) prescribe anti-fungal to be applied to fitting surface of appliance	
	Trauma from appliance components	Adjust as required	
Sore cracks at side of mouth	Angular cheilitis	(1) OHI and dietary advice (2) If marked infection or does not respond to (1) prescribe anti-fungal	

Table 23.3 Functional appliance (see also problems related to removable appliances)

Patient's presenting complaint	Possible causes	Management	Learning points
Appliance comes out at night	Appliance not retentive due to poor design	Consider adding additional clasps and/or a labial bow. If not feasible then re-make appliance with improved design	
	Clasps not retentive. NB If patient habitually clicks appliance in and out the clasps flex and become less retentive	Adjust clasps	It is advisable to warn patients when fitting appliance not to click appliance in and out
	Insufficient wear of appliance during day	Ask patient to increase daytime wear	
Teeth and jaws ache	Common occurrence during initial stages of treatment	Reassure patient	Warn patient at time of fitting that this may occur

Table 23.4 Headgear

Patient's presenting complaint	Possible causes	Management	Learning points
Face-bow comes out of tubes at night		Adjust inner arms of face-bow	Advise patients at the time of fitting that if this problem does occur they should stop wearing the headgear and contact their orthodontist
Face-bow tipping down anteriorly and impinging on lower lip	If the force vector is below the centre of resistance of the molars they will tip distally	Adjust outer arms up to raise moment of force above centre of resistance of molar to counteract tipping	Ensure movement of force acting through centre of resistance of teeth at time of fitting and check at each visit
Face-bow tipping up anteriorly and impinging on upper lip	If the force vector is above the centre of resistance of the molars they will tip mesially	Adjust outer arms down to lower moment of force below centre of resistance of molar to counteract tipping	Ensure movement of force acting through centre of resistance of teeth at time of fitting and check at each visit

Table 23.5 Miscellaneous

Patient's presenting complaint	Possible causes	Management	Learning points
Dentist fractures tooth during extraction leaving root fragment		(1) Take X-ray to investigate size of fragment (2) If large and/or will interfere with planned tooth movements refer patient for removal of fractured portion (3) If small and/or does not interfere with tooth movements keep under radiographic observation	
Appliance component missing? inhaled or ingested		(1) If airway obstructed, call ambulance and try to remove obstruction (2) If there is a risk that the component has been inhaled then refer the patient to hospital for a chest X-ray and subsequent management (give patient another similar component to aid radiologist when examining films) (3) If there is a danger that the component has been swallowed then seek the advice of the local hospital. If >6 days previously, object has probably passed through patient's system (see also Figure 23.1)	
Bonded retainer detached		If retainer not distorted and teeth still well-aligned (1) Isolate, etch, wash and dry (2) Rebond retainer with composite If retainer distorted and teeth still well-aligned, either bend up new retainer at chair-side using flexible multi-strand wire or take impression for laboratory to bond up new retainer If teeth have relapsed discuss with patient whether to monitor or re-treat	
Bonded retainer partially detached		If remainder not distorted then re-bond to remaining teeth If remainder distorted then remove and place new bonded retainer	
Vacuum formed retainer ill-fitting		If tooth alignment has not relapsed take impression for replacement retainer If teeth have relapsed discuss with patient whether or not to monitor or re-treat	
Patient/parent questions need to extract		(1) Ask why patient/parent concerned – if due to process of extraction explain and reassure (2) If due to concerns regarding perceived disadvantages of extractions – discuss rationale for treatment plan (3) Reassess if alternative approach can be used	

FA, fixed appliance; GI, glass ionomer; NT, nickel titanium; OHI, oral hygiene instruction; Quad, quadhelix; SS, stainless steel; TPA, transpalatal arch; X-ray, radiograph.

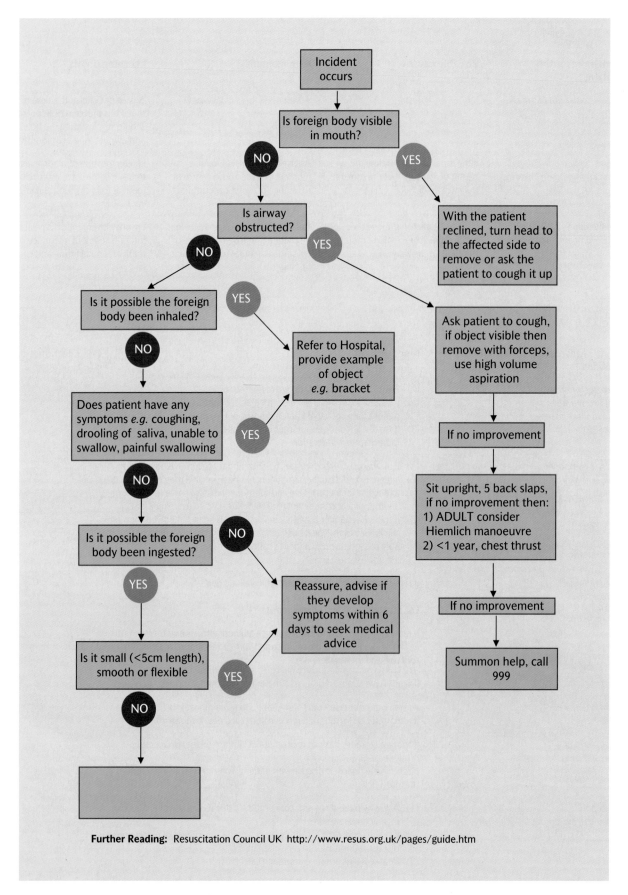

Fig. 23.1 Flow diagram showing management of missing appliance component which may have been ingested or inhaled. Produced with the kind permission of the British Orthodontic Society.

Definitions

Anchorage The source of resistance to the forces generated in reaction to the active components of an appliance.

Angulation Degree of tip of a tooth in the mesiodistal plane.

Anterior open bite There is no vertical overlap of the incisors when the buccal segment teeth are in occlusion.

Balancing extraction Extraction of the same (or adjacent) tooth on the opposite side of the arch to preserve symmetry.

Bimaxillary proclination Both upper and lower incisors are proclined relative to their skeletal bases.

Bimaxillary retroclination Both upper and lower incisors are retroclined relative to their skeletal bases.

Bodily movement Equal movement of the root apex and crown of a tooth in the same direction.

Buccal crossbite The buccal cusps of the lower premolars and/or molars occlude buccally to the buccal cusps of the upper premolars and/or molars.

Centric occlusion Position of maximum interdigitation.

Centric relation The condyle is in its most superior anterior position in the glenoid fossa.

Cingulum plateau The convexity of the cervical third of the lingual/palatal aspect of the incisors and canines.

Compensating extraction Extraction of the same tooth in the opposing arch.

Competent lips Upper and lower lips contact without muscular activity at rest.

Complete overbite The lower incisors occlude with the upper incisors or palatal mucosa.

Crowding Where there is insufficient space to accommodate the teeth in perfect alignment in an arch, or segment of an arch.

Curve of Spee Curvature of the occlusal plane in the sagittal plane.

Dento-alveolar compensation The inclination of the teeth compensates for the underlying skeletal pattern, so that the occlusal relationship between the arches is less marked.

Hypodontia This term is used when one or more permanent teeth (excluding third molars) are congenitally absent. The equivalent American nomenclature is oligodontia.

Ideal occlusion Anatomically perfect arrangement of the teeth. Rare.

Impaction Impeded tooth eruption, usually because of displacement of the tooth or mechanical obstruction (e.g. crowding or a supernumerary tooth).

Inclination Degree of tip of a tooth in the labiopalatal plane.

Incompetent lips Some muscular activity is required for the lips to meet together.

Incomplete overbite The lower incisors do not occlude with the opposing upper incisors or the palatal mucosa when the buccal segment teeth are in occlusion.

Intermaxillary Between the arches.

Intramaxillary Within the same arch.

Leeway space The difference in diameter between the deciduous canine, first molar, and second molar, and their permanent successors (canine, first premolar, and second premolar).

Lingual crossbite The buccal cusps of the lower premolars and/or molars occlude lingually to the lingual cusps of the upper premolars or molars. Sometimes referred to as a scissors bite.

Malocclusion Variation from ideal occlusion which has dental health and/or psychosocial implications for the individual. NB The borderline between normal occlusion and malocclusion is contentious (see Chapter 1).

Mandibular deviation The path of closure of the mandible starts from a postured position.

Mandibular displacement When closing from the rest position the mandible displaces (either laterally or anteriorly) to avoid a premature contact.

Midline diastema A space between the central incisors. Most common in the upper arch.

Migration Physiological (minor) movement of a tooth.

Normal occlusion Acceptable variation from ideal occlusion.

Overbite Vertical overlap of the upper and lower incisors when viewed anteriorly: one-third to one-half coverage of the lower incisors is normal; where the overbite is greater than one-half it is described as being increased; where the overbite is less than one-third it is described as being reduced.

Overjet Distance between the upper and lower incisors in the horizontal plane. Normal overjet is 2–4 mm.

Posterior open bite When the teeth are in occlusion there is a space between the posterior teeth.

Relapse The return, following correction, of the features of the original malocclusion.

Reverse overjet The lower incisors lie anterior to the upper incisors. When only one or two incisors are involved the term anterior crossbite is commonly used.

Rotation A tooth is twisted around its long axis.

Spacing Where the teeth do not touch interproximally and there are gaps between adjacent teeth. Can be localized or generalized.

Tilting movement Movement of the root apex and crown of a tooth in opposite directions around a fulcrum.

Torque Movement of the root apex buccolingually, either with no or minimal movement of the crown in the same direction.

Traumatic overbite The occlusion of the lower incisors with the palatal mucosa has led to ulceration.

Uprighting Mesial or distal movement of the root apex so that the root and crown of the tooth are at an ideal angulation.

Orthodontic Assessment Form

Patient Details

Name	Referrer:
Address	
	Reason for referral
Tel Contact:	
Date of birth:	

History

Patient's complaint	Habits
	Growth status
Medical history	Motivation
Dental History (including trauma & previous treatments)	Socio-behaviour factors

Extra-oral examination

Anteroposterior	Smile Aesthetics
Vertical	Soft tissues
Transverse	TMJ

Intra-oral examination

Teeth present:	Lower arch
Oral hygiene	
Periondontal health	Upper arch
Tooth quality	

Teeth in occlusion

Incisor relationship	*Molars* Right Left
Overjet = mm	*Canines* Right Left
Overbite	Crossbites
Centre-lines	Displacements

Index